The Reflexology Atlas

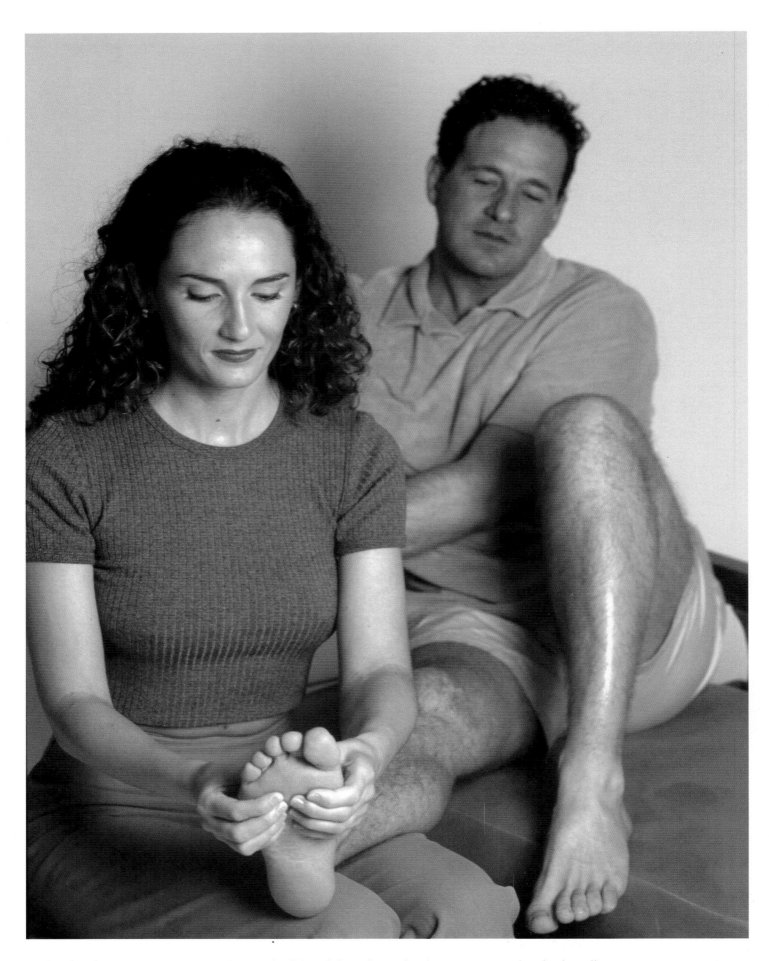

With reflexology massage, you can take your health and that of your family into your own hands—literally.

The Reflexology Atlas

Bernard C. Kolster, M.D., and
Astrid Waskowiak, M.D.

Translated from the German by Nikolas Win Myint

Healing Arts Press
Rochester, Vermont

Healing Arts Press
One Park Street
Rochester, Vermont 05767
www.InnerTraditions.com

Healing Arts Press is a division of Inner Traditions International

Copyright © 2003 Verlagsgruppe Weltbild GmbH, Augsburg
Sonderausgabe für Droemersche Verlagsanstalt Th. Knaur Nachf., München

English translation copyright 2005 by Inner Traditions International

Originally published in German under the title *Knaurs Atlas der Reflexzonen Therapie* by Verlagsgruppe Weltbild GmbH, Augsburg
Sonderausgabe für DroemerscheVerlagsanstalt Th. Knaur Nachf., München

First U.S. Edition published in 2005 by Healing Arts Press

Note to the reader: This book is intended as an informational guide. The remedies, approaches, and techniques described herein are meant to supplement, and not to be a substitute for, professional medical care or treatment. They should not be used to treat a serious ailment without prior consultation with a qualified health care professional.

Library of Congress Cataloging-in-Publication Data
Kolster, Bernard C.
  [Knaurs Atlas der Reflexzonen Therapie English]
  The reflexology atlas / Bernard C. Kolster, Astrid Waskowiak ; translated from the German by Nikolas Win Myint.—1st U.S. ed.
    p. cm.
  Includes bibliographical references and index.
  ISBN 1-59477-066-2 (hardcover)
  ISBN 1-59477-091-3 (paperback)
  1. Reflexology (Therapy)—Atlases. I. Waskowiak, Astrid. II. Title.
  RM723.R43K6513 2005
  615.8'224—dc22
                                                                              2005015512

Printed and bound in India by Replika Press Pvt Ltd.

10 9 8 7 6 5 4 3 2

Text design and layout by Priscilla Baker
This book was typeset in Minion, with Agenda used as a display typeface

Contents

Introduction

Alternative therapies for the treatment of illnesses and the alleviation of pain and chronic conditions are experiencing a growing interest. In this context, people are increasingly beginning to trust reflexology massages to further well-being.

Reflexology—Old Knowledge Rediscovered

It seems that reflexology is a very old type of therapy. We know that since ancient times, in many different regions of the world and in many different cultures, some ailments have been treated by pressure on particular zones of the body. For example, depictions from Egyptian graves show

lower extremities
upper extremities
pelvis
rib cage
spine
head
eye

kidney
bladder
ureter
gallbladder
stomach-intestinal tract
liver
heart
lungs

The auricle resembles an upside-down embryo.

the application of hand and foot massages dating back to the time of the sixth dynasty, around 2300 B.C.

If you consider the means available in ancient times for the healing of ailments, on the one hand there was therapy through external substances such as plants, minerals, and animal products. On the other hand there were the types of treatment that today we would call physical treatments—rubbing, massage, or simply the laying on of hands to influence ailments. A simple example of the latter treatment is one we are probably all familiar with: when you hurt yourself, whether through a fall or by bumping against something, you instinctively, as a reflex, rub and massage the part of the body that hurts.

Over time, people gained more knowledge about the zones of the body and their effects. This probably led to the "mapping" of zones, or the identification of those zones that can influence other parts of the body or organs. If you massage or touch such a "reflex zone" of the body, you stimulate the part of the body or organ that is connected to that zone. Through the examination of the location and order of these reflex zones, you can see that the entire human body is represented on certain parts of the body.

The example of acupuncture, one of the oldest forms of reflexology, illustrates this point very well. If you take a close look at the human ear, you can see with some imagination the outlines of an upside-down embryo. In this illustration, the earlobe corresponds to the head area. Also recognizable are the reflex zones of the legs, arms, and intestines. This spatial ordering of an embryo in the human ear is used for the selection of treatment points in ear acupuncture. For example, if the therapist wants to treat a problem like a headache, he or she will look in the head zone for one or several sensitive points, into which the therapist will carefully place a very fine acupuncture needle. This needling influences or heals the ailment.

Like reflexology, ear acupuncture is a very old therapy, dating back to Chinese sources from the first century. To this day, science has not been able to fully explain the way in which this therapy works. It is surely remarkable how reflex zones can influence body parts that are far removed. What is certain, however, is that this therapy works. Millions of patients around the world who have undergone ear acupuncture treatment can attest to the therapy's efficacy. But the ear is only one example of a reflex zone. The hands, feet, and other body parts can equally influence remote parts of the body.

Dividing the Body into Zones

In 1917, the American physician William Fitzgerald (1872–1929) published his insights into what he described as the "zone model" of humans. With this, Fitzgerald became the pioneer of the introduction of reflexology in the Western world. He had studied medicine at the University of Vermont and later practiced in Boston, London, and Vienna. In this time he specialized to become an ear, nose, and throat doctor. It remains unclear from where Fitzgerald received his research results regarding reflex therapy. Did he discover the basics in Europe and bring them to North America, or did his knowledge come from the desire to find methods of anesthesia for minor surgical procedures?

Fitzgerald noticed that patients undergoing painful procedures would instinctively grip the armrests of their chair tightly, and he began researching this phenomenon. In 1913 he shared his observations with the medical world. By this time he was the chief doctor of the ear, nose, and throat department of St. Francis Hospital in Hartford, Connecticut. He had discovered that pressure, when applied to certain parts of the body, could alleviate pain. His discoveries led to the development of a system that divided the body from head to toe into ten zones. He documented this zone model in the book *Zone Therapy*. It was by this name that reflexology became known in the early 1960s.

The Longitudinal Zones

Fitzgerald divided the body into ten zones that run lengthwise from the head to the toes. These zones form the theoretical foundations for his conclusions. They are not limited to the surface of the body but extend inside it as well. Picture the zones as dividing the body into ten long,

thin slices. The slices are demarcated by the lines, with each slice or zone running from head to foot. To properly carry out foot reflexology massages, it is necessary to deal in some detail with the bone structure of the feet and the location of the individual reflex zones. Accordingly, the following pages discuss the reflex zones as well as the anatomy of the feet.

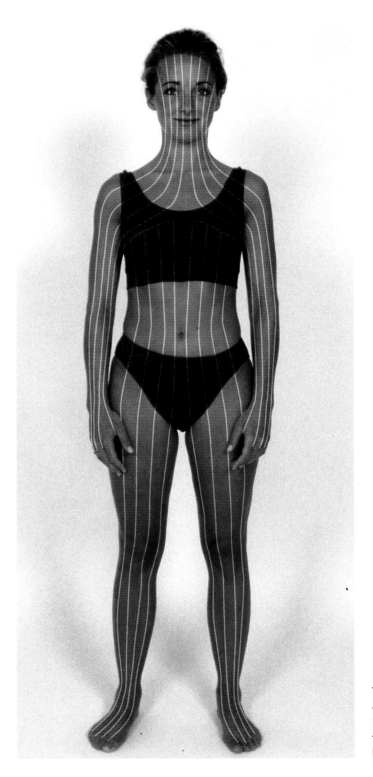

The zone model divides the body into ten zones that run from the head to the feet.

Foot Reflexology Massage

To properly administer foot reflexology massages, it is necessary to take a closer look at the bone structure of the feet and the location of the individual reflex zones.

Knowledge

In Germany, the development of reflexology is closely associated with the name Hanne Marquardt. The depiction of the zones in this book build on her knowledge.

The Feet as a Picture of the Body

As with the ear, a closer look at the foot allows you to see similarities to the outline of the human body. If you look at the illustration of an upright foot from the side, you can—with some imagination—see the outline of a sitting person. The big toe represents the head, the arched shape of the sole the S-shaped line of the spine, and the heel the buttocks.

The picture of the body can also be projected onto the soles of the feet. If you place both feet next to each other, the inner sides represent the spine. The two big toes represent the head and brain. The shoulders are inside the base (bottommost) toe joints, and the inside arches of the feet represent the chest and its organs. Beneath them, the soft parts in the middle of the feet are home to the zone of the internal organs.

Most zones that are on the soles of the feet also run along the backs of the feet. The three-dimensionality of the body, with its layers of organs, muscles, bones, and tissues, is thus represented in the three-dimensionality of the foot. As was mentioned earlier, zones apply not only to the surface of the body but to its insides as well.

Left: The profile of a sitting person has similarities to the inside profile of the foot.

Right: The body is represented on the soles of the feet.

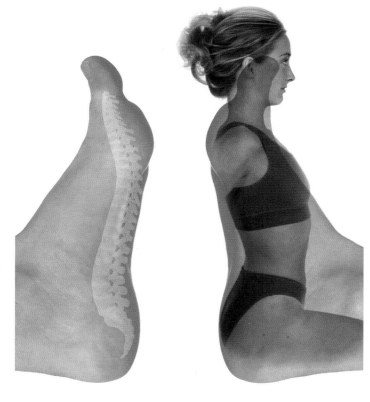

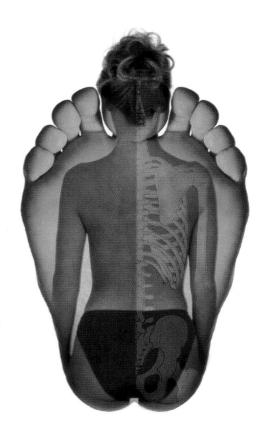

The Reflex Zones of the Feet

If you remember the projection of the human body onto the feet, it is easy to see the individual reflex zones. The right foot represents the right half of the body, and the left foot the left half. The zones of paired organs such as the lungs and kidneys appear on each of the feet, with the left organ on the left foot and the right organ on the right foot.

The zones of the spine and individual organs such as the esophagus and intestines are on the inside edges of both feet. Reflex zones of layered organs can overlap. As such, the zone of the heart is behind that of the lungs, and the zones of the major joints (shoulders, elbows, and knees) are on the outside edges of the feet. The zone of the muscles is on the tops of the feet. The zones of the shoulder, chest, and abdominal muscles run from front to back.

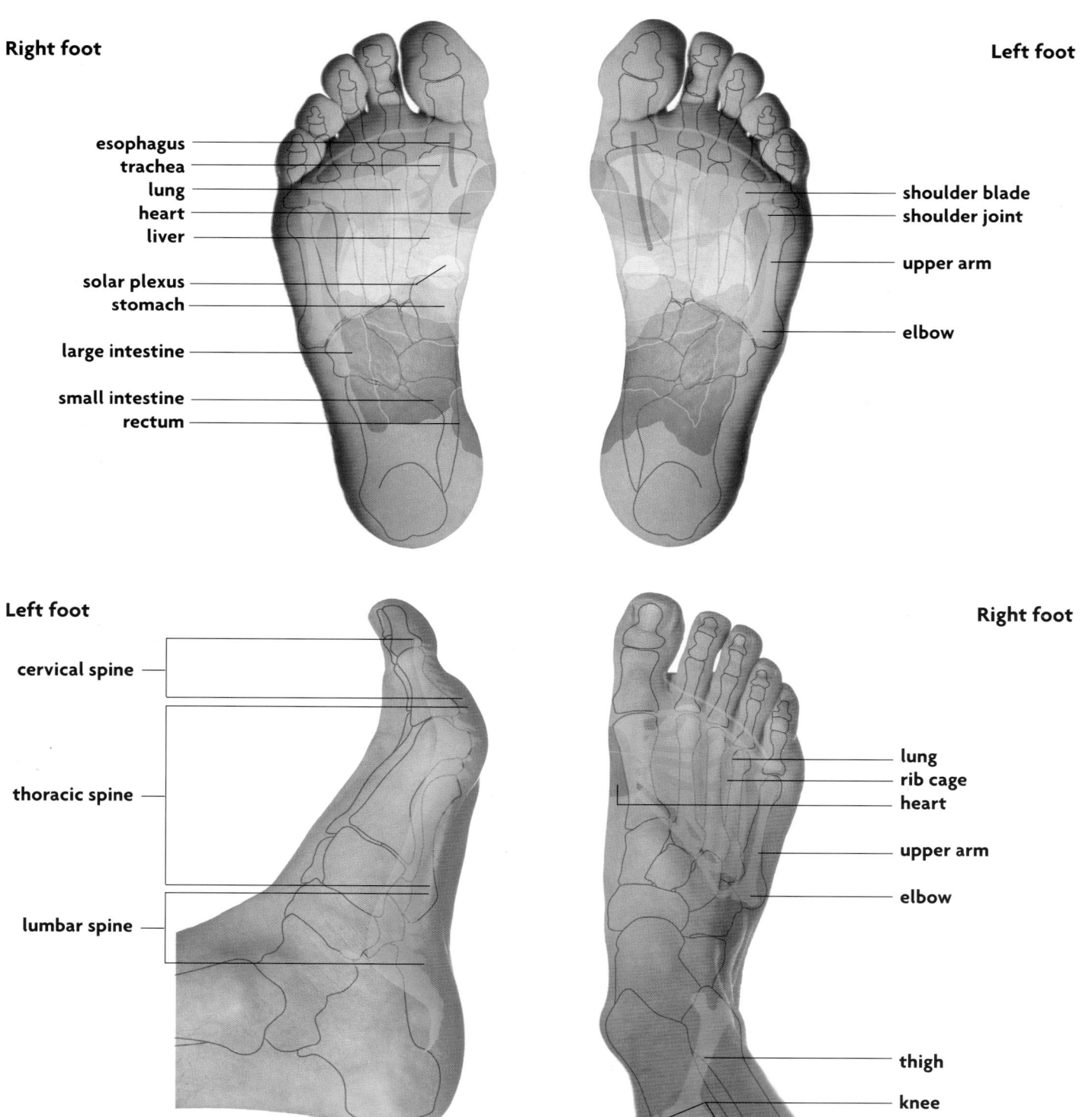

Right foot

esophagus
trachea
lung
heart
liver
solar plexus
stomach
large intestine
small intestine
rectum

Left foot

shoulder blade
shoulder joint
upper arm
elbow

Left foot

cervical spine
thoracic spine
lumbar spine

Right foot

lung
rib cage
heart
upper arm
elbow
thigh
knee

The reflex zones are on the soles of the feet (top), the sides of the feet (bottom left), and the tops of the feet (bottom right).

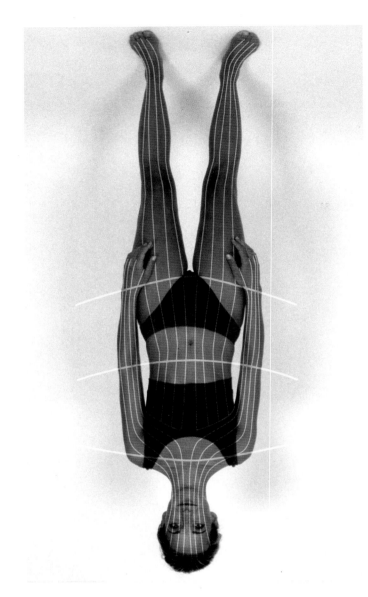

Right: The hori-
zontal zones of
the human body
are represented
on the soles of
the feet.

Left: The zone
model shows
longitudinal
(vertical) as well
as latitudinal
(horizontal)
zones.

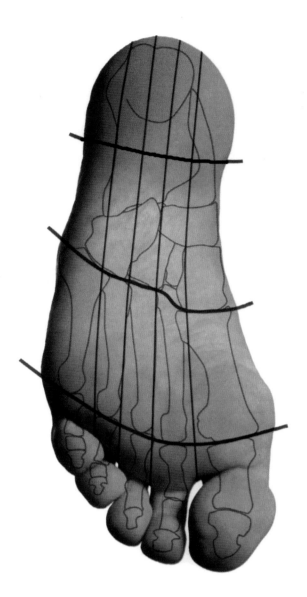

The Zones

When we look at the foot as a depiction of the whole human body, we see that the zones of the feet correspond exactly to the whole-body zone model introduced by Fitzgerald. The zone model sharpens the eye to similarities between the shape of the foot and that of the body.

The Longitudinal or Vertical Zones

Fitzgerald's zone model divides the body into ten longitudinal zones. The zones apply not just to the body surface but to the insides as well; thus we can speak of dividing the body into ten slices. Fitzgerald and his students found that the longitudinal zones of the feet offered especially effective reflex zones for organs that are in the same body zone.

The spine, for example, is located in the first two longitudinal zones of the body's middle line. If you follow these zones inside the legs down to the feet, you will see that these zones run along the inside of the feet. The foot reflex zones for the spine thus lie on the inside edges of the feet. The head zones run across the toes. The shoulder zones run across the ball of the foot in the same way in which the shoulders themselves run across the longitudinal zones of the body. In this way the entire body can be pictured on the feet, just like the embryo in the ear (see page 6).

The Latitudinal or Horizontal Cross-Zones

To improve orientation, three cross-zones can be added to the ten longitudinal zones. The upper cross-zone is in the area of the foot joints and represents the head and throat

The reflex zones on the soles of the feet are not always identical between the left and the right foot.

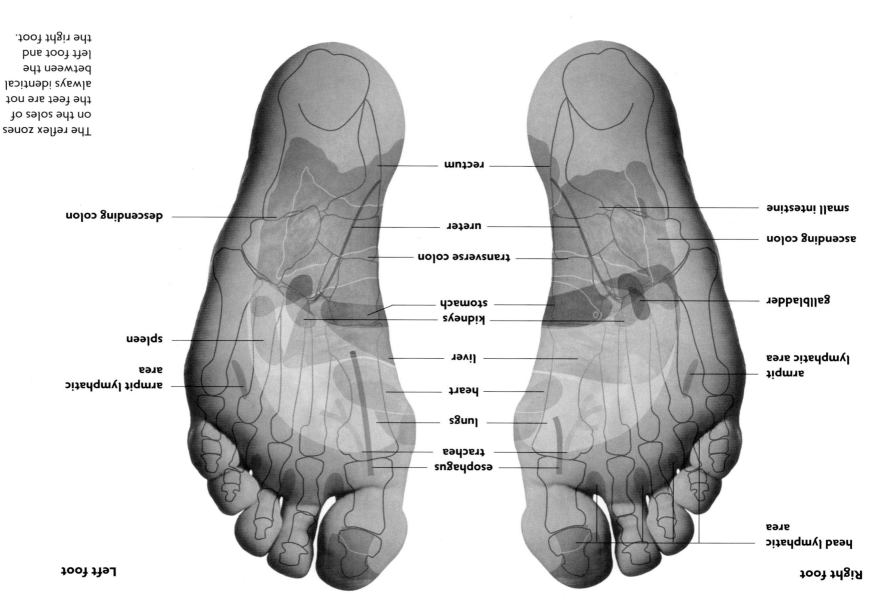

Right foot

- head lymphatic area
- armpit lymphatic area
- gallbladder
- ascending colon
- small intestine

- rectum
- ureter
- transverse colon
- stomach
- kidneys
- liver
- heart
- lungs
- trachea
- esophagus

Left foot

- armpit lymphatic area
- spleen
- descending colon

area. The second cross-zone represents the chest, with the heart and lungs and the upper abdomen. The lower abdomen and organs are found on the bottom third of the foot, or the third cross-zone. These cross-zones can be used to help locate further reflex zones on the feet. The zones for the head and throat area are thus in the toe area, the chest and upper abdomen are in the middle of the foot, and the lower abdomen and organs are on the heel near the ankle.

The Location of the Reflex Zones

The zone model can be used for the general location of the individual zones. But for practical purposes, it has been shown that the zones consist of much smaller areas. Knowledge of these areas is essential for massages. Because

some of the zones overlap, these areas are shown in different illustrations to help us pinpoint their locations.

Reflex Zones on the Soles of the Feet

The soles of the feet are home to the reflex zones of the internal organs. Take note of the varying sizes of the zones on the right and left feet. For example, the heart zone on the left foot is almost twice the size as that on the right foot.

The zones of the stomach, large intestine, and liver stretch across the soles of both feet. The zone of the large intestine starts on the right sole, corresponding to the location of the ascending colon in the body. The zone proceeds, following the sideways path of the colon, over to the sole of the left foot. From here, it follows the actual downward path of the descending colon.

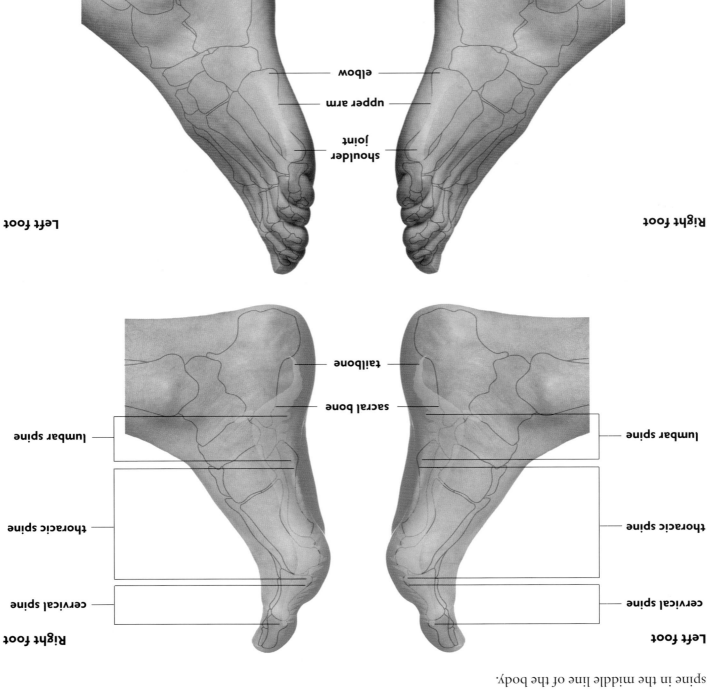

The zones of the shoulders, upper arms, and elbows are on the outside edges of the feet.

Left foot

Right foot

elbow
upper arm
shoulder joint

The zone of the spine extends along the inside edges of the feet.

tailbone
sacral bone
lumbar spine
thoracic spine
cervical spine

Right foot

Left foot

lumbar spine
thoracic spine
cervical spine

Reflex Zones on the Outside Edges of the Feet

The outside edges of the feet correspond to Fitzgerald's fifth longitudinal zone. This zone represents the regions of the body located on its sides, among them the zones of the shoulder joints, upper arms, and elbows.

Reflex Zones on the Inside Edges of the Feet

The zone of the spine is on the inside edges of the feet and runs from the big toes to the heels. It runs along the first longitudinal zone according to Fitzgerald's zone model. This position on the feet corresponds to the location of the spine in the middle line of the body.

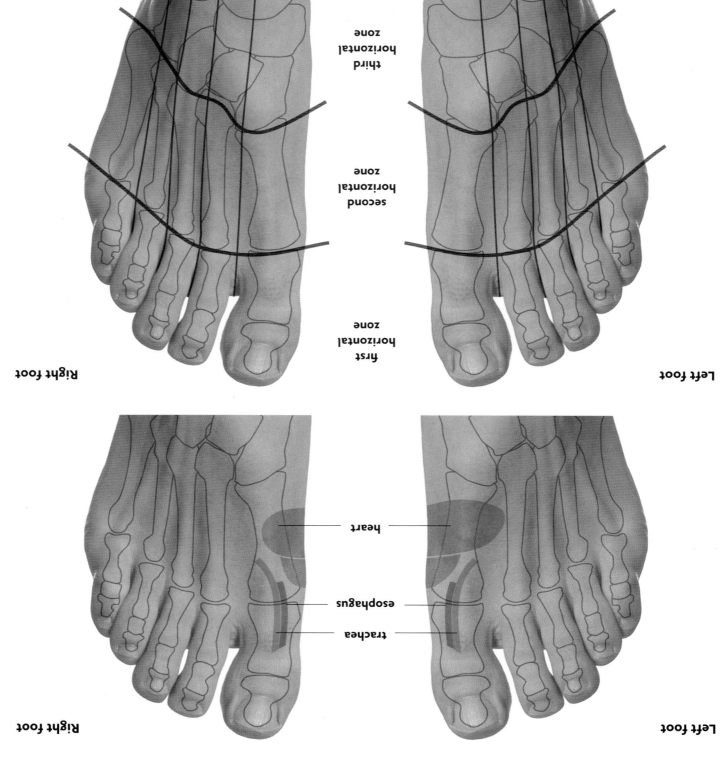

Right foot   **Left foot**

first
horizontal
zone

second
horizontal
zone

third
horizontal
zone

You can locate
zones on the tops
of the feet using
the longitudinal
and latitudinal
lines.

Right foot   **Left foot**

heart

esophagus

trachea

Reflex Zones on the Tops of the Feet

It is easy to locate the individual zones on the tops of the feet by recalling the zone model. Zones run from the middle line of the body outward. Thus, in the first zone you will find all the body parts and organs that are located in the body's center. The horizontal zones offer further

orientation. They divide the body into three areas: head and throat, chest and upper abdomen, and lower abdomen. Once you know the longitudinal and latitudinal zones of the body, you can transfer them to coordinates on the feet.

Our Feet—Load Carriers and Heavy Workers

In the course of foot reflexology, you will have occasion to take a closer look at the feet. Our feet are load bearers and heavy workers. They usually do their duties unnoticed and without complaint. But during summer heat or after standing for long periods, you start to feel your feet: they feel swollen and may even hurt. How do the feet manage to carry our body weight day in and day out on their small surface? To do this job reliably and over time, the feet have to be robust and have a stable build. But the skin of our sturdy feet is extremely sensitive to the touch. While soft and fleeting sensations are registered as tickling, gentle pressure is experienced as a pleasant sensation and a foot massage creates a feeling of relaxation that extends beyond the feet themselves.

The Anatomy of the Foot

The intricate construction of the feet is what allows us to move about upright and to be able to walk and climb over obstacles of all kinds. From the outside, the anatomy of the foot can be divided into three areas: the front of the foot, including the toes up to the ball of the foot; the middle of the foot; and the back of the foot, including the heel. These areas correspond to the horizontal zones discussed above.

Looking at the bones of the foot, you see a supporting construction that consists of twenty-six individual bones. From the side, these bones form an arch. This structural arch is important for the overall function of the foot, in the same way that the arch of a bridge can support heavy loads with a minimum of material.

The big toe consists of two joints; the other toes have a base, middle, and end joint. The middle of the foot, also

heel bone

ankle

anklebone

navicular bone

inner cuneiform bone

metatarsal bone

base joint

end joint

heel bone

navicular bone

middle cuneiform bone

inner cuneiform bone

metatarsal bone

base joint

end joint

cuboid bone

outer cuneiform bone

base joint

middle joint

end joint

Each foot is supported by a construction of twenty-six individual bones.

known as the metatarsus, has five metatarsal bones, which run along the top of the foot and are easily felt. The tarsus, or the bones of the back of the foot, connects to the metatarsus. It consists of the anklebone, the heel bone, three cuneiform bones, the cuboid bone, and the navicular bone. This complicated construction is held together by ligaments, tendons, and muscles. Muscles that run both lengthwise and widthwise are in a way the support beams of the construction. There are two groups of foot muscles: The calf muscles, at the back of the lower leg, run past the ankle joint down to the heel bone. Their job is to move the foot downward and to tighten the foot construction. The front muscles are found to the left and right of the shin and run across the top of the foot up to the toes. Their job is to move the foot upward. Further muscle groups are found between the sole of the foot and the toes. They run with accompanying tendons up to the tips of the toes and allow the spreading

> **Note**
>
> Obesity, weak tendons, or genetic predisposition can cause the arch of the foot to be flat. In this case, the middle part of the sole of the foot, which normally does not touch the ground, is lowered and may touch the ground. The term *flat-footed* refers to a person for whom the entire sole of the foot touches the ground.

of the front of the foot as well as the curling of the toes.

Because of their constant use, most foot muscles are tight and hardened. You can change this with a foot massage of stroking and kneading movements. This type of massage is also an ideal introduction to the foot reflexology massage.

You have now seen the feet as robust and sensible body parts and learned about their construction. The following pages will discuss how reflexology works.

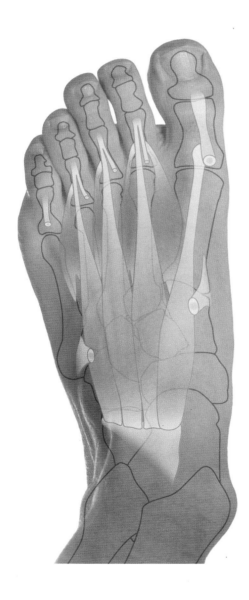

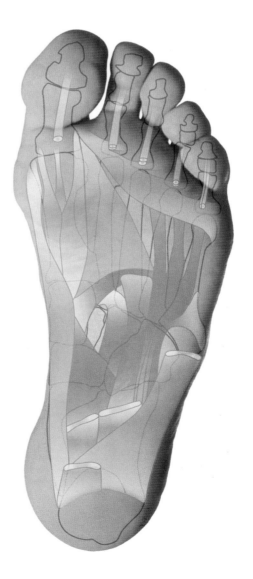

Left: The supporting construction of the individual bones is held together by ligaments, tendons, and muscles. The muscles on the top of the foot pull the foot upward.

Right: The muscles on the sole of the foot allow the spreading of the front of the foot and the curling of the toes.

How Reflexology Works

Up to now we have not discussed how the reflex zones of the feet are connected to their respective body parts and organs. In this context, the term *reflex* is misleading. In medical language, a reflex is a reaction of the body to a stimulation, transmitted via a nerve. One example is the knee-jerk reflex, in which a light tap on the tendon below the knee leads to an immediate tension of the large quadriceps muscle of the thigh, which results in the knee moving from a bent to a straight position, lifting the lower leg. This reflex is transmitted via a certain nerve. Such a direct connection has up to this point not been shown for the reflex zones.

Reflexology via the Skin

The British neurologist Sir Henry Head (1861–1940) described skin zones, called Head zones, on the human body that correspond to specific internal organs. Illnesses of these organs cause the associated skin zones to "coreact." Reactions can take shape as pain or sensitivity to touch in the respective skin area. Conversely, problems of the organs, especially pain, can be influenced via these areas. Therapeutic treatment can be massages, applications of heat, or injections.

There is a scientific explanation for the relationship between organs and the skin. The skin contains blood vessels and a dense network of nerves. These nerves come as a bundle from the spine. They run not only to the skin but also to the muscles and organs. Thus, in a simplified manner, skin, muscles, and organs are connected with one another via nerves. These connections can be illustrated anatomically and provide an explanation for why organs can be represented as skin zones and why skin zones can influence organs. For example, gallbladder problems can take the form of shoulder or back pain. Pain in the left arm sometimes indicates problems of the heart. Patients with strokes often describe a pain in the left arm.

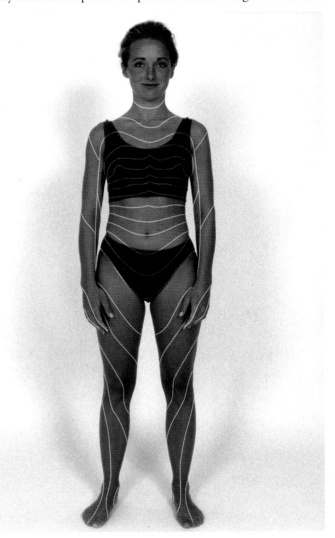

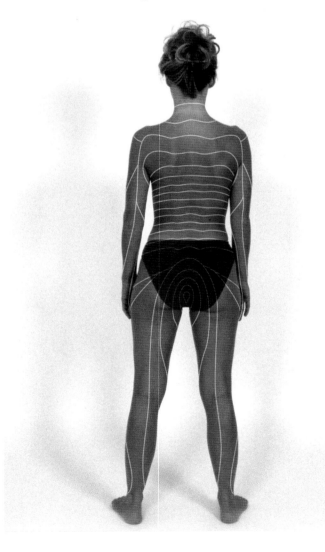

The reflex zones of the organs are also projected onto the skin.

Foot Reflexology from the Perspective of Acupuncture

While there is a concrete, verifiable scientific explanation for the Head zones, no similar explanation has been found for foot reflexology as of yet. No nerves have been found by which effects are transmitted between the feet and the rest of the body. However, many observations collected over the years have shown the effectiveness of reflexology.

Perhaps foot reflexology can be explained via the basic principles of Eastern healing methods. The oldest and probably most successful type of reflex therapy is acupuncture. It is based on the principle that the entire body is covered by a network of energy pathways. These energy paths, or meridians, have certain routes along the body surface and by way of these can be influenced through pressure on the body's surface. In a healthy person, life energy passes through the net of meridians without obstacles.

According to this concept, pain or illness of an organ or body part is an expression of energy disturbance. Thus the

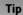

Tip

The stomach zone is located one hand-width below the sternum on the left side of the thorax. In the case of acute or chronic stomach pain, this zone can be sensitive. In this case, place a hot water bottle wrapped in a towel on this zone for 20 to 30 minutes. This measure will alleviate pain. However, if the pain recurs, consult a doctor.

basic tenet of Chinese acupuncture views illness as a result of energy imbalance. A disruption or illness can be caused by too much or too little energy in a particular area. A therapist restores the energy balance through his or her treatment and thus resolves the disturbance at its root. Once the energy balance has been restored, the patient recovers.

It is a similar process in the case of foot reflexology. An illness or disturbance in a certain part or area of the body is translated into a painful or especially sensitive zone in the foot. If this zone is then massaged in the proper manner, the symptoms improve or disappear in the respective body part or area.

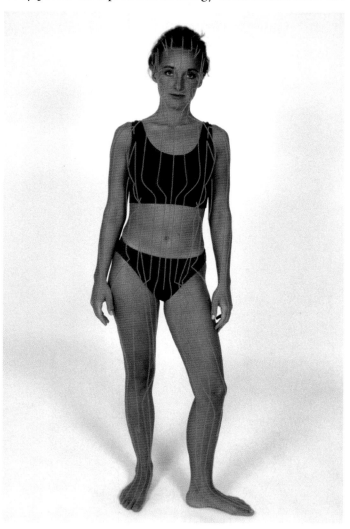

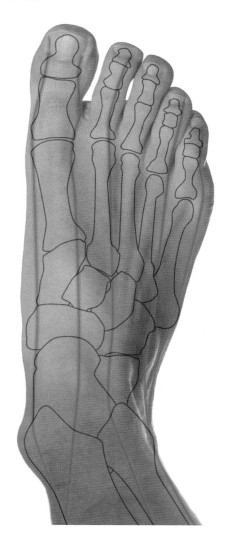

An interesting parallel can be drawn between acupuncture and foot reflexology. Six of the fourteen main meridians begin or end in the feet. This means there are many acupuncture points on the feet that can influence the meridians.

Restoring Balance in the Body

To understand the way in which foot reflexology works, it is useful to discuss the causes and origins of illnesses.

Causes of Illnesses and Ailments

The two terms *functional illness* and *functional disturbance* are often used as synonyms. A functional illness or disturbance occurs when symptoms exist but even the most modern diagnostics are unable to show signs of physical damage to the body. One example is stomach and intestinal problems: Many people suffer from recurring stomach pains whose causes remain unclear even after a colonoscopy. Despite the fact that no medical causes can be found, the patient suffers from these symptoms. There are many types of such functional illnesses, many of which have pain as a common symptom. Such symptoms always need first a medical investigation, and only when no physical cause is found does the problem become categorized as a functional illness.

But what are the causes of problems that can have significant effects on the quality of our life but for which there seems to be no clear scientific explanation? Many disturbances are the result of harmful life situations. Bad working conditions, relationship problems, unhealthy eating habits, excessive consumption of alcohol, cigarettes, or

Stress Factors
• Constant overexertion
• Lack of sleep
• Unrealistic expectations
• Psychological problems
• Unhealthy eating habits
• Excessive consumption of alcohol, nicotine, or other drugs

drugs, and even too little sleep all have something in common: If they exist for prolonged periods of time, they place stress on our body. Stress in this sense means that the body loses the ability to recover after prolonged and damaging stimulation. Too much stress can lead to high blood pressure, constriction of blood vessels, and stroke.

As described above, stress has many faces. Continued stress via a chain of different reactions causes a lack of oxygen in certain organs. Oxygen is a life necessity for all body cells. Continued lack of oxygen basically leads to the starvation and dying off of cells and thus to a reduced functioning of the attached organs. This often leads to an illness. Of course, the body is able to regenerate to a certain degree—that is, to deal with the consequences of the unhealthy stress. But at a certain point the balance is so disrupted that the body's ability to compensate is no longer sufficient. The result is the development of illness.

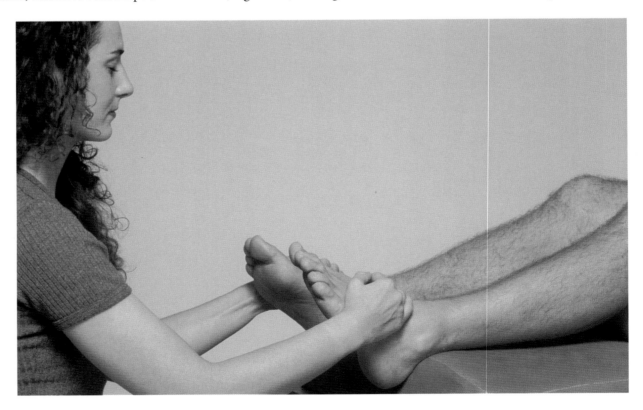

Soft strokes and grips help restore the balance of the body.

The First Step—Finding the Root Causes

To resolve a functional disturbance, you have to find its root causes. Often there will be one or more factors in your environment that are bringing your body out of balance. Only when you know these factors will you be able to restore your body's balance.

The Second Step—Bringing About Harmonization

Finding a permanent balance is the key to solving all health problems.

A foot reflexology massage can counteract the effects of stress. Through the reflex zones of the foot, the massage brings about a relaxation of and increased circulation in the damaged body part or parts. In this way, the foot reflexology massage leads to the restoration of a healthy balance.

There are a number of other easily learned techniques that help reduce stress and bring about harmonization. Not every method is suited to all people. The many possibilities allow individuals to find the way that is best suited to them. In that process, you should follow these basic principles:

1. Choose from among the procedures presented in this book those that work for you.
2. When you begin a new procedure, start with a low load.

3. Try to spend a few minutes each day on the procedure that you have selected for yourself.

> **Tip: Additional Relaxation Measures**
>
> Sports
> Cardiovascular sports such as walking, jogging, cycling, rowing, and swimming encourage a reduction of physical tension through steady and continuous activity without demands for sudden spurts of energy. A pleasant side effect of these types of sports combined with a diet low in fats is a small and steady weight reduction. Those who are new to these sports should begin with a light regimen of activity and steadily increase it. The right dosage is your own well-being.
>
> Relaxation Measures
> There are many relaxation measures:
> - Progressive muscle relaxation, according to Edmund Jacobson, who invented the technique, is very effective and easy to learn.
> - Autogenic training is the classic relaxation technique. It is a little more difficult to learn; the most important thing is to practice it regularly.
> - Different types of yoga offer the possibility of finding relaxation through physical exercises. Exercises should be learned under instruction. Many yoga courses are now offered.
> - Tai chi is a Far Eastern method of relaxation focused on the fluid movement of the body. These movements strengthen muscles and tendons. Tai chi can be learned only from an instructor.

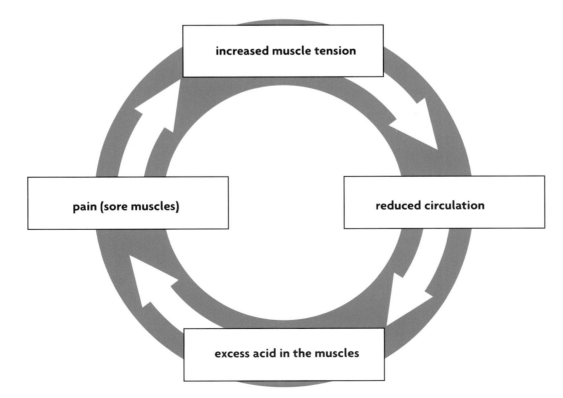

Increased muscle tension leads to a vicious cycle: reduced blood circulation and biochemical processes lead to sore muscles, which in turn cause muscles to become more tense.

The Possibilities of Foot Reflexology

Foot reflexology massage is an effective way to look after your health. A regular massage of the reflex zones harmonizes the flow of energy in your body. When practiced regularly, it provides good protection against a wide range of ailments.

Areas for Applying Foot Reflexology

A massage of the reflex zones can be used in the case of all functional disturbances (those illnesses for which no physical root cause can be found). One of the pioneers of natural healing processes, Dr. Horst Ferdinand Herget (1929–2001), described the treatment spectrum of reflexology therapies with this core statement: "Reflexology heals what is disturbed; it does not heal what is destroyed." Up front, it needs to be understood that foot reflexology massage cannot be the only medicine for the illnesses described on the following pages—but it can be a good accompanying measure.

Sleep Disorders, Nervousness, Stress, and Anxiety

In the case of sleep disorders, a massage of the appropriate reflex zones helps bring about a calm and deep sleep. Moreover, it alleviates nervousness—for example, before exams or during difficult situations. At the same time, it serves to reduce stress. Even anxiety and minor depressions can be positively influenced through foot reflexology in conjunction with other types of therapy. Moreover, reflexology can be effective in remediating all psychosomatic illnesses.

Ailments in the Head Area and Nerve Pains

Western medicine often treats headaches and migraines with strong medicine. These medications can have significant side effects. The goals of reflexology are to extend the intervals between attacks, to alleviate acute pain, and to thus reduce the consumption of medication. Burning nerve pains are probably something that everyone is familiar with. Here, too, medical school teachings are limited to a range of medications. When applied properly, foot reflexology can alleviate the symptoms and be used to extend the intervals between them.

Digestive Problems

Digestive problems, from chronic stomach pain to constipation and diarrhea, are common physiological occurrences. Here, too, the principle applies: If the basic illness has been diagnosed and no physical problems are found, reflexology can help.

Hormonal Disturbances and Menstrual and Pregnancy Problems

There are those days before menstruation or the time before menopause when a number of unpleasant symptoms severely impair the quality of life for those affected.

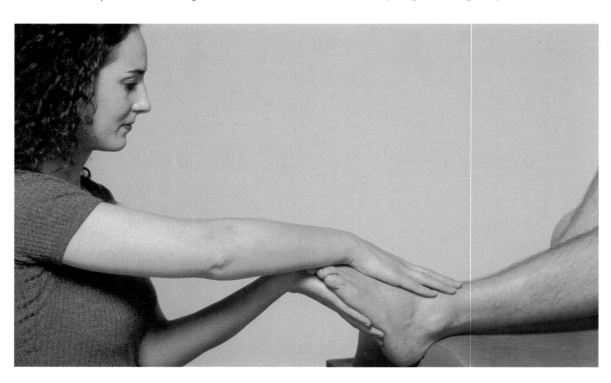

Reflexology massages are especially effective for functional ailments.

These symptoms, which are caused by hormonal changes, respond especially well to foot reflexology. The same is true for the nausea often experienced by women during the first three months of pregnancy: in a simple and effective way, reflexology can help.

Illnesses of the Breathing Passages

Breathing problems caused by asthma or hay fever are also good candidates for relief via foot reflexology. Here, the basic illness should be diagnosed and the prescribed medication taken, accompanied by foot reflexology.

Rheumatic Illnesses

There are a number of illnesses of the rheumatic type, for which the common symptom is pain. Foot reflexology can alleviate this pain and thus, after consultation with a physician, lead to a reduction of the medication taken.

Joint Pain

Joint pain often occurs because of improper stress or as a result of so-called overuse. It limits range of motion, and while reflexology cannot enable the production of new bones or bone marrow, it can effectively alleviate accompanying problems such as muscle pain.

Skin Problems

Skin problems such as neurodermatitis, psoriasis, and acne are very stressful for their sufferers because of their visible effects as well as their sometimes painful symptoms, such as itchiness. In combination with other therapy, foot reflexology can provide relief.

Allergies

According to the basic understanding of naturally oriented medicine, allergies are caused by disturbances in the energy balance. Aside from medication and possible sensitization treatment, homeopathic medicine is often prescribed. Together with these types of therapy, foot reflexology can be used with much success.

Problems of the Urinary Tract and Genitals

Because of the differences between their anatomies, genitourinary infections tend to affect women more than men. They are painful and unpleasant and are usually treated with antibiotics. A foot reflexology massage (the feet should be warmed first) is pleasant and reduces the pain.

Accompanying Therapy for Severe Illnesses

Serious illnesses such as tumors have many effects on overall well-being. Aside from physical pain, psychological symptoms such as fear and depression as well as exhaustion are frequently observed. Treatment is usually based on medication and is directed at specific organs. Complementary reflexology helps patients regain their inner balance.

Accompanying Measures

Foot reflexology can be combined with other natural healing treatments. For example, it can be used together with hand, ear, or head reflexology or with shiatsu, acupressure, or acupuncture. These methods can complement one another and lead to increased effectiveness. There are a number of other treatment possibilities that can be combined with foot reflexology and traditional therapies.

For functional illnesses of the stomach and intestines, for example, under medical supervision an intestinal cleansing or fast might be helpful. Allergic illnesses and skin problems can also be treated through intestinal cleansing, homeopathic methods, or blood therapy.

A strengthening of the immune system can be achieved through balneological methods such as treading water, through hot and cold water treatments, or by taking herbal supplements such as echinacea. Physical therapy, strengthening of the muscles, and endurance training can help with joint problems. Illnesses of the breathing passages can be treated through certain types of breathing therapy in combination with reflexology.

Indications
- Sleep problems, nervousness and stress, fear
- Ailments in the head and neck area
- Digestive problems
- Hormonal disturbances, menstrual problems, or problems in pregnancy
- Illnesses of the breathing passages
- Rheumatic illnesses or joint pains
- Skin problems
- Allergies
- Problems of the urogenital system
- As accompanying therapy for severe illnesses

The Limits of Reflexology

Foot reflexology can be used effectively to treat a variety of ailments. The restoration of the energy balance of the body alleviates or even eliminates symptoms. But reflexology should not be used for self-treatment of ailments. Talk with your doctor or therapist about whether the use of reflexology in addition to ongoing treatment could be useful. Treating acute new illnesses with reflexology without consulting a physician carries the danger that symptoms will become unclear or that more immediately necessary medical treatment will be delayed. Do not try to diagnose yourself or treat yourself or others using the knowledge gained here. This can do more harm than good.

Indications That Foot Reflexology Is Not Appropriate

Foot reflexology aims to restore the body's energy balance. This balance, however, cannot be restored if tissue is already destroyed. In this case, reflexology is not only ineffective but also dangerous. These contraindications are all based on the maxim "Reflexology heals what is disturbed, not what is destroyed."

Varicose Veins in the Foot or Calf

A massage near varicose veins can lead to blood clots and can have dangerous side effects such as infection and thrombosis (the formation of a blood clot in a blood vessel).

Wounds, Infections, or Tumors on the Foot or Calf

Areas on the foot or calf with a tumor, infection, or broken or lacerated skin should not be touched. These types of injuries always indicate the need for medical therapy, and a massage should be carried out only after the area has healed completely and in consultation with the attending physician.

Severe Infection and Fever

Severe infections and fever pose a high degree of stress to the human body. Thus, only medical symptomatic treatments can be carried out in these cases. When fever and severe infection are present, reflexology is of no use.

Illnesses That Require Surgery

Of course, illnesses such as acute appendicitis cannot be treated with reflexology. Immediate examination and treatment by a specialist is required.

After Surgery on the Foot or Calf

After surgery has been performed on the bones or tissue of the foot, reflexology should be done only after consultation with the attending physician.

Coliclike Ailments

Colic, caused by mechanical obstacles that prevent the exit of secretions (bile, urine) or intestinal contents, is characterized by increasing, severe pain. Because of the resulting complications, colic always poses an emergency that requires immediate medical attention.

High-Risk Pregnancies

High-risk pregnancies exist in the case of previous miscarriages, premature contractions, or any other ailment not typical to pregnancy. Foot reflexology is not advisable during a high-risk pregnancy.

One exception is morning sickness, which—in consultation with the attending physician—can be treated with foot reflexology.

Severe Depression

Severe depression requires treatment by a specialist. Foot reflexology can lead to a blurring of symptoms and may even make symptoms worse.

In general, if you are unsure, consult with your physician to find out whether foot reflexology can be applied.

Contraindications
- Varicose veins in the foot or calf
- Infections, tumors, or wounds on foot or calf
- Acute illnesses such as severe infections, fever, and colics
- Illnesses that require surgery
- Recovery after surgery on the foot or calf
- High-risk pregnancies
- Severe depression

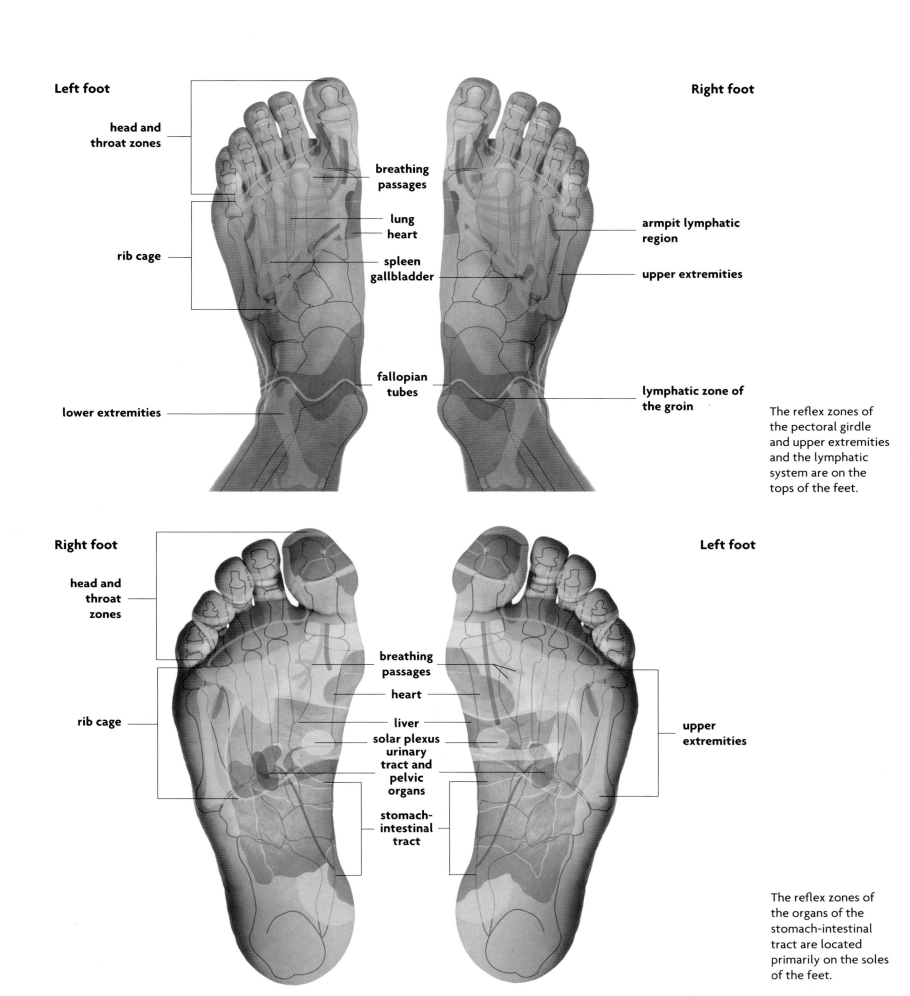

Left foot

head and throat zones

rib cage

lower extremities

breathing passages

lung
heart

spleen
gallbladder

fallopian tubes

Right foot

armpit lymphatic region

upper extremities

lymphatic zone of the groin

The reflex zones of the pectoral girdle and upper extremities and the lymphatic system are on the tops of the feet.

Right foot

head and throat zones

rib cage

breathing passages

heart

liver

solar plexus
urinary tract and pelvic organs

stomach-intestinal tract

Left foot

upper extremities

The reflex zones of the organs of the stomach-intestinal tract are located primarily on the soles of the feet.

Learning Foot Reflexology Massage Step by Step

A good foot reflexology massage relaxes and calms the recipient. Aside from good technique, many factors need to be considered for the success of the massage treatment. Here are a few helpful points.

The Golden Rules of Massage

An appealing ambience is important for a good treatment. This means that the massage should take place in a well-ventilated room with a pleasant temperature and that the recipient should be in a comfortable position. The recipient's feet, calves, and, if possible, legs should be free of clothing. If the recipient's pant legs are simply pushed up, make sure that they are not tight, or else they will restrict circulation below the knees, reducing the flow of energy. The massager's clothing should be comfortable and not restrictive.

For the massager, comfortable body position is important. Consider that a full foot reflexology massage will take 30 to 45 minutes. If you become tense during this time because of your own body position, you will have little fun giving foot reflexology massages.

The massage is usually done with the thumbs and tips of the fingers. Make sure that your fingernails do not extend beyond your fingertips, since the massage can otherwise become an unpleasant experience for your partner. Do not give a massage with cold hands. The recipient is likely to experience cold hands as being unpleasant. This leads to tension, which in turn nullifies any beneficial effect of the massage.

The feet of the recipient must be warm and dry. Cold feet are the most common reason for the failure of a foot reflex-zone massage. If the recipient's feet are cold, warm them either with a heat lamp (common to the trade), a warm footbath, or a hot water bottle wrapped in a towel.

Massage gently. Start the massage with a few introductory strokes over the whole area before you begin addressing the individual zones.

Keep eye contact with your partner. By looking at your partner, you will know immediately how your massage is being received. Ask your partner about his or her

The Eleven Golden Rules

- Have a pleasant environmental ambience.
- Wear comfortable clothing.
- Assume a comfortable position.
- Make sure your fingernails do not extend past your fingertips.
- Make sure your hands are warm.
- Make sure the feet of the recipient are warm and dry.
- Begin the massage with gentle strokes.
- Maintain eye contact with your partner and note how he or she is feeling.
- Allow 30 to 45 minutes for the massage.
- Don't use oils or lotions during the massage.
- Allow for a rest period of 30 minutes after the massage.

sensations. It is important that you communicate during the massage and give your partner the opportunity to ask questions. But do not make diagnoses or suppositions about illnesses if certain zones are sensitive.

Allow a full 30 to 45 minutes for a massage. Should you or the recipient be under time constraints, it is advisable to reschedule the massage rather than abbreviate it. Do not use oils, creams, powders, or other lubricants during the massage, since they make the skin slippery and will prevent you from massaging individual zones. However, applying skin-care products at the end of the massage might make for a pleasant finish.

Foot reflexology massage leads to optimal relaxation. To fully appreciate the blessing of this relaxation, the recipient should plan on a resting period of 30 minutes following the massage.

Posture during Massage

Your body posture is very important during massages. Consider that a good treatment requires about 45 minutes. It is almost impossible to massage for this length of time in an unsuitable position without afterward requiring a good back massage yourself. Good posture is characterized by an upright upper body and relaxed shoulders. Ideally, the recipient will be resting on a low bed, with his or her feet accessible from all sides. The massager sits on a stool, with his or her upper body straight and upright. The massager's lower arms can rest on the bed, while the shoulders should be relaxed.

Body Posture during Self-massage

The advantage of self-massage is that it can be done anytime and at any place. For self-massage of the feet, you can sit either in a chair or on the floor with your legs crossed. Simply try the two positions and then decide which one is more comfortable for you.

Foot Massage Sitting on a Chair

Use a chair with a high backrest but no armrests (armrests can get in the way during the massage). Place your feet on the ground shoulder-width apart. The soles of your feet should touch the ground and your knees should be slightly bent. If it makes you more comfortable, you can also lean back a little bit. Place one foot on the thigh of the opposite leg. You can pull the foot a little closer to your body if that creates a more comfortable position. Now you can comfortably massage the sole of that foot with both hands.

Foot Massage Sitting Cross-legged

People who are adequately flexible can perform a foot massage while sitting on the floor. Sit cross-legged on a soft surface, either a thick carpet or a rubber or foam pad. Place one foot over the thigh of the opposite leg. In this position you can comfortably massage your foot with both hands.

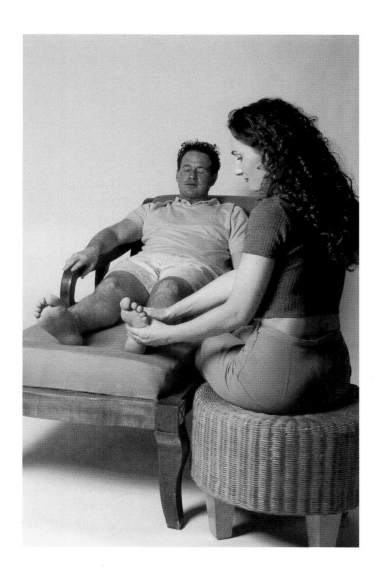

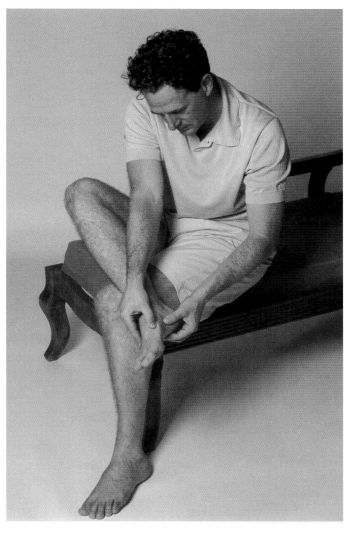

Left: Be sure to keep your upper body straight and your shoulders relaxed.

Right: You can massage yourself either while sitting on a chair or while sitting on the floor with your legs crossed.

Preparing the Hands

During a foot reflexology massage, you will work a lot with the tips of your thumbs. They apply a dynamic pressure, but they are also sensitive to touch and are thus able to sense knots and tensions in the individual zones. Your fingernails, especially those of the thumbs, should be short. They should not extend past the fingertips, to avoid giving the recipient unpleasant sensations during the massage.

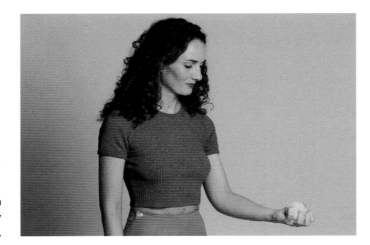

Loosen and warm up each hand by squeezing a ball.

> **Tip**
> Instead of a ball, you can use a balloon filled with flour. Get a good-quality balloon (for example, from a toy store) and use a funnel to fill it with flour. Tie a knot in the balloon. You now have a smooth and flexible cushion that you can use to build up strength in your fingers.

Strengthening, Loosening, and Warming Up Your Hands

Carry out a few strengthening and stretching exercises for your hands before you begin the massage. These will prepare your hands for the exertions of a massage. A simple strengthening exercise can be done with a small ball. Take the ball in one hand and squeeze it. Try to keep up the tension on the ball for 7 seconds, and then slowly release it and relax your hand. The relaxation phase should be three or four times as long as the contraction phase. In other words, if you keep up the tension for 7 seconds, you need 21 to 28 seconds to relax your hand. Repeat five to seven times. Then carry out the same exercise with your other hand.

During and after the exercise, you will feel how warm and flexible your hands are. When you have finished the strengthening exercise, you're ready to stretch the muscles

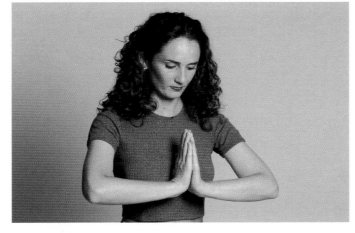

Place your hands together in front of your chest.

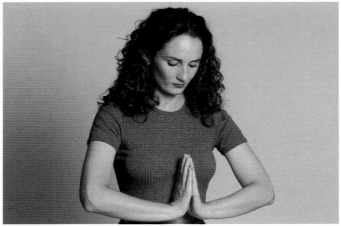

Pressing your hands together and down in front of your chest is a simple and effective stretch for your hand muscles.

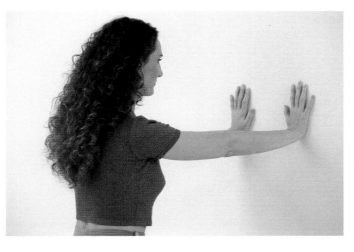

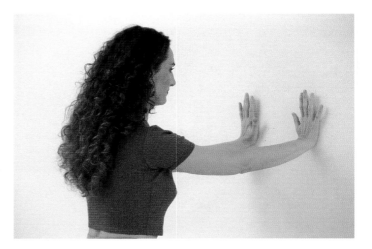

Left: You can stretch your arm muscles by first placing your hands flat against a wall.

Right: Lift your fingers to lengthen the stretch, and then return them to rest.

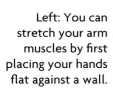

of your hands. Place your hands in "prayer position" with your palms together in front of your chest, fingertips pointing up and elbows pointing out. Slowly and consciously move the heels of your hands toward the ground, keeping your hands in prayer position. Move the hands downward until you feel a noticeable pull in the backs of your hands. Keep them in that position for 20 to 30 seconds. Repeat this exercise two or three times.

You can also stretch your hand and lower-arm muscles with a different exercise. Standing in front of a wall, place the palms of your hands flat against the wall at shoulder level, with your fingers pointing up. Stretch and spread your fingers. In your lower arm you will notice a pronounced but not painful pull. You can increase the stretch by slightly lifting your palms and fingers away from the wall, keeping the heels of your hands against the wall. Stay in this position for 20 to 30 seconds, then relax. Repeat this exercise two or three times.

The Energy of the Hands

After you have finished these exercises, your hands will be warm and loose. The following perception exercise can heighten the sensitivity of your hands.

Perception Exercise

Make sure that your hands are warm before beginning this exercise. Take slow and regular breaths. Close your eyes. Keep your shoulders relaxed. Now place your hands in front of your body, with the palms facing one another but not touching. Concentrate your attention on your palms. Try to feel the warmth that emanates from each palm to the other.

Now imagine this feeling of warmth as a flow of energy that passes between your hands. Once you start perceiving this flow, begin to play with it. Make small, slow circular movements with your hands in opposite directions. Also increase the distance between your hands, but only to the point where you can still sense the energy or warmth flowing between your hands. Do this exercise a few times.

Over time, your sensitivity to the warmth and energy between your hands will increase. When you are performing a foot reflexology massage, imagine that you are passing this flow of energy on to your partner through your hands.

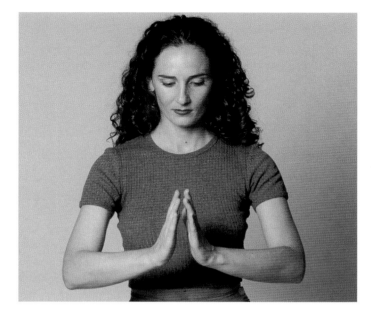

Feel the flow of energy between your hands. Make sure your hands are warm.

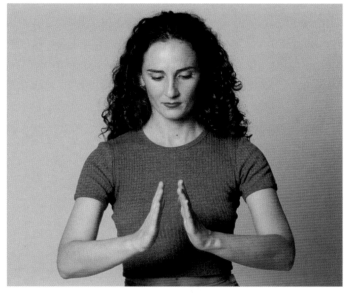

Move your hands as far apart as you can while still feeling the energy between them.

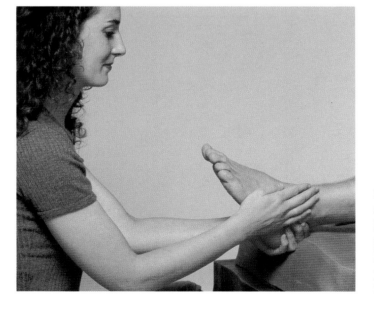

Focus your attention on your hands and their perceptions. Feel how the skin of your partner's feet feels.

> **Caution**
>
> If your partner's feet have been injured, the skin of the feet is irritated, or the feet suffer from any other illness, you should not carry out a foot reflexology massage.

Sensing the Other

In the previous sections you have practiced the strengthening, loosening, stretching, and sensitizing of your hands. Perhaps you are already feeling the energy that lies within your hands. Your hands are now warm and sensitive, and you can turn to massaging your partner.

Begin by making contact with your partner's feet. For this, simply place your hands on the tops of your partner's feet and let them rest there for a little while. This gives your partner the opportunity to feel the skin contact. Try seeing with your hands instead of with your eyes. Close your eyes and focus all of your attention on your hands. Concentrate on their perception, and find out how the skin of the feet feels: is it warm or cool, moist or dry, rough or smooth?

Moist and/or cool feet can indicate tension in your partner. As mentioned above, the feet should be warm and dry for a massage.

Cold Feet Not Wanted

Performing a foot reflexology massage on cold feet is one of the most common causes for the lack of success. Foot reflexology massages are given with the goal of getting energy streams to flow by activating the foot zones. Coldness causes these energy streams to freeze. Indeed, water is a good analogy for illustrating this problem: When warm, it flows freely; when cold, it forms a solid and rough mass. Cold feet must be warmed before they are massaged. This is easiest to do by giving the recipient a warm footbath or by placing a hot water bottle wrapped in a towel against his or her feet.

> **Administering a Footbath**
>
> For a footbath, you will need a small tub that is tall enough that about two thirds of the calves will be covered with water. You can also administer a footbath in a regular bathtub. First fill the tub with lukewarm water (about 95 degrees Fahrenheit [35C]), put feet in the tub, then slowly add hot water until the temperature rises to 102 to 104 degrees Fahrenheit (39 to 40C). To avoid scalding the feet, it is best to pour in the hot water along the edge of the tub. After 10 to 15 minutes, remove feet from the tub and rinse with cooler water. Pat dry.

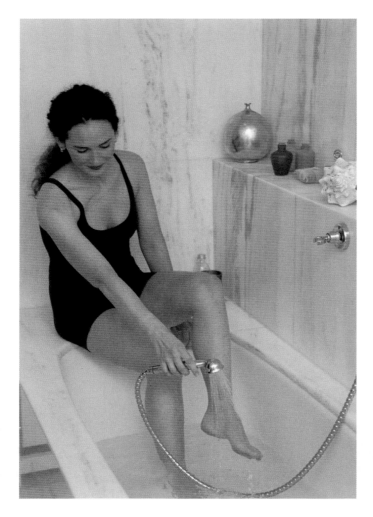

Warm your feet or your partner's feet with a footbath or a hot water bottle.

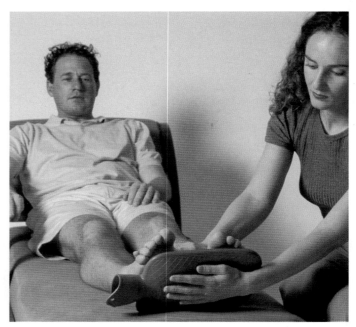

Loosening the Foot Muscles

A further preparation for the foot reflexology massage is the loosening of the recipient's foot muscles. You can loosen tense muscles in each foot with a few effective moves.

Stroking the Top and Sole of the Foot

Take the foot into your hands, with one hand lying flat against the sole and the other resting against the top of the foot. Now slide both hands together, keeping them parallel, toward the toes. Repeat this stroking motion three or four times.

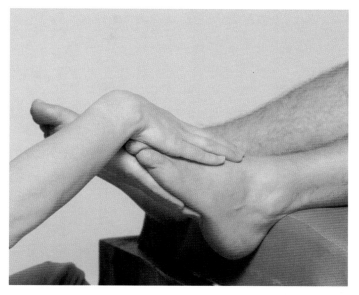

Stroke the foot with both hands.

Moving the Metatarsal Bones

First find the five metatarsal bones. They are located in the upper third of the foot and are easily identified by their pipelike structure. Hold the first metatarsal bone with one hand, and with the other hand move the other four metatarsal bones up and then down. The range of motion here is very small. Then hold the first and second metatarsal bones and move only the remaining three bones up and down. Then hold the first three bones and move the remaining two. Finally, move the fifth metatarsal bone against the others.

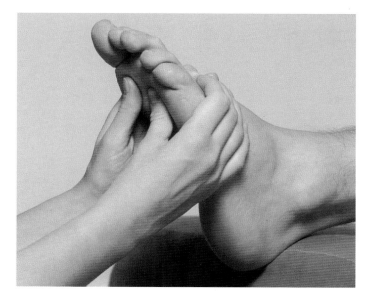

Move the metatarsal bones against each other.

Stretching the Toes

Using your thumb and index finger, grasp the big toe at its base. With slight pressure, pull your fingers up the toe. Repeat this stretch on the other four toes.

Final Stretches

After you have stretched all the toes, do a few final stretches. Resume the initial position of placing one hand against the sole of the foot and the other against the top of the foot. With slight pressure, move your hands from the heel over the foot and up to the toes. Repeat several times for each foot.

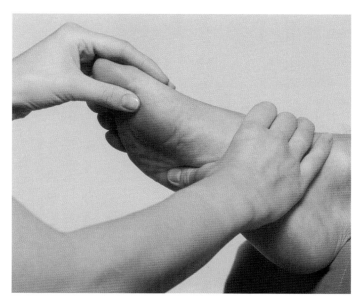

Gently pull your fingers up each toe.

Painful Zones and Their Meaning

Reflexology stimulates zones along the soles of the feet that have a relationship with the organs, muscles, and joints of the body. Using massage, you encourage the harmonization of circulation in the parts of the body that are connected to the zones you are massaging, and thus you support the energy balance as well as the well-being of the recipient. Your massage, at the same time, encourages the dissolution of stress-related tensions, causing a feeling of deep relaxation. However, it is possible that you may touch your partner in places where he or she is especially sensitive, perhaps causing unpleasant sensations and even pain. Most often, these unpleasantly sensitive areas indicate energy problems. Usually they disappear after a few massages. Nonetheless, it is important for you to know what to do when you come upon a sensitive zone.

First, you must respect the points that are sensitive and painful to the touch. Massage gently; do not try to "massage away" a sensitive zone with increased effort. Definitely do not make premature comments to the recipient about a possible illness in the corresponding part of the body. Instead, calm your partner and explain to him or her that painful or sensitive areas are usually not a sign of illness. But if a zone remains unchanged or if your partner has the feeling that something is indeed wrong, suggest that he or she seek medical advice.

Significance of Painful Zones

Areas with heightened sensitivity to pressure indicate an energy blockage. The sensitivity of these zones will usually disappear during the massage. Respect these areas and massage them very gently. Explain their presence to your partner, but do not make guesses about illnesses they may indicate.

What Reactions Can You Expect during or after the Massage?

Aside from unpleasant sensitivity, a number of more common, body-wide reactions can occur during a massage. Sometimes a feeling of deep sleepiness appears during or after the massage. This is actually one of the desired effects, as it indicates the transition from a tense to a relaxed state, brought about by your massage. In fact, your partner may even fall asleep during the massage. This too shows you how relaxing your massage is. These sleepy feelings should be welcomed. Inform your partner about these possible reactions and ask him or her to simply let go and give in to these feelings of drowsiness or relaxation, and not to focus on trying to stay awake. Plan for a rest of about 30 minutes after the massage.

Respect zones that are sensitive to pressure, and don't guess about problems they may indicate in the corresponding body part.

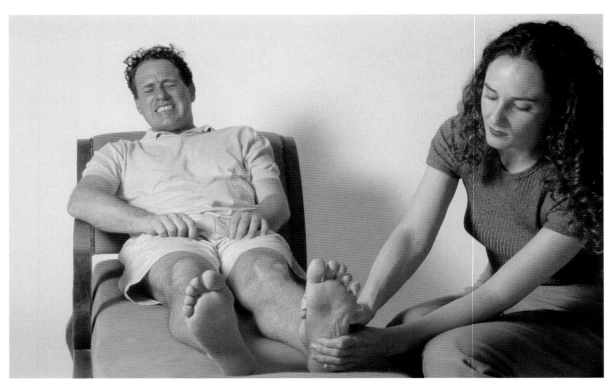

Dealing with Special Situations

The following section offers advice on dealing with special situations.

Blocked, Painful Zones

During the massage treatment, you will occasionally encounter a zone with heightened sensitivity to pain. Your partner might even feel a pulling or sharp pain when you touch one of these areas.

Deal with such a zone in the following way: First gently place your thumb on the painful spot. Then bend the thumb at the base joint, leaving the tip of the thumb perpendicular to the painful area, and apply as much pressure as the pain sensitivity of your partner allows. Keep the thumb in this position without movement until the pain subsides noticeably. This could take up to 20 to 30 seconds.

General Anxiety

In exceptional cases, you might notice anxiety or even fear in your partner. This feeling is expressed through tension in the muscles of the feet, a drop in the skin temperature, or cold sweat on the skin. Calm your partner and explain that these feelings can appear during the course of a massage. Take his or her heels into your hands and slightly stretch the muscles by pulling on the heels. This stretch reduces muscle contractions and improves circulation. Then, on each foot, perform a few sandwich strokes (see page 38) from the heel and back of the foot up to the tips of the toes. During these strokes, cover the foot with your hands, ensuring good skin contact, and carry out these movements very slowly. Repeat three times for each foot. Then you can resume the focused massage on individual parts of the foot.

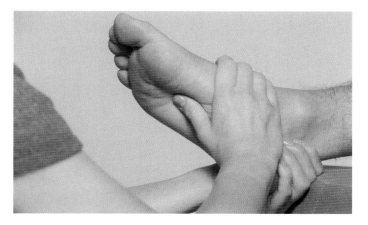

Place your thumb, without pressure, on the painful area.

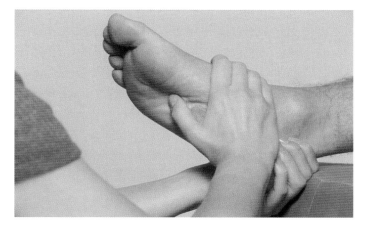

With the thumb bent so that the tip is perpendicular to the foot, apply as much pressure as is acceptable to your partner until the pain subsides.

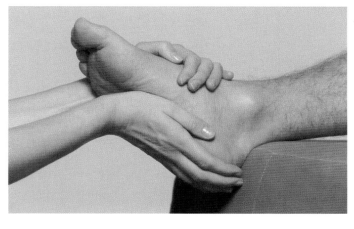

Take the foot in both hands . . .

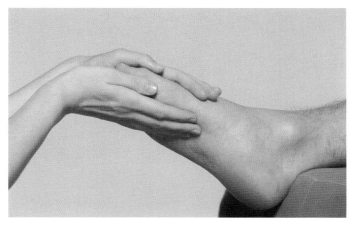

. . . and stroke it from the heel to the toes.

> **Note**
>
> For the massage giver:
> - Short fingernails
> - Soft fingertips
> - Upright posture
> - Warm, relaxed hands
> - Attention to pain
>
> For the massage recipient:
> - Warm feet
> - Rest after the massage

Reactions between Massages

Massage recipients may report that existing ailments actually get worse after the first massage. This is a normal physical reaction. Natural-healing therapists call this the "initial worsening." It is a positive sign and shows that the body is reacting to the massage treatment. These symptoms usually wane quickly, but you should nonetheless explain this possibility to your partner. It is also common for recipients to experience an overall sense of slowing down in response to treatment. An increased need for sleep and even a feeling of depression can be among the possible reactions and do not pose a need for worry.

Massage Aids

A number of aids for healthy feet and the stimulation of foot reflex zones are available. You can safely forget about all of them. You can neither replace nor support your

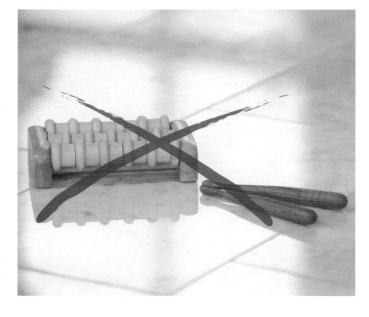

Do not use any aids during the massage.

hands during the massage. The entire sensitivity of your hands and your body is needed for foot reflexology. Definitely avoid instruments such as massage sticks, foot rollers, and other massaging aids. Salves, lubricants, and oils are also not suitable for foot reflexology. There is no reason not to apply oils or lotions after the massage; on the contrary, most recipients perceive this as pleasant. However, these substances are not recommended for use during the massage because they make it easier for your fingers to slip, thus keeping you from using the appropriate techniques on certain spots.

Duration of the Massage

The massage movements that are used for reflexology will probably be tiring and unfamiliar at first. This is true especially for the continued exertion of pressure with the tip of the thumb and the thumb itself (see page 40). Thus the duration of the massage is limited by your own endurance. Massage only for as long as you can without undue exertion, especially if you are just beginning to learn foot reflexology. For a full massage of the zones of both feet you need about 45 minutes. With sufficient endurance and experience, you won't have any problem carrying out a full massage. The frequency of treatment depends on the goal you set. If the focus is on relaxation and reducing stress, these massages can be done daily. Long-term positive effects for overall well-being can be attained with two or three massages a week. So-called therapeutic massages should be given every two or three days. But the exact frequency should be decided mainly according to your own desire and that of your partner.

> **Important Reflexology Facts**
> - Very old form of therapy, initiated around 2330 B.C.
> - Aims to re-create the energy balance inside the body
> - "Reflexology heals what is disrupted; it cannot heal what is destroyed"
> - Longitudinal zones and cross-zones, according to Fitzgerald, and Head zones are the basic foundations of reflexology
> - Images of the entire human body can be superimposed on the sole of the foot and the auricle
> - Disruptions in certain body parts appear as painful zones on the foot
> - Illnesses in different body regions can be positively influenced through massages of the ears, head, hands, and feet

Perfect Feet

Tight shoes and the rubbing of the balls and heels of the feet in shoes lead to unappealing, sometimes rather thick calluses. Thick calluses are sometimes responsible for limiting the effects of reflexology and may need to be removed or reduced. If the recipient's toenails are polished, the polish should be removed, if possible using a natural product that contains healing or conditioning substances.

> **Checklist for Foot Care**
> - Nail polish remover
> - Bath salts
> - Small scissors
> - Nail file
> - Pumice stone
> - Scraper for callused skin
> - Rosewood sticks for the cuticles
> - Towel
> - Lotion or oil

Pleasant Footbath

To begin the path to perfect feet, treat them to a footbath. Fill a tub or container with warm water and add bath products of your choice. A footbath should take 10 to 15 minutes, after which you should towel-dry your feet, paying special attention to the skin between your toes.

Removing Calluses

After the footbath, any calluses will be soft. Smaller parts can be rubbed off with a pumice stone. For bigger calluses near the heel or the base of the big toe, you may need to use a callus scraper. Wet the pumice before use, and wash your feet well after removing the calluses. As after the footbath, dry your feet carefully.

Nail Care

The preceding footbath will have softened and smoothed the nails and the skin around them. Carefully push back the skin around your nails with a soft stick made for this purpose, which can be bought in drugstores and pharmacies. Excessive skin can be carefully cut off using small scissors. Please be very careful not to injure the nail bed.

The toenails should be cut straight and the edges slightly rounded off with a nail file. Cutting nails straight prevents ingrown toenails. If you already have ingrown toenails, you should contact a foot care specialist.

Massaging and Putting Lotion on the Feet

To finish off your foot care, give yourself a foot massage. Sit on a soft rug or pad on the floor. Beginning with either foot, knead the sole of the foot with your thumb. Start at the heel and slowly work your way up to the ball of the foot. Then use your thumb and index finger to knead each toe. Next, stroke along the top of the foot up to the toes. Finally, take your foot between your hands, press your palms against the foot with slight pressure, and make small circular movements. These movements will loosen the joints and metatarsal bones. Then massage the other foot. Apply lotion to your feet afterward.

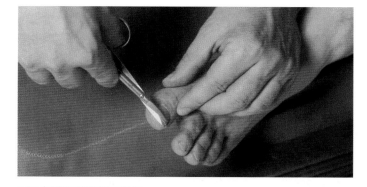

Cut the nails straight, then round off the corners using a file.

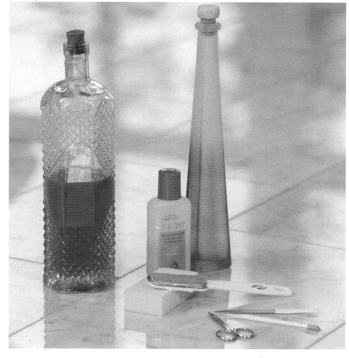

When purchasing tools for foot care, make sure they are of good quality.

Administering Foot Reflexology Massages

The preceding section has demonstrated the fundamentals of foot reflexology. This section will now introduce you step by step to the administration of foot reflexology massages. We will start with the most important basic techniques that you will need for every massage. Afterward, you will learn how to massage individual zones using these techniques.

Preparing for a Reflexology Massage

A pleasant ambience supports the relaxing and harmonizing effects of a foot reflexology massage. You as the massage giver and your partner as the recipient should mentally prepare yourselves for the upcoming massage. Time pressure and restlessness are factors that may jeopardize the success of the treatment.

Room and Atmosphere

A quiet room with a pleasant temperature is ideal for giving the massage. An inviting atmosphere is supported by indirect and soft light. Infusers with scented oils also further relaxation. Some people find that calm music deepens the mood; others opt for silence and isolation. Ask your partner what seems preferable to him or her. Take the proper time for the massage and try to make sure that you won't be disturbed by telephone calls or other interruptions. Wear light, comfortable, loose clothing for the massage.

Tip: Recipe for a Relaxing Scent	
Rosemary oil	2 drops
Neroli oil	2 drops
Melissa oil	2 drops
Lavender oil	2 drops
Add these oils to a full water bowl of an infuser.	

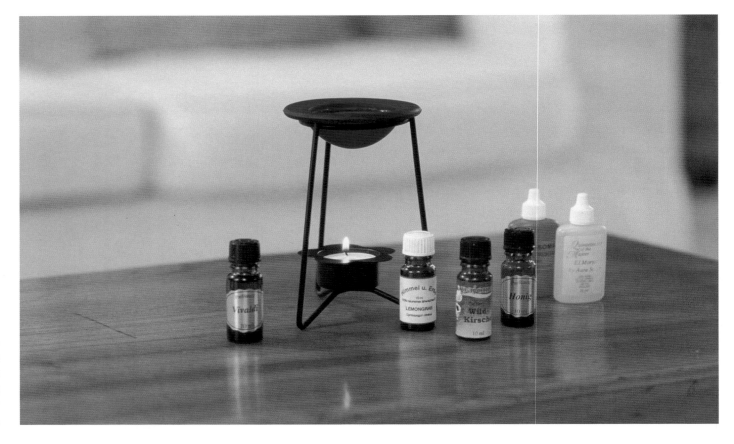

An infuser with essential oils helps create a pleasant atmosphere for relaxation.

The Position

A decisive factor in the success of a massage is the relaxed position of your partner. Lying down allows all muscles to relax, and your partner can thus fully open him- or herself to the massage. A massage chaise is ideal. Your partner lies on his or her back, with both knees slightly raised by resting on a rolled-up blanket or a cylindrical cushion. A large, firm cushion under your partner's upper body can also be helpful. The upper body rests in a slightly raised position while the arms lie loose next to the body. The cushion under the knees leaves the legs slightly bent in the knee and hip joints. This position allows all the leg muscles to relax while keeping your partner's back straight. Finally, the feet have to be easily accessible from all sides. If your partner's feet are between the level of your chest and abdomen, you have located the ideal height. You can now massage with your arms bent at right angles without having to pull up your shoulders.

One alternative to the rather rare massage chaise is a mat. Here, too, the legs should be well supported and the feet should be in a convenient position. Your partner can then lean back during the treatment and enjoy the massage.

Eye contact with your partner is another important component of the position. By watching your partner's face, you will get immediate feedback on the effects of the massage. You can perfectly moderate the tightness of your grip by aiming for a relaxed facial expression on your partner. Although it may be obvious that your partner's feet will have to be bare for the massage, you should still prepare your partner for this circumstance before the first massage. If your partner has simply pushed up his or her pant legs, check how tight they are; if pant legs are too tight, they may

Preparation

- Room is at a pleasant temperature
- Recipient is in relaxed position lying on the back, with feet around the level of the massager's chest and abdomen if possible
- Recipient's feet and calves are bare
- Massager makes eye contact during the massage

impair circulation. In that case, your partner should take off his or her pants.

To protect the legs against the cold, you can wrap them down to the feet in a warm blanket.

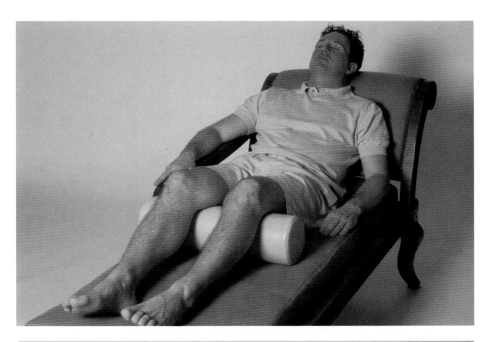

A pillow under the knees relaxes the leg muscles.

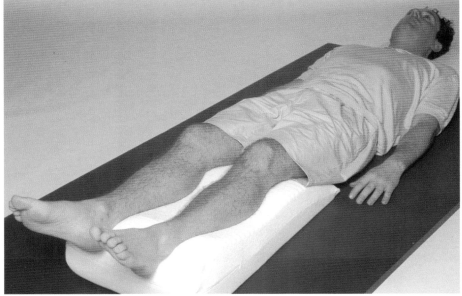

If you are using a mat as a surface, slightly elevate the calves and feet.

> **Note**
> Those parts of the foot where bones and tendons are located directly under the skin are usually much more sensitive than areas with plenty of muscle tissue. Adjust your pressure based on the sensitivity of your partner and the area you are massaging.

Massage Techniques

An effective and relaxing foot reflexology massage can be done with a few simple moves. These moves are described individually on the following pages. You will notice quickly which ones feel good for your partner.

Choosing the Right Pressure Technique

The massage techniques presented here have different ways of applying pressure. The pressure technique used depends on what the reflex zone is like. Is it small and circular or does it extend along a line or across a larger area? A further factor in choosing the pressure technique is the pain sensitivity of a zone.

The Sequence of the Massage

Begin by systematically working through all areas of the feet, touching each of them. Remember any sensitive zones you may notice. During your second run-through,

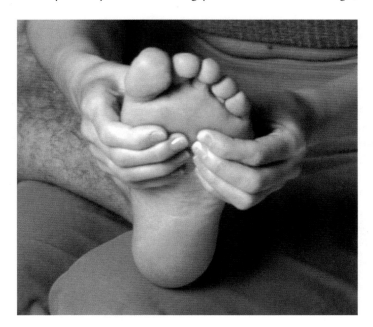

Always adjust your pressure to the sensitivities of your partner.

address these zones very carefully and comprehensively. If the unpleasant sensations do not disappear after the first or second round of massage moves, massage the feet again after two or three days. Remember, especially when you encounter sensitive zones, that the massage should be pleasant for your partner. For this reason, the pressure you apply should always depend on the well-being of your partner.

The Techniques

There are many different techniques and moves in foot reflexology. Generally, however, a few will suffice. The following section presents a rather large spectrum of techniques, so that you can choose those with which you feel most comfortable. It is not necessary to know many moves; rather, it is better to fully master a small number of techniques.

The moves can be divided into three categories: strokes and stretches, pointed-pressure exertions, and balancing touches. Strokes are used for the introduction and closure of the massage. They have a relaxing and harmonizing effect. Pointed pressure is used to massage the individual zones on the foot. Pressure can be applied with the tip of your thumb or with your fingers. Balancing moves are used when you notice a so-called autonomic reaction in your partner, such as anxiety, sweating, or cold feet.

Placing Your Hands on the Feet

Placing your hands on the feet is not a technique or move in the strict sense. It serves mainly to make the initial contact and help your partner relax. Placing your hands on the tops of your partner's feet for a few moments mentally prepares both you and your partner for the massage. It is best to start every massage this way. After you have placed your hands on the feet, close your eyes and take a few deep and conscious breaths. Focus your attention on your hands and imagine collecting all your energy in them. Then try to feel the flow of energy between your hands and the feet of your partner. Your resting, warm hands should calm and relax your partner.

Strokes and Stretches

Ideally, you would use strokes to begin and end a massage. Strokes are also used during the massage to give closure to the massage of certain zones. Stretching the calf and foot muscles helps the massage recipient relax and get full benefit from the session.

Begin with Stroking Hands

Much as with the initial placing of the hands on the feet, strokes introduce and set the mood for the massage. Place both hands flat on one leg, to either side of the knee. Now slide your hands downward over the shins and the top of the foot up to and beyond the toes. Imagine yourself almost pulling tension out of the foot with these movements. Make sure that the whole palm of your hand stays in contact with your partner's skin, and carry out this movement slowly and harmoniously.

Repeat these strokes several times for each leg.

Afterward, stroke each leg separately by sliding one hand after another from the knee to the tips of the toes. Before the first hand is finished stroking the toes, the second hand should begin at the knee.

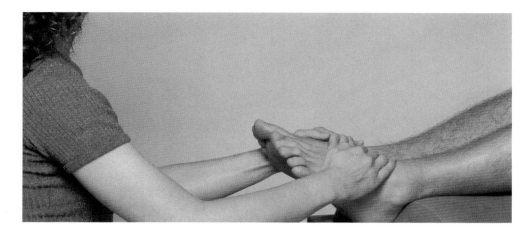

Placing your hands: Place your hands on the tops of the feet and concentrate on your breathing.

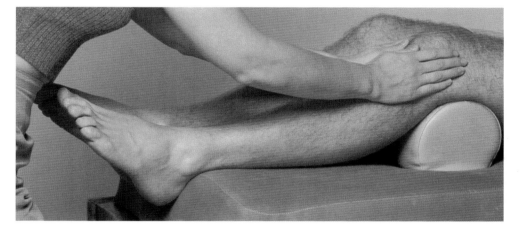

Stroking the legs: Place your hands on either side of one of your partner's knees, making contact with the skin.

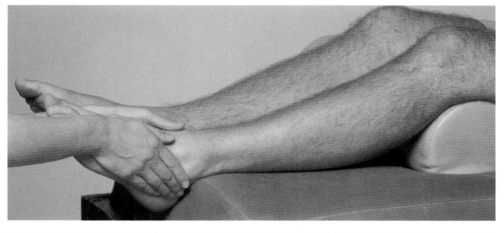

Now slide your hands downward toward the foot with steady pressure.

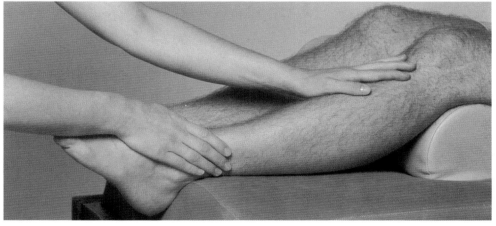

Stroke each leg using both your hands one after the other.

Stroking Fingers

Stroking with your fingertips is a good move for massaging the spaces between the metatarsal bones on the top of each foot. You can feel the metatarsal bones between the base joints of the toes and the tarsus (the bones at the base of the foot). Between these pipelike bones are muscles that are difficult to reach, but with your fingertips on the top of the foot, you can access them. Touch the spaces between the bones at their base, close to the tarsus, and with one fingertip in each space, slowly glide your hand over the spaces, with steady pressure, up to the base joints of the toes. The nonmassaging hand forms the counterbalance, supporting the foot while the fingers of the other hand are making their gliding movement.

You can also stroke these muscles one at a time with one finger; the principle is the same, but you are able to apply more pressure. Again, supporting the foot with one hand, put the index finger of your other hand in the metatarsal space and with steady pressure glide down between the two bones to the base joints. Stroke each space in this way.

Sandwich Strokes

Sandwich strokes are another variation of soft and calming strokes. Do these strokes between the different massage stages to give closure to the zone you have finished.

The name *sandwich stroke* refers to the way in which you hold the foot with your hands. Take the foot between your palms, with one hand on the top of the foot and the other on the sole. Now pull both hands with steady pressure toward and beyond the toes. Repeat this stroke several times.

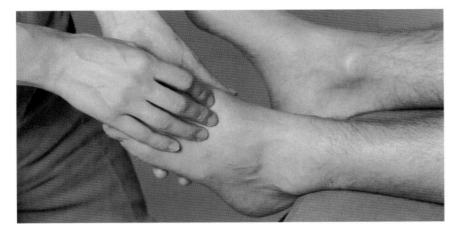

Finger strokes: Place your fingertips close to the tarsus in the spaces between the metatarsal bones . . .

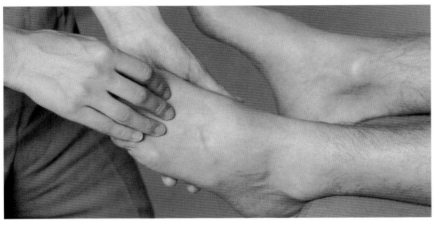

. . . now glide your fingers along these spaces to the base joints of the toes.

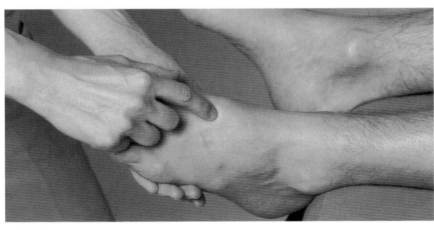

You can also do the finger stroke using just one finger.

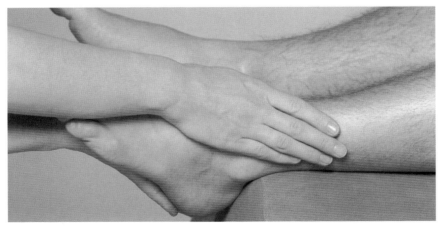

Sandwich stroke: Take the foot between your hands . . .

Stretching the Heels

A stretch of the calf and foot muscles can be done as a gentle opening or end to a massage. It can also be used during the massage, especially in cases where the partner is anxious. Slow stretches done in the rhythm of the recipient's breathing are wonderfully relaxing; they loosen and relax the calf and foot muscles.

Cup your hands around the heels from the outside, steadying the heels between the heels of your hands on one side and your fingers on the other side. Make sure that you are holding the heel bone, rather than the Achilles tendon.

Now pull both legs slowly and steadily. Try to follow the breathing of your partner: Slightly strengthen the pull during the exhalation and relax it a little during the inhalation. Pull along the same axis that the legs are in, with the knees remaining on the surface. Do not lift the legs during the stretch.

You can also stretch the heels one at a time. For this, again take the heel in one hand and now place the other hand flat against the sole of the foot. Again, pull the heel along the axis of the leg but in addition, apply just a small amount of pressure with the other hand on the ball of the foot. Stretching the heels one at a time with both hands in this manner also stretches the short muscles of the soles of the feet.

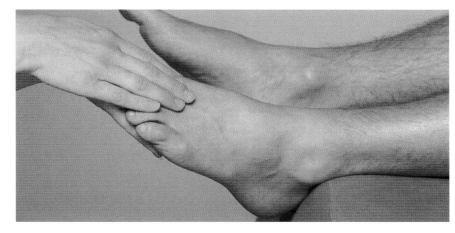

. . . and glide down to the toes in one fluid movement.

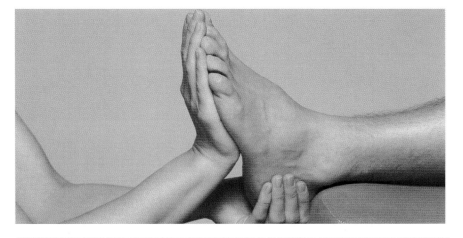

Introductory stretch: Grasp the heels and stretch the legs without lifting them.

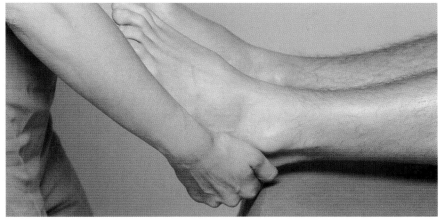

Heel stretch: Take the heel bone in one hand and place the other hand on the ball of the foot . . .

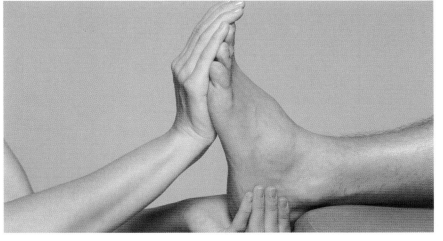

. . . then lightly pull on the heel and at the same time gently press against the ball of the foot. Carry out this movement in synchrony with your partner's breathing.

Pointed-Pressure Techniques

The actual massage of individual zones is done using different pressure techniques that use the fingertips, especially the tips of the thumb and index finger.

Pressure can be applied in two ways: a steady pressure or one that moves through a zone point by point.

A Source of Error

Make sure that your pressure is not circling, bouncing, or weak but rather steady and applied with a perpendicular thumb.

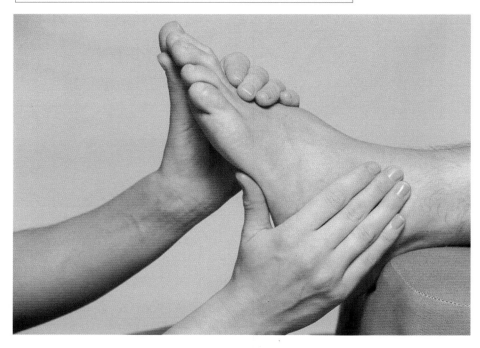

Thumb or caterpillar walk: Place the top joint of the thumb flat on the area without applying any pressure . . .

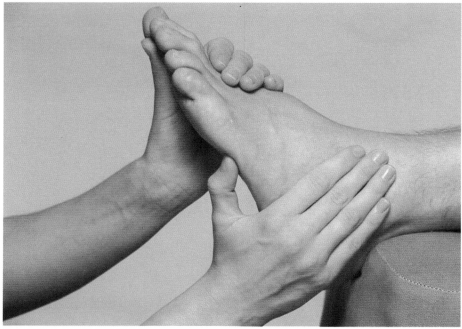

. . . then bend the thumb so that it is perpendicular to the skin and apply pressure.

The Thumb or Caterpillar Walk

The thumb or caterpillar walk is one of the most commonly used moves in foot reflexology. Pressure is applied vertically on the tissue, and the following release and small movement of the thumb onto the next point is reminiscent of the walk of a caterpillar. The thumb, however, is not simply a tool used to apply pressure but also a sensitive instrument for detecting tension in the tissue. The art of foot reflexology is in the relationship between properly applying pressure and perceiving tension and the quality of the tissue.

The thumb walk consists of several phases that are initially best visualized separately. Once you are familiar with all the phases, you can turn them into a flowing movement of pressure, relaxation, perception, pressure, and so forth.

In the first phase, you place your thumb flat on the skin without applying any pressure.

In the second phase, you bend your thumb at its last joint, which brings the tip of the thumb into contact with the skin. The tip of the thumb is now perpendicular to the area you are going to massage. By bending your thumb, you also start applying pressure. The maximum pressure is applied when the thumb is exactly vertical to the skin.

In the final phase, you release the pressure and straighten your thumb so that the tip of the thumb is again flat on the skin. Now the next cycle begins. During the transition from touching and applying pressure to releasing, you will work through the tissue millimeter by millimeter. As mentioned, this cycle of motion can be visualized by imagining the movements of a caterpillar. Exert the pressure point by point, with the points lined up immediate next to each another, like pearls on a necklace.

While you are exerting pressure with your thumb, a counterbalance is needed, which is provided by the fingers. From the side, your hand looks like it is curving or forming a U shape around the foot.

The Right Pressure

For how long should pressure be applied? The answer to this question cannot be generalized. The strength and the duration of the pressure depend on the condition of your partner—it is an individual dosage. Try to work in the breathing rhythm of your partner, with the pressure phase taking place during exhalation and the relaxation phase during inhalation. Make sure that your thumbnails do not extend beyond the tip of the thumb, since they will otherwise cause unpleasant sensations for your partner. Also keep in mind that pressure is applied with the tip of the thumb and not its flat part.

Before you perform this move on your partner, visualize the individual phases and try them on your own hand. The steady and point-oriented pressure is the essence of reflexology. Avoid all circular, tipping, or bouncing movements with your thumb. The American pioneer of foot reflexology, Eunice D. Ingham, described the motions and feeling as similar to those of crushing sugar crystals in your palm with the tip of your thumb. Practicing this move on your own hand will help you become comfortable with it. When you later apply the thumb walk to the foot of your partner, you will feel the exertion after a few minutes. Keep in mind that this is a movement your body is not used to and will have to build up strength for. With increased practice, you will notice that you can use your thumb longer without any problem. But do not overexert

yourself at the beginning, or you will lose the joy of foot reflexology. Keep loosening your hands by doing one of the stroking movements after this pointed massage with the thumb.

> **The Thumb Walk**
> - Place the top joint of your thumb flat on the surface.
> - Bend the last joint.
> - Apply pressure with the tip of your thumb.
> - Roll off the thumb and return it to its initial position.

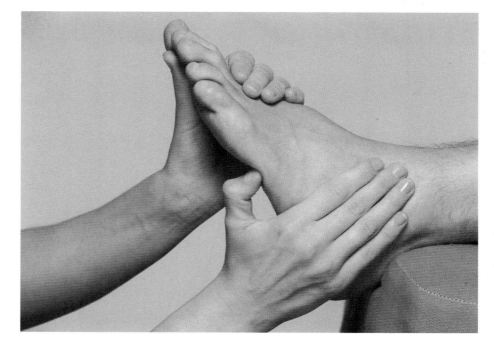

The thumb is now perpendicular to the skin. Maximum pressure is applied, and the pressure is directed straight against the tissue.

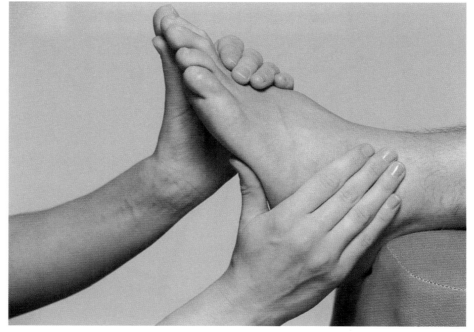

After you have exerted pressure, roll the thumb back down to its top joint, and thus initiate the next pressure cycle.

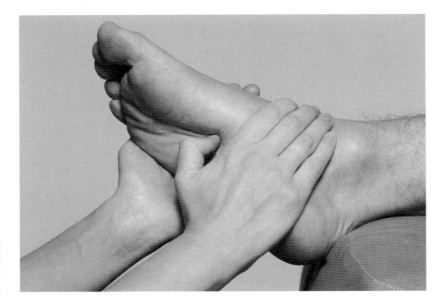

Painful zones can often be resolved using steady thumb pressure.

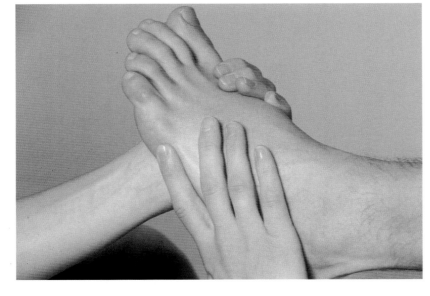

Caterpillar walk with the index finger: Place the top joint of the index finger flat on the skin without applying pressure . . .

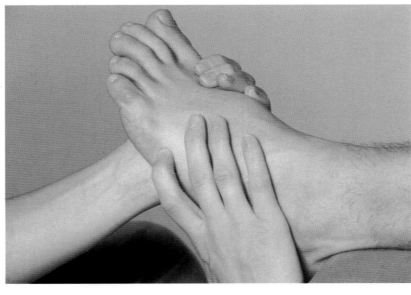

. . . then bend the index finger in both its joints, so that its tip is perpendicular to the skin, and apply pressure.

The Technique of Steady Pressure

For painful or especially sensitive zones, you can use steady pressure with the thumb. The movement of the caterpillar is skipped and instead pressure is applied exactly to the sensitive or painful spot and kept steady for a longer period. Again, place your thumb flat on the targeted area, bend your thumb, and in this position apply a steady pressure.

The duration of the pressure can be from 1 to 2 minutes. Here, too, the previous rule applies: The intensity and the duration of the pressure depend on the needs of your partner. Steady pressure will often resolve the painful zones. But definitely respect the pain limits of your partner. If the sensitivity of the zone does not decrease, you can massage the zone again in a later pass.

The Caterpillar Walk with the Index Finger

You can massage by "walking" with your index finger just as you can with your thumb. This variation of the caterpillar walk is especially good for zones that because of their sensitivity do not respond well to strong pressure. It is used primarily on the top of the foot, since there are bones and tendons directly under the skin in this area. As with the thumb walk, the caterpillar walk with the index finger can be split up into several phases. In the first phase, you place the index finger flat on the skin without applying any pressure. In the second phase, you bend the finger in its middle joint and, as you bend it, start applying pressure to the tissue. Here, the thumb is the counterbalance. In the final phase, you release the pressure and roll the tip of the finger until it come to a rest flat against the skin, again not applying any pressure. From this position, you can begin the next pressure movement. As with the thumb walk, with the index-finger walk you work point by point through the selected zone.

The Tweezers Move

In the tweezers move, you work with the tips of the thumb and the index finger. With this move you will reach the "swimming skins," or membranes between the toes. Take the skin between the flat parts of your thumb and index finger and slightly pull it out in the direction of the toes. This helps the circulation in these zones. The pull as well as the pressure applied is steady. Switch between pull and relaxation in rhythm with the breathing of your partner.

With the tweezers grip you can also massage the individual toes point by point. Beginning at the base of the toe, apply pressure for a moment, then release it. Work point by point from the base of the toes to the tips.

Balancing Touches

This section introduces two other helpful moves that you can apply in special situations. Remember that it's better to be good with a select few moves than to know a large number of moves less precisely.

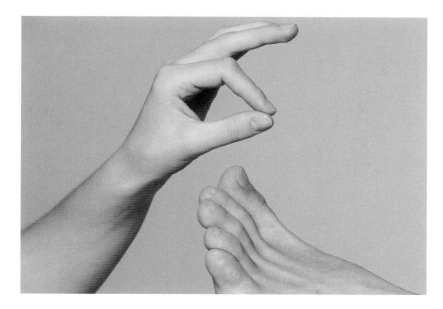

Tweezers grip: In the correct basic position for the tweezers technique, the thumb and index finger form an O.

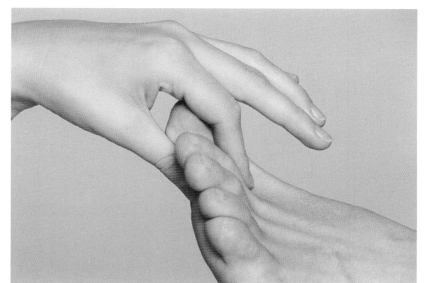

Tweezers move: Take the skin between the toes between the thumb and index finger. Apply light pressure between your partner's inhalations.

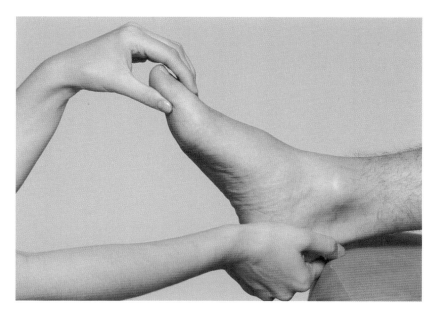

You can massage the toes using the tweezers grip.

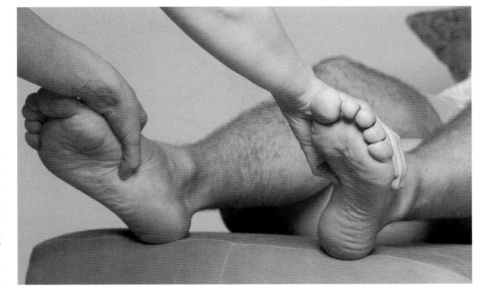

Technique to relax breathing: Place the hands over the inside edges of the feet and put the thumbs on the middle of the feet, below the balls . . .

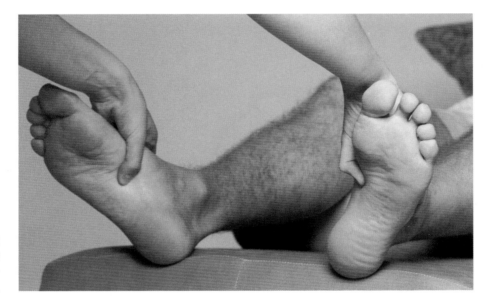

. . . now bend the feet upward as your partner inhales.

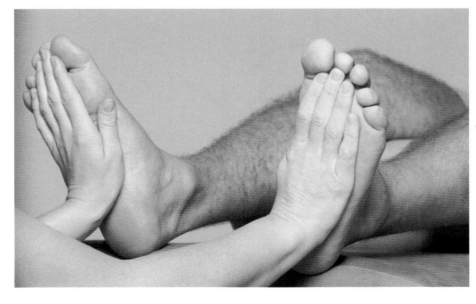

Supporting the sole: Cover as much of each sole as possible with your hands.

Move to Relax Breathing

Anxious or tense people tend to breathe shallowly and quickly. In this case, you can use a move to relax their breathing. Put your hands on the inside edges of the feet, with the tips of your thumbs in the middle of the feet, just past the balls of the feet.

Now use the tips of your thumbs to move the feet of your partner upward in the ankle joint. Hold this position for one or two breaths, and then relax the tension with your partner's exhalation. Repeat this cycle for several breaths; you will notice that your partner's breathing slows down and becomes deeper.

Supporting the Soles of the Feet

This move is simple and practical. You can use it at the beginning or the end of the massage. Place your entire palms in contact with the feet of your partner. Rest in this position for 1 or 2 minutes. While touching your partner's feet, visualize the energy of your hands flowing into his or her feet.

At the same time, your hands will receive information about your partner's physical and mental state. Warm and dry feet suggest good relaxation; cold and moist feet are an indication that your partner is tense.

Summary

In the preceding pages you have learned a number of grips, strokes, and stretches. In the following summary you will see a selection of techniques. Choose those that work for you and try to perfect some of these through frequent application. Only when you are able to massage without becoming tired or tense during a 45-minute session will you be able to enjoy foot reflexology. Some of these techniques you can practice on and apply to yourself.

Techniques at a Glance

STROKES AND STRETCHES

Placing Your Hands on the Feet
Close your eyes and breathe deeply. Focus your attention on your hands and feel the energy in them.

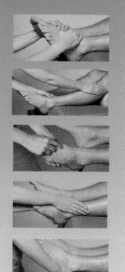

Stroking Hands
Place your hands on the legs, to the sides of the knees. Stroke slowly, smoothly, and harmoniously downward over the shins to the toes and beyond.

Stroking Fingers
Feel the spaces between the metatarsal bones. With one finger in each space, stroke with steady pressure from the point closest to the tarsus up to the base joints.

Sandwich Strokes
Place one hand on the back of the foot and the other on the sole of the foot. Pull both hands with steady pressure toward the tips of the toes and beyond.

Stretching the Heels
Place your hands around the heels from the outside and steady them between the heels of your hands on one side and your fingers on the other. Apply a steady pull to both legs.

PRESSURE TECHNIQUES

Thumb or Caterpillar Walk
Apply pressure point by point, with the points immediately adjacent to one another like pearls on a necklace.

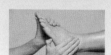

Steady Pressure with the Thumb
Place the top joint of your thumb on the painful zone, bend your thumb, and apply steady pressure.

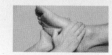

Caterpillar Walk with the Index Finger
Place the top joint of the index finger flat on the skin. Bend the finger and apply pressure. Release pressure and roll the fingertip back until it rests on the skin without pressure.

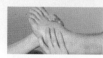

Tweezers Move
Take the webbed skin between the toes between your thumb and index finger. Pull the skin in the same direction as the toes. You can also use this grip to massage the toes point by point.

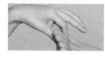

HARMONIZING TECHNIQUES

Move to Relax Breathing
Place the top joints of the thumbs in the middle of the arches of the feet, close to the balls of the feet. Move the feet up into the ankle joint, toward the head.

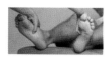

Supporting the Soles of the Feet
Place your palms flat against the soles of the feet. Picture the energy being transferred from your hands to your partner's feet.

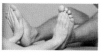

Massaging the Foot Reflex Zones

The following pages describe different parts of the body and their reflex zones on the feet. The goal of foot reflexology is to increase well-being.

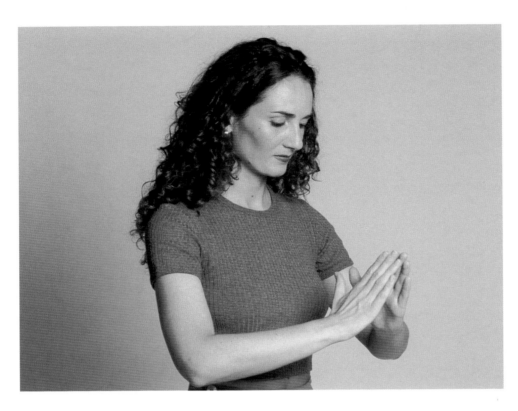

Concentrate on the flow of warmth and energy between your hands.

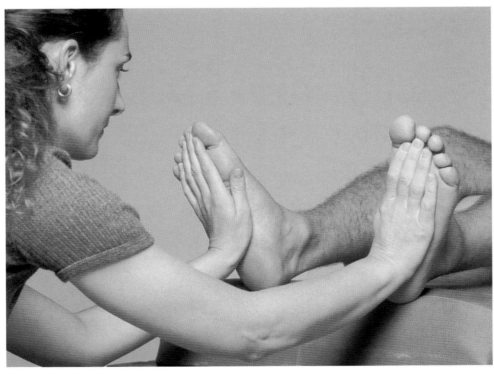

The sole technique is good for making initial contact.

Things to Note before the Massage

In classical foot reflexology, each reflex zone on the two feet is treated in turn. For example, after you have finished massaging the head zone on the right foot, you follow by massaging the head zone on the left foot. This helps you notice different sensitivities of the zones in the right and left feet.

However, if the focus of your reflexology is harmonizing the bodily balance and helping the recipient relax, it makes more sense to first massage all the reflex zones of one foot and to then switch over to the other foot. Moving back and forth between the two feet in this case would be disruptive to the flow of the massage.

Take a lot of time for your massage. Plan on spending 45 to 60 minutes for a first massage. Setting the right mood is especially important. Give your partner enough time to reach a relaxed, meditative mood. The external ambience can help with this. Also make sure that you are not disrupted by phone calls or other events during the treatment.

The massage treatment should be done a few times. The frequency depends on how necessary and pleasant you and your partner see the massage to be. As a point of reference, three to six treatments is generally sufficient.

Pay attention to the reactions of your massage partner. Respect his or her pain limits, and for touches that he or she enjoys especially, add a few extra strokes.

The Introduction

The actual reflexology massage is preceded by an introduction. Your hands should be pleasantly warm, as should the feet of your partner. Concentrate on the energy of your hands, and, to this end, carry out the exercise described on page 27.

Now make contact with the feet of your partner by placing your hands on them. Feet that are dry and warm signal that your partner is relaxed. Cold or moist feet suggest internal tension. If this is the case, warm the feet with a hot water bottle before the massage.

Soft strokes are an ideal opening for the massage. Perform a few sandwich strokes on each foot with both hands. Then put your hands under the heels and hold them. Simply holding the feet helps your partner relax and warms the feet.

You can now begin massaging the individual zones.

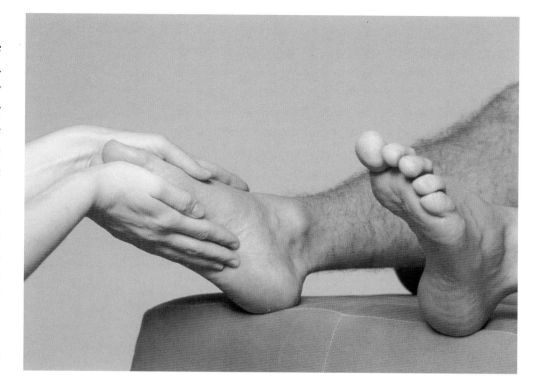

Using both hands, cover the sole and the back of the foot with your hands and slowly pull them toward the toes.

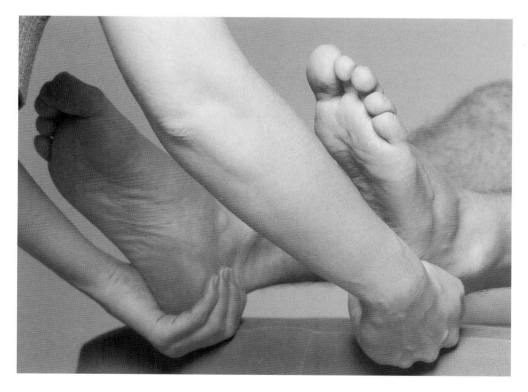

Simply holding the heels warms and relaxes the feet.

The Head

The head is the nerve center of the body and the most important area for the conscious reception, processing, and dissemination of information. It houses the brain as the central point that processes information and gives consciousness to processes. Moreover, sensory organs such as the ears, eyes, nose, and tongue are also in the head area. With the upper breathing organs—the nose and the mouth—we receive life-giving oxygen, and with the upper digestive organs we take in fluids and food. Most of the stimulations of our environment are processed in our head. Stress and external influences disturb our bodily balance and often translate into problems in the head area—from tension headaches to illnesses of the upper breathing passages.

Note

The range of motion in the upper part of the cervical spine corresponds roughly to the range of motion of the base joint of the big toe. You can test this on your partner. Take his or her big toe and carefully carry out some circular movements. Movement that is restricted or that rubs can indicate problems in the neck area. Test this if necessary by asking your partner to get up and move his or her head in all directions.

Locating the Reflex Zones of the Head

The reflex zone of the head is located on the toes. The head is unusual in that it is represented twice: Fitzgerald, who described the zone model (see page 7), divided the body into ten longitudinal zones. These are all represented on the big toe, so that each of the two big toes is divided into five zones. For this reason, the big toes are one zone for the entire head, but in addition, detailed smaller zones for

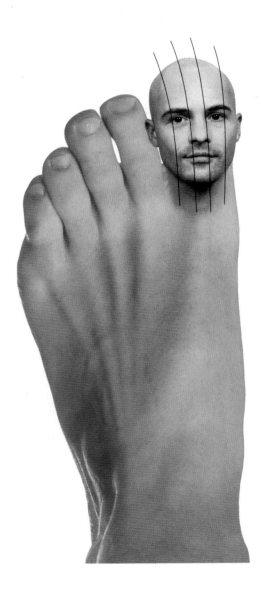
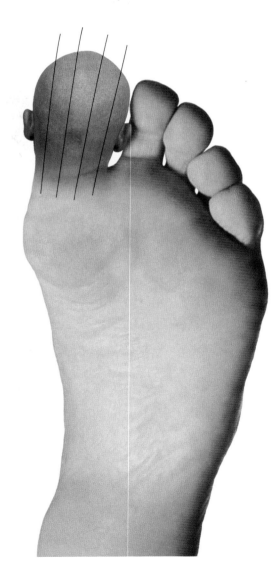

Left and right: The ten zones of the body are represented as ten zones on the big toes.

the individual areas of the head are spread out over all the toes. The facial zones are represented on the top surface of the toes. These include the zones for the forehead, sinuses, temples, eyes, jaw joints, nose-throat area, and ears. Note that the zones for the teeth are on the top surface of the big toe as well as on the second to fifth toes. The bottom sides of the toes, known as toe berries, correspond to the back of the head. The brain zone is in the middle of the berry of the big toe. On its side is the zone of the pituitary gland. This critical gland is the "command center" for many other glands in the body. Above the brain zone is the zone of the skull. The eyes zones are between the base and middle joints on the second and third toes. The zones for the ears are on the fourth and fifth toes.

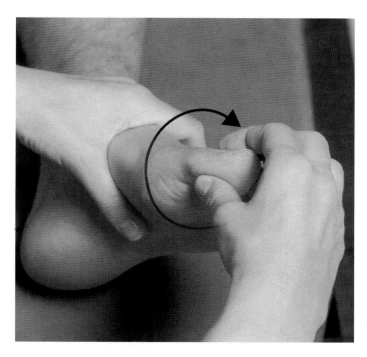

Before you begin the massage, loosen the toes with circular movements.

Right foot

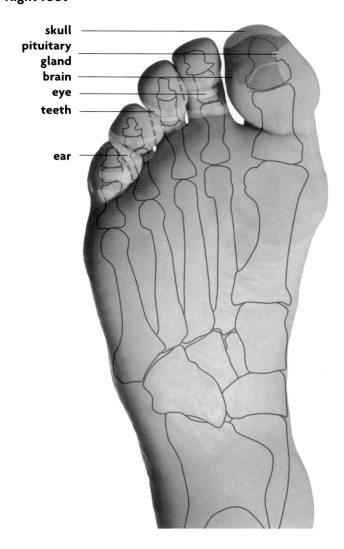

skull
pituitary gland
brain
eye
teeth

ear

Right foot

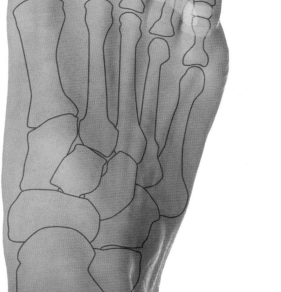

brain
temple
sinus
eye
jaw joint
nose-throat area
teeth
ear

Left: The zones of the head and the brain are represented on the bottoms of the toes.

Right: The zones of the face are represented on the tops of the toes.

Massaging the Head Zones

Massage the main head zones with the tweezers grip, using the tips of your thumb and index finger. Begin with the big toe. Use the base joint as your starting point and move from there point by point up to the tip of the toe. This sequence massages the zones of the neck, the brain (including the pituitary gland), and the roof of the skull. Be sure to pay attention to the reactions of your partner when massaging the toes. The skin between the toes is very thin, and too much pressure can easily be painful or unpleasant.

Massaging the Big Toe Point by Point

With the tweezers grip, apply pressure point by point with the tip of your thumb. The big toe can be massaged from the tip down along several different treatment lines, corresponding to the five separate zones found on each big toe.

Massaging the Undersides of the Small Toes

You will also use the tweezers grip to massage the undersides of the small toes. Again, start with the base of the toes. For the small toes, one path is enough. Follow the natural line of the toes, and don't try to straighten the toes.

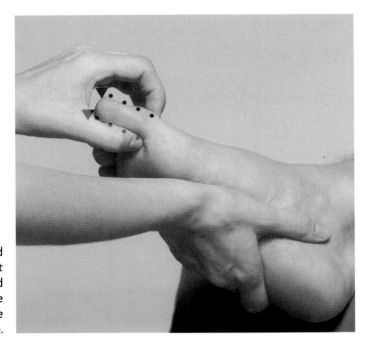

The right hand supports the foot while the left hand massages the toe using the tweezers grip.

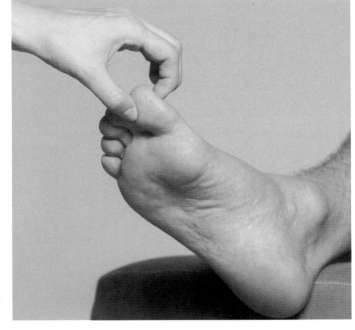

Far right: The zones of the scalp, brain, neck, eye, ear, and teeth are located on the bottoms of the toes.

The massage is done point by point. In this picture, the thumb is resting at the zone of the brain.

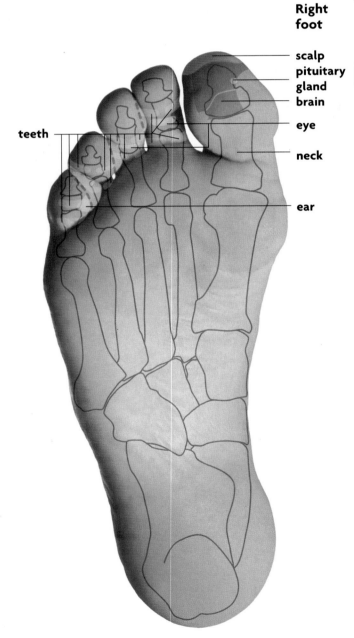

Right foot

scalp
pituitary gland
brain
eye
neck
teeth
ear

Massaging the Frontal Head Zone

Massage this zone with the tweezers grip. The zones for the forehead, sinus, jaw joint, and nose-throat area are on the big toe. The eye zone is between the second and third toes, and the ear zones are on the fourth and fifth toes. The zones for the teeth are represented on the tops as well as the bottoms of the toes.

Massaging the Facial Zones

Starting from the base of the toes, now massage the frontal facial area—the zones for the nose-throat area, jaw joint, forehead, and sinus—point by point. Support the foot

with your free hand. Make several lines of treatment along the underside of the big toe, following the dotted lines pictured in the illustration on the facing page.

Massaging the Zones for the Teeth

These zones are off to the side of the middle joints. You can reach these zones by massaging the each of the four small toes point by point, beginning a little bit to the side of the base.

When you have finished massaging the head zones, perform some strokes as a transition for moving to the next zone.

Right foot

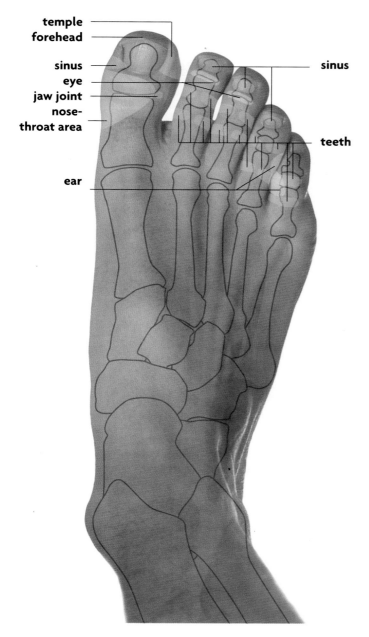

temple
forehead
sinus
eye
jaw joint
nose-throat area
sinus
teeth
ear

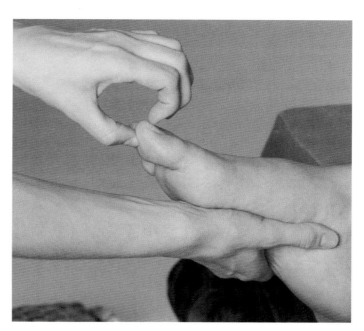

Far left: The zones of the forehead, sinus, jaw joint, nose-throat area, eye, ear, and teeth are located on the big toe.

The zones of the face are located on the toenail.

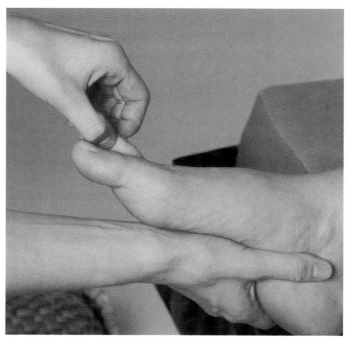

Start massaging the zones of the teeth at the base of the toes.

Massaging the Zones for the Neck, Shoulders, and Chest

The shoulder girdle connects the chest with the arms. Arms and shoulders are connected to the torso only by muscles and tendons. This allows the arms to have a large range of motion. Tension that originates in the neck, arms, or upper back leads to a hardening in the area of the shoulder muscles. Prolonged activities in which the arms must be raised, poor posture, and ergonomically unhealthy workplaces are some of the most common causes of painful ail-ments in this area. A proper foot reflexology massage leads to a relaxation of the shoulder muscles.

Locating the Reflex Zones

The zone of the shoulder girdle extends from the base joints of the toes over the entire foot. The upper arm is projected onto the fifth metatarsal bone. This bone and the upper-arm bone in a smaller scale have a similar shape. The zone of the entire chest cavity covers the area of the

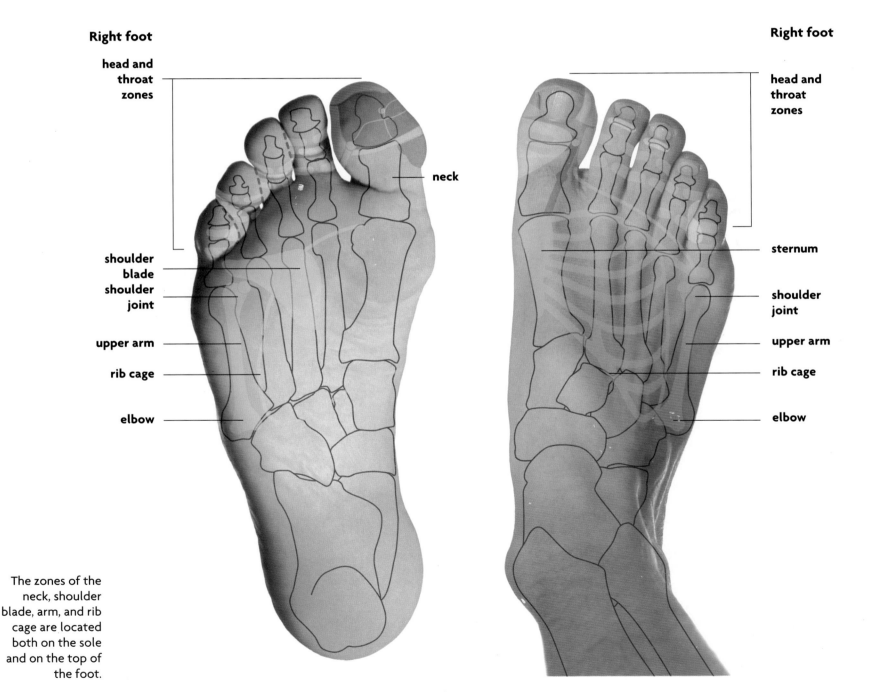

Right foot

head and throat zones

neck

shoulder blade
shoulder joint

upper arm

rib cage

elbow

Right foot

head and throat zones

sternum

shoulder joint

upper arm

rib cage

elbow

The zones of the neck, shoulder blade, arm, and rib cage are located both on the sole and on the top of the foot.

first four metatarsal bones. The neck zone runs from the base to the end of the first big-toe bone.

Locating the Reflex Zones on the Top of the Foot

The zone of the sternum is on both sides of the foot in the first zone and covers almost the entire length of the first metatarsal bone. The zone of the collarbone, which is the bone bridge from the arms to the torso, runs along the ridges of the base joints of the toes. The upper-arm bone is projected onto the fifth metatarsal bone. The zones of the ribs and the bones of the chest cavity extend from the zone of the sternum to the first four metatarsal bones.

Locating the Reflex Zones on the Sides of the Foot

The zone of the upper-arm bone follows almost entirely the fifth metatarsal bone. For problems with the sides of the upper arms, this area should be treated point by point with the thumb or index finger.

Left foot

Left foot

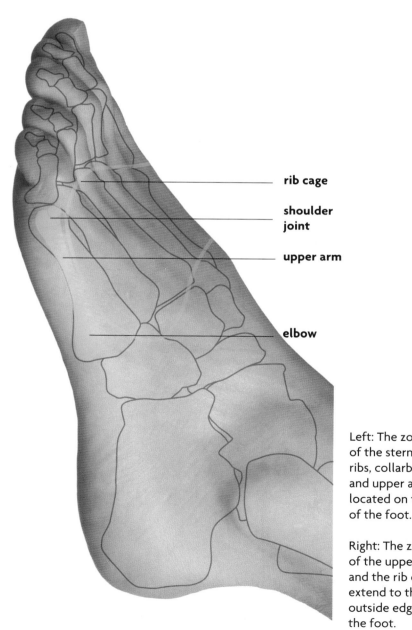

collarbone
sternum

shoulder joint

ribs

upper arm

elbow

rib cage

shoulder joint

upper arm

elbow

Left: The zones of the sternum, ribs, collarbone, and upper arm are located on the top of the foot.

Right: The zones of the upper arm and the rib cage extend to the outside edge of the foot.

Massaging the Neck, Shoulder, and Chest Region

Massage the zones for the neck, the shoulder girdle, and the chest cavity on the sole of the foot with the thumb walk. Apply pressure point by point with the tip of the thumb.

Start the massage in the middle of the foot's side and then move upward step by step. Circle the neck zone, which extends past the first joint of the big toe, with several treatment lines. Make sure that the individual treatment lines run closely next to each other.

Afterward, you can massage the base joint from left to right or right to left point by point.

Massaging the Neck Zone

The neck zone is in the area of the first joint of the big toe. Pay special attention to this zone by massaging it in several rotations along lines running closely parallel.

Massaging the Shoulder Zones

These zones should be massaged from top to bottom or vice versa in parallel lines. Pay special attention to the gaps around the metatarsal bones. You may want to exert stronger pressure in this area, as there are often calluses here. As always, adjust the pressure of your touch based on the sensitivity of your partner.

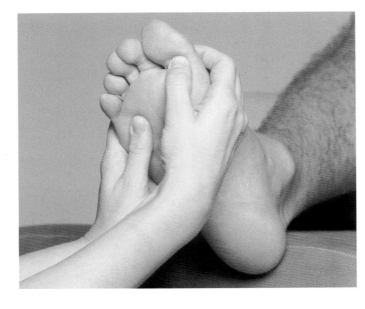

The tip of the thumb rests in the neck zone, which is massaged in several paths from top to bottom and from bottom to the top.

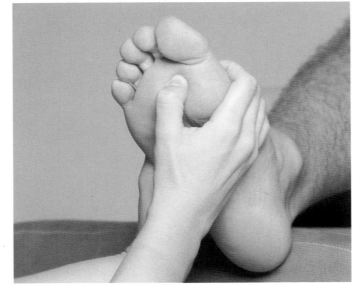

Far right: The zones of the neck, shoulder blade, upper arm, and chest are located on the sole of the foot.

The shoulder zones are massaged in the area of the ball of the foot.

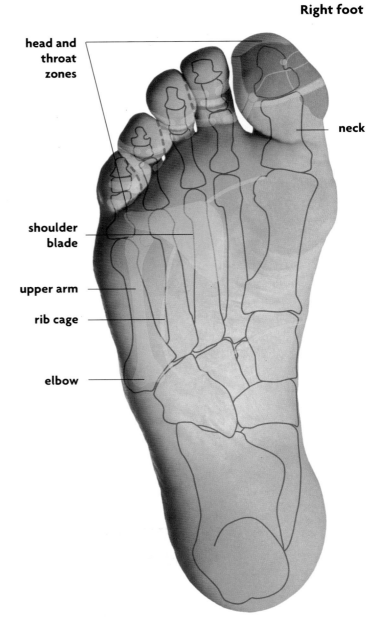

Right foot

head and throat zones

neck

shoulder blade

upper arm

rib cage

elbow

Massaging the Upper Arm and Sternum

The zones on the top of the foot are best massaged with your index finger. Here, too, massage individual spots and work up or down step by step. Note that on the top of the foot, the metatarsal bones are immediately under the skin. The bones are surrounded by very sensitive bony tissue, so avoid applying strong pressure around the bones. Pay special attention to the area between the toes and massage these point by point.

The Caterpillar Walk on the Top of the Foot

Use your index finger to locate the first metatarsal bone. Place the tip of your finger in the gap between the first and second metatarsal bones. Apply pressure to the gap, and then move upward step by step. Do the same for the gaps between the other metatarsal bones.

Shaking the Front of the Foot

After you have massaged the zones on the sole and the top of the foot, it is good to conclude with loosening the entire shoulder girdle zone. To do this, take the front of the foot in both hands and perform slight shaking and stroking movements. When done properly, these movements spread over the whole body and cause a pleasant and relaxed sensation. This loosening of the shoulder girdle zone is also an ideal transition to the massaging of the next zone.

Right foot

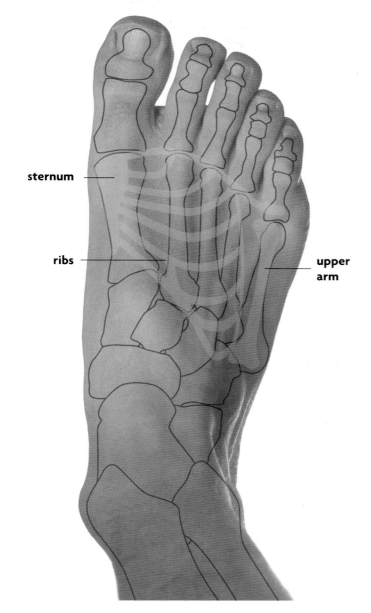

sternum

ribs

upper arm

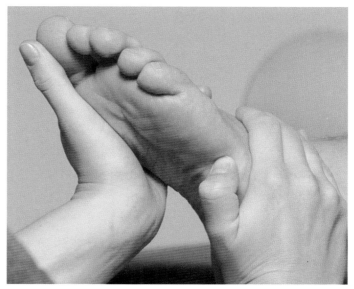

The upper-arm zone can also be massaged on the sole of the foot.

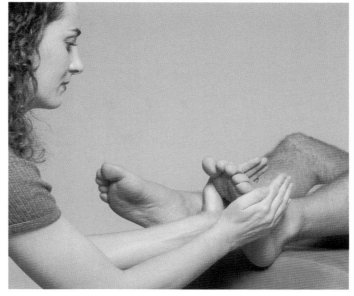

Far left: The zones of the sternum, ribs, and upper arm are located on the top of the foot.

Shaking the shoulder girdle zone creates a pleasant and relaxed feeling.

The Spine

The spine is the scaffolding of bones that enables us to carry our torso erect. It forms a safe canal inside which the spinal cord runs The spinal cord is the main line of nerves connecting the brain to the rest of the body. Between the individual vertebrae, pairs of nerves extend from the spinal cord to either side, supplying the corresponding organs with neural impulses from the brain.

The complicated construction of the spine allows a range of motion in many directions. Looking at the spine from the side, you notice that it has the shape of a double S. This S-shaped bend is used to dampen the impact of bumps and jarring movements.

The cervical or upper spine is made up of seven individual vertebrae. These vertebrae are more slender and frail in their structure than the other vertebrae. The range of motion is largest in this area. Our ability to turn and incline our heads and to look to the sides is made possible primarily by these seven neck vertebrae.

The thoracic or chest spine consists of twelve individual vertebrae. Motion in this part of the spine is much more restricted. The thoracic vertebrae are notable for their flexible connection to the ribs. Together with the ribs and the collarbone, the thoracic spine offers a stable yet elastic protection for the fragile chest organs such as the heart and lungs.

The five vertebrae of the lumbar or lower spine are much more stable than the others, as they have to carry more weight. The space between the fourth and fifth lumbar vertebrae is the most vulnerable point of the lumbar spine. Stress or strong pressure leads to the wearing down of the disks that serve as a buffer between the individual vertebrae. Once injured, disks cease to cushion the vertebrae properly, which sometimes allows the vertebrae to shift, putting painful pressure on the nerves that extend from the spine. Another weak point of the spine is the transition from the cervical spine to the thoracic spine. This region experiences a special stress because it forms the top of the first bend.

Left: A vertebral segment consists of the bone (vertebra), the disk, and the spinal nerves emerging in pairs from the spinal cord.

Right: The spine is divided into several segments.

transverse process

spinal nerve

disk

vertebra

dorsal process

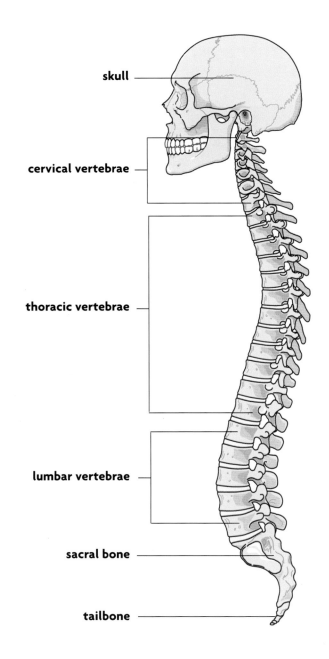

skull

cervical vertebrae

thoracic vertebrae

lumbar vertebrae

sacral bone

tailbone

The lumbar spine extends into the sacrum. The sacrum is made up of vertebral segments that are fused together, and it forms the foundation of the spine in the pelvis. The sacrum is followed by a few small tailbone, or coccyx, vertebrae, which are also fused. The muscles and tendons that make up the pelvic floor are attached to the coccyx vertebrae.

The spine's complex construction makes it highly susceptible to certain injuries. Back pain, encouraged by a sedentary lifestyle, has become a common ailment. Massaging the zones of the spine on the feet relaxes the associated back muscles, alleviates pain, and, combined with a back-friendly lifestyle, is an excellent injury-preventive measure.

> **Note**
>
> Restriction in the range of motion of the big toe and the first metatarsal bone may indicate problems in the area where the cervical spine transitions to the thoracic spine.

Locating the Spine Zones

The spine zones are located along the inner edges of the feet in the first zone (see page 9). The zone of the cervical spine runs along the first base joint. Next to it is the zone of the thoracic spine, which follows the outer edge of the first metatarsal bone. The transition from the base joint of the toe to the first metatarsal bone is the zone marking the point of transition from the neck to the chest part of the spine. The lumbar spine is represented in the area of the tarsal bones (the cuboid bone and the navicular bone). The sacrum is reflected on the inside rim of the heel.

Left foot   **Right foot**

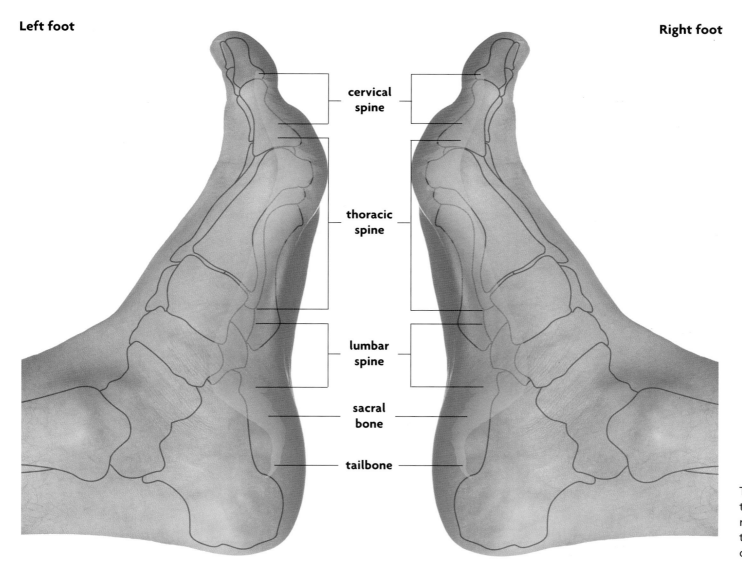

cervical spine

thoracic spine

lumbar spine

sacral bone

tailbone

The segments of the spine are represented on the inside edges of the feet.

Left foot   **Right foot**

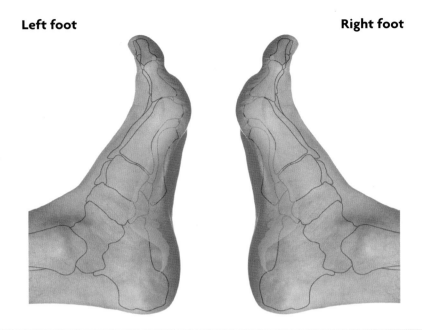

The zones of the spine segments are located on the inside edges of the feet.

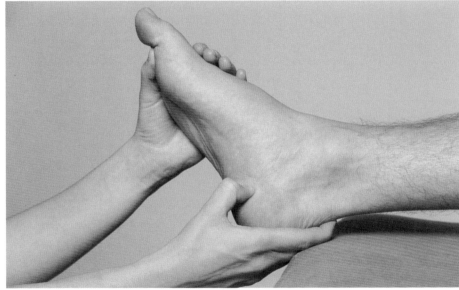

The tailbone zone can be felt at the edge of the heel bone.

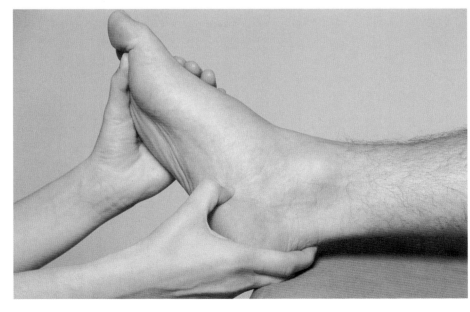

The sacral bone zone is located a little deeper in the foot, so you should use more pressure when massaging it.

Massaging the Spine Zones

The zones of the spine are massaged lengthwise. The massage can begin at the top or at the bottom.

Note that painful areas are frequently located inside these zones.

Massage the zones with steady pressure as outlined on page 42. Place the tip of your thumb on the painful area, apply as much pressure as your partner can tolerate, and maintain pressure for 1 to 2 minutes.

Massaging the Coccyx Zone

To massage the spine zones from bottom to top, begin the massage with the zone of the coccyx. In the side of the heel area, feel for the edge of the heel bone and apply pressure with the tip of your thumb, supporting the foot with your free hand. Massage point by point toward the big toe.

Massaging the Sacrum Zone

The zone of the sacrum is also located on the outer edge of the heel bone but a little more toward the toes. Apply pressure with your thumb and continue massaging point by point in a lengthwise direction. Because the sacrum zone is located deeper and a little more toward the middle of the foot, you can work with greater pressure in this area.

Massaging the Lumbar Spine Zone

The zone of the lumbar spine is located at the edge of the navicular bone and the medial cuneiform bone. This zone, too, can be massaged with your thumb.

Very painful zones are often located in this area. You can work on these using steady pressure for a duration of 1 to 2 minutes. The amount of pressure depends on the sensitivity of your partner.

Massaging the Thoracic Spine Zone

The zone of the thoracic spine runs along the edge of the easily felt first metatarsal bone. Massage this zone point by point. The transition from the thoracic spine zone to the cervical spine zone is located at about the bottom of the joint at the base of the big toe.

This area, too, is frequently the site of painful zones.

Massaging the Cervical Spine Zone

This zone begins at about the bottom of the base joint of the big toe. It, too, can be found on the upper and outer edge of the bone. Massage this zone point by point.

Because this zone is usually somewhat sensitive, adjust your pressure to the sensitivity of your partner.

To bring closure to this part of the massage, carry out a few soft strokes to prepare your partner for the next stage.

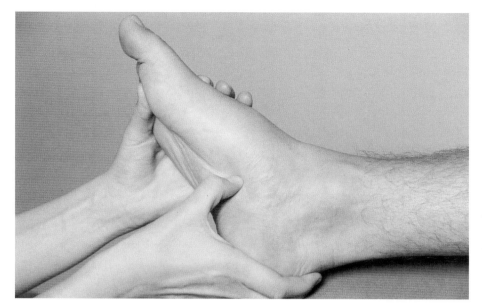

The lumbar spine zone begins at the edge of the navicular bone and the inner cuneiform bone.

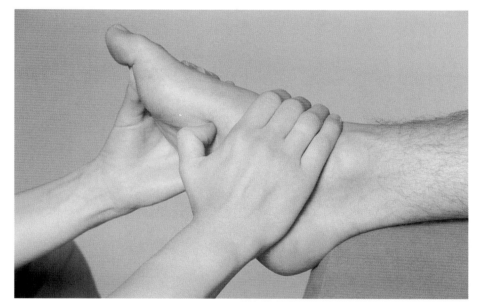

The thoracic spine zone runs along the first metatarsal bone.

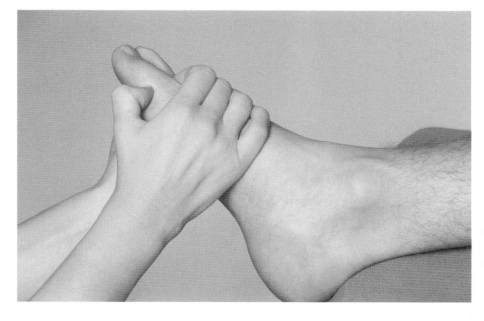

The cervical spine zone begins at the bottom of the base joint of the big toe.

The Digestive Tract

Picture the digestive tract as a long hose running through the body. This hose begins in the mouth and ends in the anus. Aside from the mouth, esophagus, stomach, and various intestinal tracts, there are three important organs in the digestive system: the pancreas, the liver, and the gallbladder. The function of the digestive system is to break up food into its smallest components, which can be absorbed into the blood in the intestines and thus provide the body with the energy and nutrients necessary for life. The leftover parts are excreted through the rectum. A massage of the reflex zones of the digestive system harmonizes and stimulates all the functions relating to the digestive system.

The enormously large surface of the digestive tract is in direct contact with our surroundings via the food we eat. When you consider that the food we eat is not always sterile, you can imagine what an important role the digestive tract plays in fending off infections. The intestines house the largest immune system of our bodies. Numerous "islands" of lymphatic cells (called Peyer's patches) are embedded in the intestinal membrane and fend off bacteria. The digestive system also produces toxins that the body has to dispose of.

When the didestive tract, with its different functions, is not working properly, any number of illnesses can result. The basic precondition for a healthy digestive tract is a balanced and regular diet. A healthy digestive tract helps prevent illnesses. Foot reflexology massage can assist in the stimulation and balancing of the entire digestive tract."

Locating the Reflex Zones

The zone of the mouth cavity is located on the inner edge of the big toe. On the sole of the foot, the esophagus zone extends from the base joint of the big toe along the first metatarsal bone. On the left foot, it reaches the stomach zone. On the right foot, it is shorter, ending in the ball of the foot. The zones of the mouth cavity and the esophagus are also found on the tops of the feet, the mouth zone at the joint between the first and second big-toe bones, and the esophagus zone extending from the middle of the first big-toe bone into the top of the first metatarsal bone. The gallbladder zone is on the sole of the right foot at the base of the third metatarsal bone. The zone of the liver extends over both soles; the larger part is located on the right sole, along the breadth of the first four metatarsal bones. Below the liver zone are the zones for the pancreas and the stomach.

The zone of the digestive tract is represented on the soles of the feet. The stomach zone is found primarily on

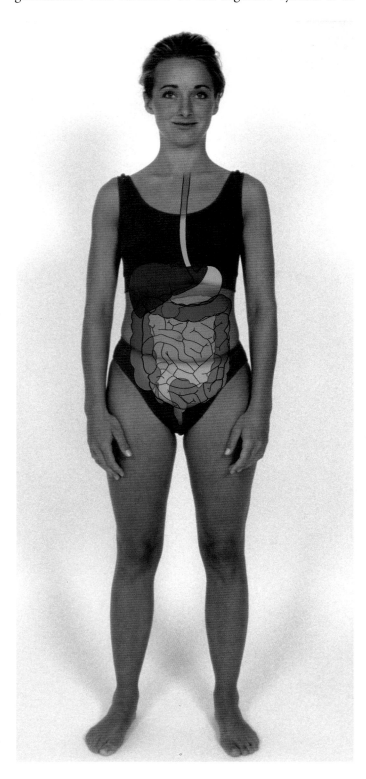

The digestive system breaks down food into its smallest components.

the left foot; it extends sideways over the base of the first two metatarsal bones. The zone of the large intestine, or colon, and its three components starts in the right foot on the base of the heel bone and runs toward the toes up to the base of the fourth metatarsal bone. It then turns right and runs across the left foot to the base of its fourth meta-tarsal bone. From here it runs downward to the heel bone and then back to the inner edge of the foot, where on both feet the rectum zone is located. The rectum zone extends to the outer edges of the heel bone. The large intestine zone thus to some degree frames the small intestine zone, which is located on both soles.

Right foot

Left foot

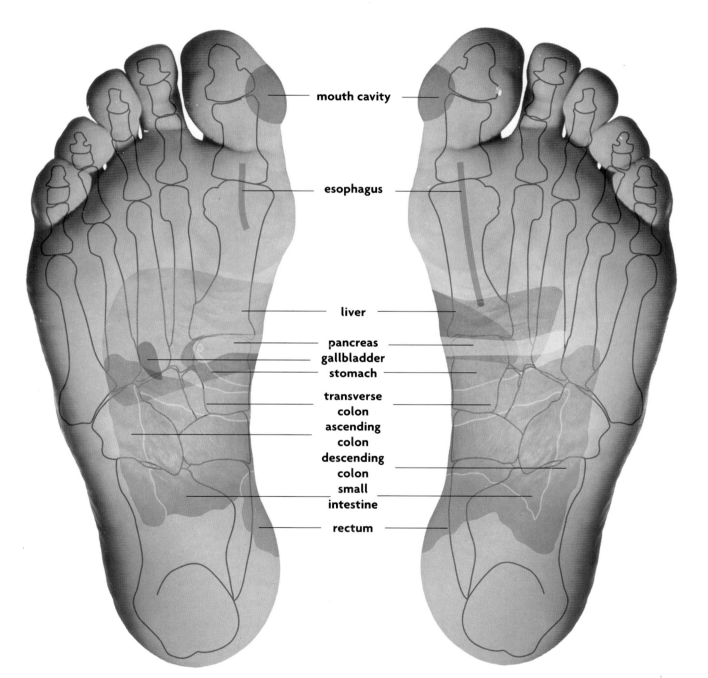

mouth cavity

esophagus

liver

pancreas
gallbladder
stomach
transverse
colon
ascending
colon
descending
colon
small
intestine
rectum

The zones of the digestive tract are located on the soles of the feet.

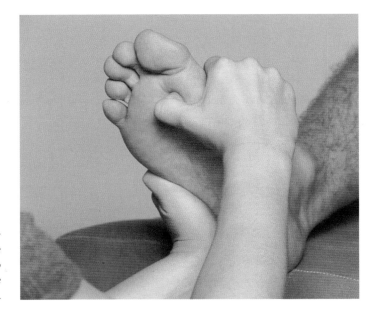

Apply point-by-point pressure with your thumb tip to massage the esophagus zone.

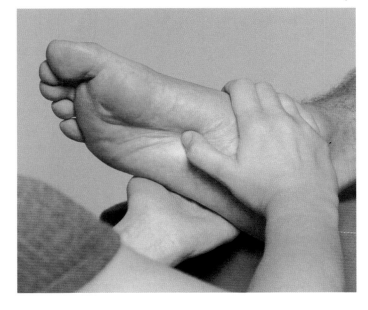

Massage the stomach and small intestine zones both lengthwise and crosswise. Support the foot with your free hand.

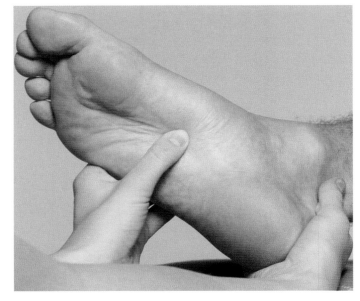

The liver zone, too, should be massaged both lengthwise and crosswise. Use steady pressure for the most sensitive points.

Massaging the Zones of the Digestive Organs

Begin the massage of the digestive zones with a few sandwich strokes. For each foot, place one hand on the top of the foot and the other on the sole and with both hands stroke from the base of the foot up to the toes.

Massaging the Mouth and Esophagus Zones

The mouth and esophagus zones on the tops of the big toes can be massaged with the tip of your index finger.

The esophagus zones on the soles of the feet should be massaged point by point with the tip of your thumb, running down from the big toe toward the middle of the foot.

Massaging the Stomach and Small Intestine Zones

You can reach the stomach and small intestine zones best by turning the foot you are working on slightly outward. Support the foot with your free hand and work the zones with the tip of your thumb both lengthwise and crosswise.

Massaging the Liver and Gallbladder Zones

The liver zone runs on the inside edges of the feet. Massage the liver zone on each foot both lengthwise and crosswise. The gallbladder zone is found on the sole of the right foot at the base of the third metatarsal bone. This zone can be very sensitive. Rest here for a moment, applying steady pressure at a level acceptable to your partner, for 1 to 2 minutes.

Massaging the Large Intestine Zone

The large intestine can be divided into several parts: the ascending colon, transverse colon, and descending colon. At the end of the large intestine zone is the rectum zone, which is located along the inside edge of the sole at the heel on both feet. Massage in the direction of the large intestine—that is, starting with the ascending colon and ending at the rectum.

Massaging the Zone of the Ascending Colon

The zone of the ascending colon, in the right foot, is massaged lengthwise with the tip of your thumb. Start in the heel and massage point by point up to the fourth metatarsal bone.

Massaging the Zone of the Transverse Colon

This zone runs from the base of the fourth metatarsal bone in the right foot across to the same position in the left foot. Follow this path across the feet, massaging the zone point by point.

Massaging the Zones of the Descending Colon and Rectum

The zone of the descending colon begins at the base of the fourth metatarsal bone in the left foot.

Massage downward, parallel to the outer edge of the foot. Then move to the inside edges of the heels to massage the rectum zone point by point, moving toward the toes.

Left foot

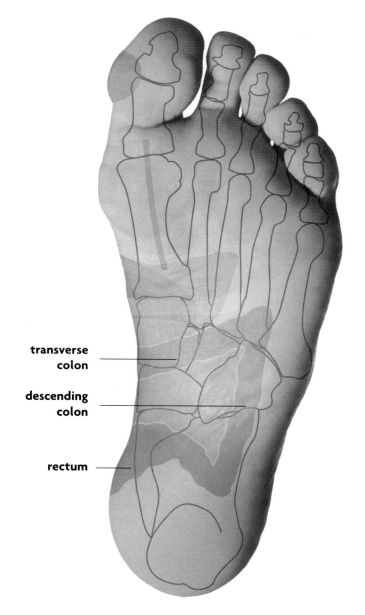

transverse colon

descending colon

rectum

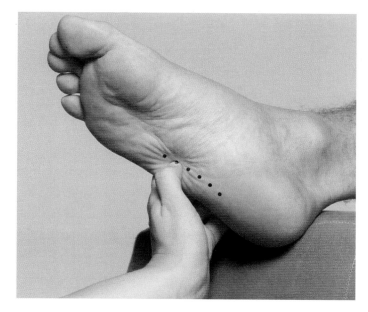

Massage the zone of the ascending colon on the right foot with the tip of your thumb point by point from the heel to the bottom of the fourth metatarsal bone.

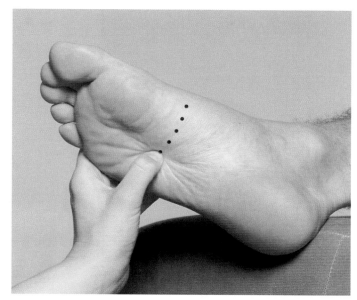

Massage the zone of the transverse colon point by point across the feet.

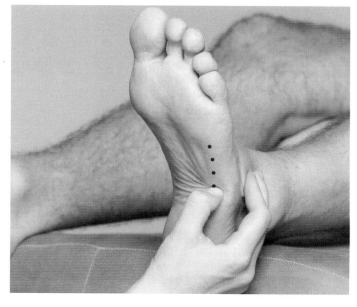

Far left: The zones of the large intestine and the rectum are located on the soles of the feet.

Massage the zone of the descending colon parallel to the outside edge of the left foot.

The Lymphatic System

The lymphatic system consists of small vessels that cover the cells of the body like a fine net. They merge to form large lymphatic ducts that eventually connect to the circulatory system.

We draw a distinction between the primary, central lymphatic organs (the thymus and bone marrow) that support the formation, development, and maturation of the lymphatic cells and the secondary, peripheral lymphatic organs such as the lymph nodes, the spleen, and the lymphatic tissue of the skin and mucous membranes (the tonsils and lymphatic intestinal tissue). Lymph is the watery fluid in the lymph vessels, which is collected from the tissue fluids. It is high in protein and nutrients and also contains lymphatic cells that support the body's defenses. This fluid is filtered through a system of vessels and ducts connected by lymph nodes and returns back to the blood via the thoracic duct.

The lymph nodes function essentially as filters, removing and eliminating from the lymph substances foreign to the body.

Lymph nodes are surrounded by a capsule of connective tissue that becomes tense when the lymph nodes swell, causing pain. Swollen, painful lymph nodes are a sign of maximum lymphatic-system activity and indicate that immune processes are taking place.

A functioning lymphatic system enables the filtering of cellular debris and foreign substances from the body and ensures a smooth circulation of lymph. When parts of the lymphatic system are injured, massive lymph collections are the result (for example, the lymphedema that forms in the arm after surgical removal of the lymph nodes of the armpit).

Massaging the zones in the feet associated with the lymphatic system activates and supports the lymphatic system in its functions and thus supports the body's immune defenses.

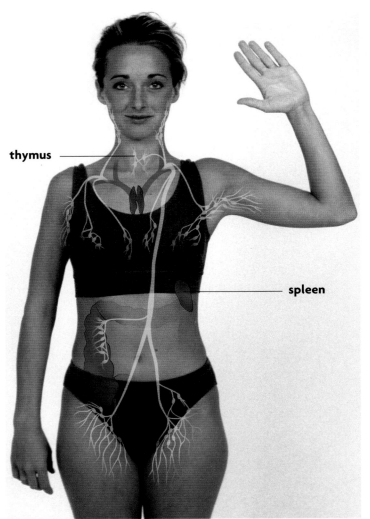

thymus

spleen

The lymphatic system is made up of lymphatic vessels and ducts, lymph nodes, the spleen, and the thymus.

Primary Lymphatic Organs	Function
bone marrow, thymus	formation of lymphocytes

Secondary Lymphatic Organs	Function
lymph nodes	filtration of lymph by lymphocytes, removing pathogens and foreign substances
tonsils	deflection of infections in the nose-throat area
spleen	decomposition of old or damaged blood cells
lymphatic cells of the intestines	defense against and destruction of pathogens and foreign substances

The Thymus Gland

The thymus is located behind the collarbone. Its maximum activity takes place from childhood up to puberty. With sexual maturity, this gland begins to shrink; by age forty it is as small as it was at birth. The thymus forms the T cells (T = thymus), lymphocytes that are important for immune-system defenses.

The Spleen

The spleen is not an essential organ for adults, as its functions can be taken over by the liver, bone marrow, and other lymphatic organs. The spleen is located in the left half of the body behind the stomach. It is important for breaking down old and damaged blood cells and for maintaining the body's defenses.

Locating the Reflex Zones of the Lymphatic Organs

The zone of the lymphatic system in the head and throat is in the "webbed" skin between the toes. The thymus zone is below the base joint of the big toe, slightly off to the side on the first metatarsal bone. On the same level, between the fourth and fifth metatarsal bones, is the zone of the armpit lymphatic system. The spleen zone is located at the base of the fourth and fifth metatarsal bones in the left foot.

The zones of the lower body's lymphatic system are found on the top of the feet. They extend in a band across the arches of the feet near the ankle joints. The zone of the lymphatic system of the backs and sides of the upper thighs runs along the bottom sides of the calves and merges on the arches of the feet with the zone of the groin lymphatic system.

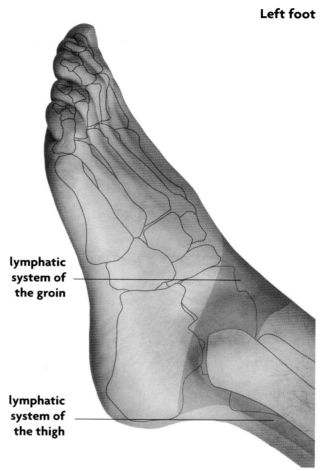

Left foot

lymphatic system of the groin

lymphatic system of the thigh

The zone of the groin lymphatic system connects with the zone of the thigh lymphatic system across the arch of the foot.

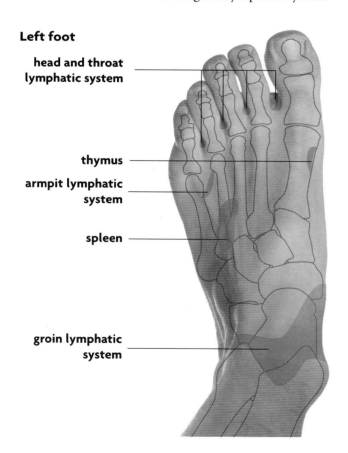

Left foot

head and throat lymphatic system

thymus

armpit lymphatic system

spleen

groin lymphatic system

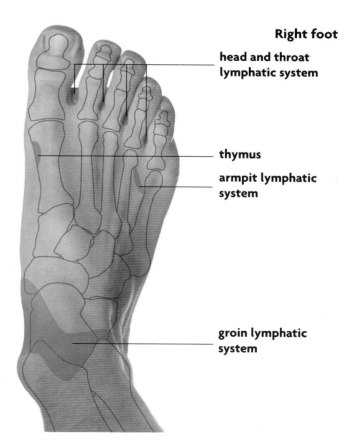

Right foot

head and throat lymphatic system

thymus

armpit lymphatic system

groin lymphatic system

The zones of the lymphatic system are present mostly on the tops of the feet and the ankle regions.

Massaging the Zones of the Lymphatic System

Massaging the zones of the lymphatic system harmonizes that system and increases its activity. It thus offers good prevention against ailments that are caused by a weak lymphatic system. These include increased susceptibility to illnesses caused by viruses, bacteria, or fungi. The zones of the lymphatic systems of the head, throat, armpit, and thymus on the arch of the foot are best massaged with the fingertips. The webbed skin between the toes can be massaged using the tweezers grip.

Massaging the Zone of the Head's Lymphatic System

The zone of the head's lymphatic system is massaged on the back of the foot with the tweezers grip. Place your thumb and index finger at the base joint and move them toward the toes until you are grasping the webbed skin between the toes with the tips of your thumb and index finger. Carefully stretch this zone downward toward the sole of the foot, using the tip of your thumb as a fulcrum. Then stretch it in a similar way toward the back of the foot, using the tip of your index finger as the fulcrum. Repeat until you have massaged the skin between all the toes.

Massaging the Zone of the Armpit Lymph Nodes

The zone of the armpit lymph nodes is located between the fourth and fifth metatarsal bones. Use your index finger to massage this zone point by point, heading toward the toes.

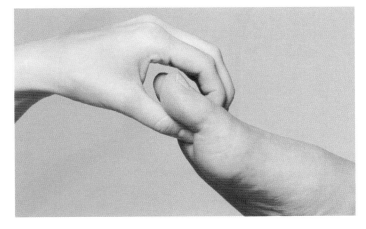

Grasp the webbed skin using the tweezers technique and carefully stretch it up and down.

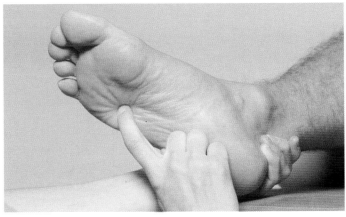

Massage the zone of the armpit lymph nodes point by point in the direction of the toes.

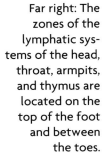

Far right: The zones of the lymphatic systems of the head, throat, armpits, and thymus are located on the top of the foot and between the toes.

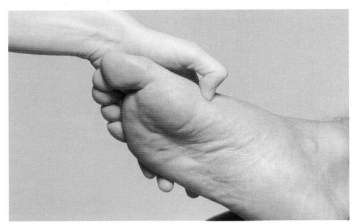

Massage the zone of the thymus on the top of the foot moving toward the heel.

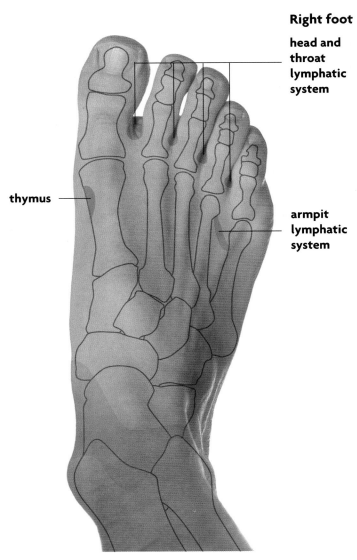

Right foot

head and throat lymphatic system

thymus

armpit lymphatic system

Massaging the Thymus Zone

The thymus zone is located below the base joint of the big toe on the outer edge of the first metatarsal bone. Massage this zone from the top to the bottom, moving from the toes toward the heel.

Massaging the Zone of the Lower-Body Lymphatic System

The zone of the lymphatic system of the legs and pelvis is located around the ankles. It overlies the zone of the groin lymphatic system.

The zone of the lower-body lymphatic system is massaged first from the inside edge of each foot. Begin with strokes in the lower third of the calf, below the shin, using the base of your thumb or your index and middle fingers to stroke toward the heel. Use your fingertips to massage around the heel up to the arch of the foot. Use your free hand to hold and support the foot at the heel.

The calf and outer edge of the foot are easiest to reach with the fingertips of your middle and index fingers. Using

these fingers, stroke below the calf in the direction of the heel, then use the base of your thumb to massage around the heel toward the arch of the foot.

Massaging the Zone of the Armpit Lymph Nodes

The armpit lymph nodes zone also appears on the sole of the foot, between the fourth and fifth metatarsal bones just below the base joints of the toes. Using the tip of your thumb, massage this zone with gentle pressure in the direction of the toes.

Finish massaging the zones of the lymphatic system with gentle strokes.

Left foot

lymph region of the groin

lymph region of the thigh

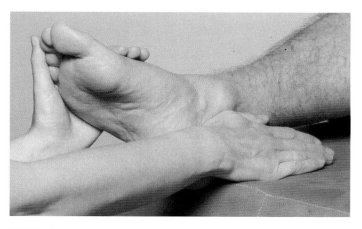

Using the base of your thumb, stroke the lower third of the calf toward the heel and then around the ankle.

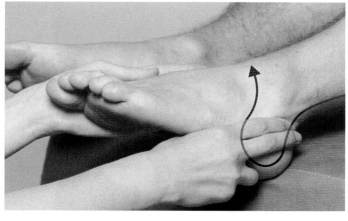

Massage the calf down to the heel and then around the heel using your index and middle fingers.

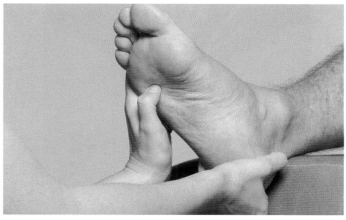

Far left: The zone of the lower-body lymphatic system is located around the ankles.

Use your thumb to massage the zone of the armpit lymphatic system in the direction of the toes.

The Urinary Tract and Pelvic Organs

The urinary tract consists of the kidneys, ureter, and bladder. The two kidneys are located on each side of the spine, slightly below the last ribs. They are the most important organs of elimination of the body. Each day, they filter waste particles from about 1,500 liters of blood. Via the urine and the ureter, these particles are passed on to the bladder and then excreted via the urethra. Each day the kidneys produce between 1.5 and 2 liters of urine. They are also involved in many other functions of our body: the regulation of the water content of the blood, the formation of red blood cells, and—by way of the adrenal glands—the regulation of blood pressure, to name but a few. If both our kidneys were to fail at the same time, we would die within a short period if we did not receive immediate medical attention.

The urine formed in the kidneys reaches the bladder via the ureter. The ureter is composed of muscle strings that are about 30 centimeters long and end in the bladder.

The bladder itself is located in the pelvis behind the pubic bone. It is a muscular, hollow organ that can contain between one-quarter and one-half liter of liquid. The bladder muscle seals the urethra and prevents urine from exiting the body.

The pelvic area also houses the sexual organs: for women, the ovaries, fallopian tubes, and uterus, and for men, the prostate, testicles, and spermatic duct.

Locating the Reflex Zones of the Urinary Tract and Pelvic Organs

The kidney zone is shaped like the kidney itself. The zone is about the size of a bean and is located at the base of the third metatarsal bone. The zone of the ureter runs from the kidney zone across to the inside of the heel.

The bladder zone is about two finger-widths below the bottom edge of the ankle, toward the heel. Farther toward the heel is, in men, the zone of the sexual organs: the prostate, penis, and testicles. In women, the zone of the uterus is directly below the bladder zone but more toward the sole of the foot. On the outside edge of the foot, about two finger-widths below the ankle and more toward the heel, is the zone of the ovaries. The zone of the fallopian tube or vas deferens wraps around the top of the foot.

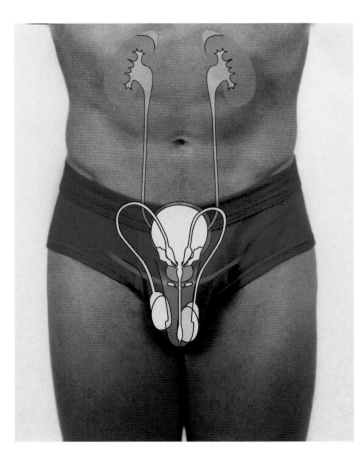
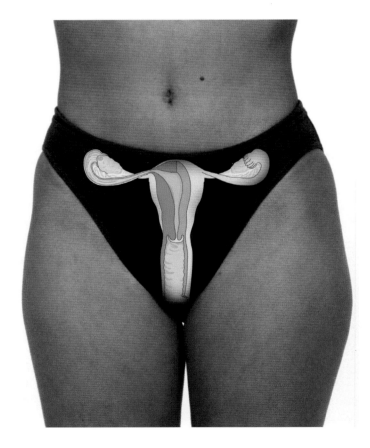

The genitals are located in the pelvic area.

Left foot

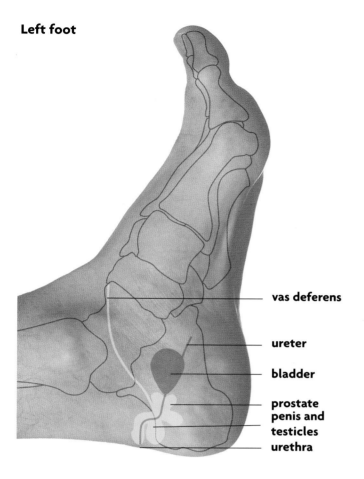

- vas deferens
- ureter
- bladder
- prostate penis and testicles
- urethra

Left foot

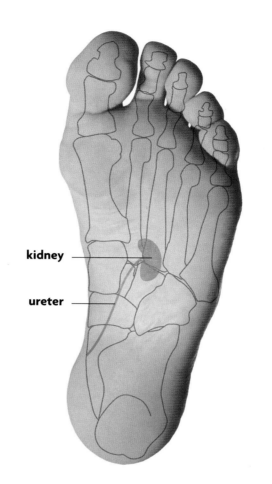

- kidney
- ureter

Left: The zones of the male genitals are located below the inside of the ankle.

Right: The ureter zone connects to the kidney zone.

Right foot

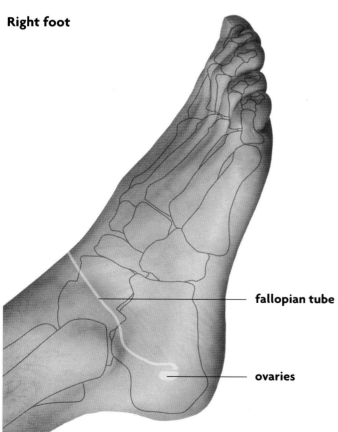

- fallopian tube
- ovaries

Right foot

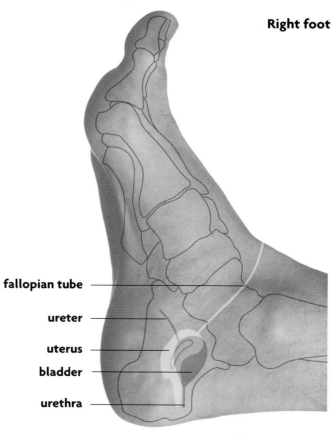

- fallopian tube
- ureter
- uterus
- bladder
- urethra

Left: The zones of the female genitals extend from the outer side of the foot . . .

Right: . . . to the inside edge of the foot below the ankle.

Massaging the Zones of the Urinary Tract and Pelvis

The kidney zone is a very small zone that is best massaged with the tip of the thumb. The same goes for the very thin zone of the ureter, which runs across the foot from the kidney zone to the edge of the heel. The skin in the middle of the sole is thinner than that of the heel or under the toes. Start your massage here very carefully, and make sure your fingernails are short.

Massaging the Kidney Zone

The kidney zone is located at the base of the third metatarsal bone, roughly in the middle of the foot, slightly toward the outer edge. Find the space between the second and third metatarsal bones on the top of the foot and run the tip of your index finger along this space until you notice a bump. Now place the tip of your thumb opposite the tip of your index finger on the sole of the foot and exert steady pressure on this point in keeping with your partner's comfort level.

Massaging the Ureter Zone

The ureter zone is a fine line that originates from the kidney zone and runs to the middle edge of the heel. Massage this zone point by point with your thumb tip in the direction of the urinary tract—that is, from the kidney zone toward the heel.

Right foot

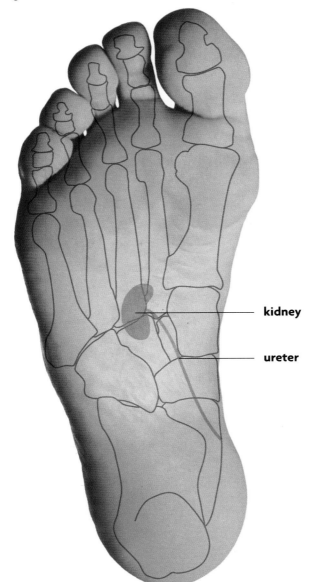

kidney

ureter

Left: The bladder zone and the ureter zone are massaged with the tip of the thumb.

Top right: The kidney zone, too, is massaged with the tip of the thumb.

Bottom right: Massage the zone of the ureter in its natural direction.

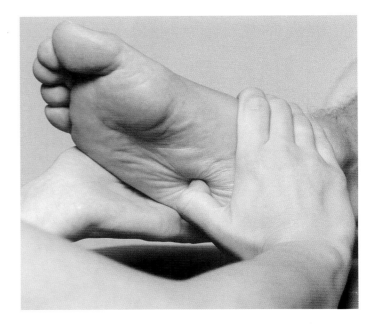

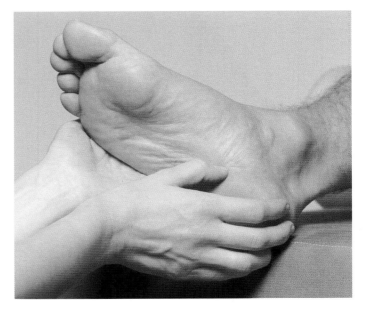

Massaging the Bladder and Genital Zones

The genitals zone and the bladder zone are located close together on the inside of the foot below the ankle. The uterus is slightly more toward the sole of the foot, while the male genital organs are located more toward the heel.

Massaging the Bladder Zone

The bladder zone is also a very small zone. It should be massaged with the thumb tip, point by point, from top to bottom. Especially in cases of urinary tract infections, this zone can at times be very painful. When you come upon a painful spot, apply steady pressure at a level acceptable to your partner, and keep up the pressure for 1 to 2 minutes.

Massaging the Genital Zones

Because they are located so close together, when you massage the bladder zone you usually also massage the zone for the sexual organs. Note that for men the zone is located more toward the heel, while for women the zone of the uterus is located slightly below the bladder zone and the zone of the ovaries is at the level of the bladder zone. Massage this area in several treatment lines.

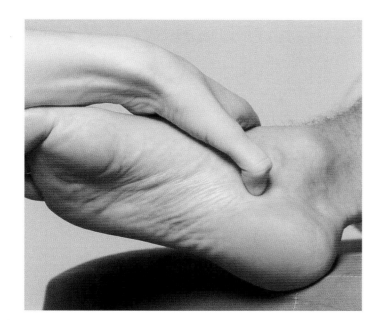

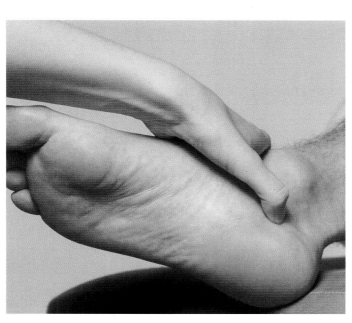

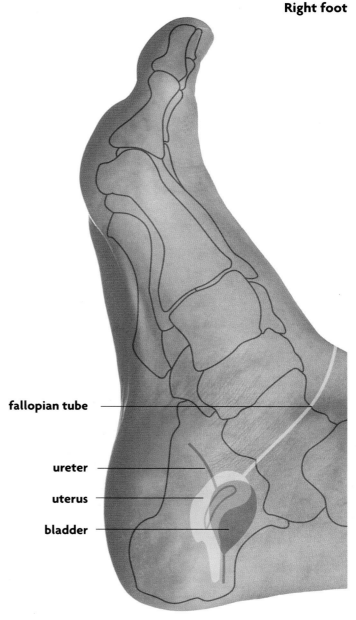

Right foot

fallopian tube

ureter

uterus

bladder

Top left: If the bladder zone is very sensistive to pain, apply steady pressure.

Bottom left: The zones of the bladder, male reproductive organs, and uterus are massaged point by point using the thumb.

Right: The bladder and genitals zones are located close together and are massaged at the same time.

The Organs of the Rib Cage and the Solar Plexus

The ribs and muscles of the rib cage surround and protect the lungs and heart as well as the large blood vessels that originate in the heart. Air reaches the lungs from the nose and throat area via the trachea and bronchi. In the lungs, gases are exchanged between air and blood: oxygen from the air is transferred into the blood, while carbon dioxide is transferred from the blood into the air. The oxygen-rich blood then reaches the prechamber of the left heart, where it is distributed to the entire body via the aorta. As the body uses up the oxygen in the blood, oxygen-poor blood passes from the body through the vena cava into the prechamber of the right heart, from where it goes via finely divided and heavily branched vessels to the lungs, where the gas exchange

takes place and the cycle of blood circulation starts anew.

The chest cavity is separated from the abdominal area by the diaphragm. The diaphragm is a flat, cupola-shaped muscle that supports breathing by lowering during inhalation, which expands the chest area, and rising during exhalation, which contracts the chest area. In a highly simplified analogy, the diaphragm functions like a piston in a pump: when the piston moves upward, volume is reduced and pressure is released. When the piston is pulled down, space increases and air is sucked in. The function of the diaphragm and with it our breathing is to some degree autonomic, directed as a reflex by the brain and not by our will.

When we are at rest, we carry out approximately eight breathing cycles per minute. During athletic exercise and periods of tension or stress, our breathing rate increases.

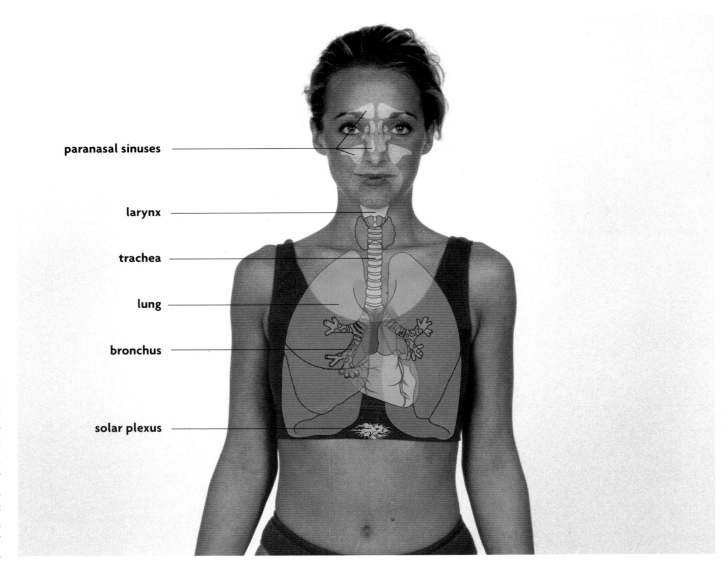

paranasal sinuses

larynx

trachea

lung

bronchus

solar plexus

The rib cage envelops and protects the sensitive heart and lungs. The solar plexus, located under the diaphragm, directs autonomic processes, especially digestion.

Breathing rate is a good way to judge a person's state. Calm, deep, regular breaths indicate a balanced state; shallow, rapid, irregular breathing indicates tension.

The solar plexus is a large collection of nerve cells located close to the diaphragm in the frontal pit of the abdomen, in front of the aorta. The solar plexus is partly responsible for the functioning of the autonomic nervous system. All processes in our body that we cannot consciously direct, such as breathing, heart rate, and digestion, are directed by the solar plexus. Massaging the zone of the solar plexus is thus especially harmonizing and relaxing for the autonomic nervous system.

Locating the Reflex Zones of the Organs of the Rib Cage and the Solar Plexus

The nose-throat zone extends from the front of the big toe around its base. The lung zone encompasses the area of the second, third, and fourth metatarsal bones. The trachea zone runs across the base joint of the big toe into the lung zone. The heart zone extends from the inside edge of the foot across the middle of the first metatarsal bone. The diaphragm zone runs along the base of the first four metatarsal bones and continues at the inside edge of the foot in the area of the medial cuneiform bone. The solar plexus zone is located at the base of the first metatarsal bone and on the edge of the medial cuneiform bone.

Left foot

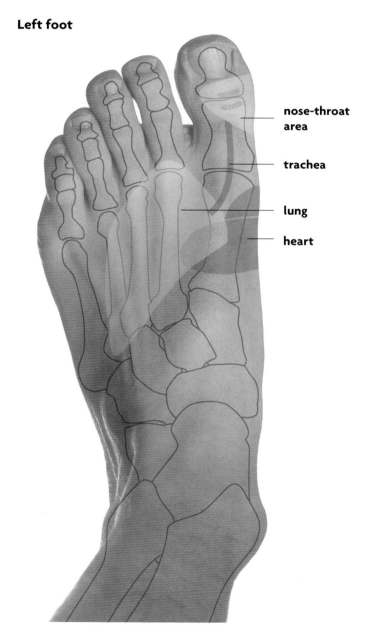

- nose-throat area
- trachea
- lung
- heart

Left foot

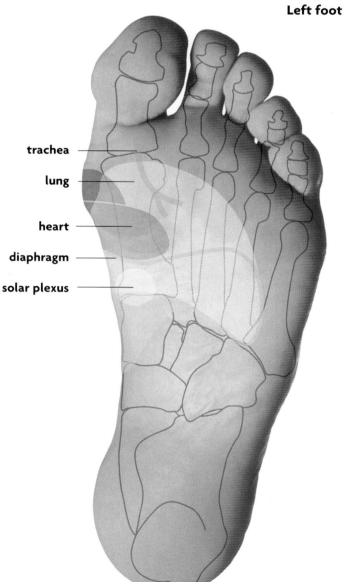

- trachea
- lung
- heart
- diaphragm
- solar plexus

Left: The zones of the nose-throat area, trachea, lungs, and heart are located on the top of the foot.

Right: The zones of the trachea, lungs, and heart, as well as the zones of the diaphragm and the solar plexus, are located on the sole of the foot.

Massaging the Zones

Massage the zones for the nose-throat area, the organs of the rib cage, and the solar plexus on the top of the foot with your index finger and on the sole of the foot with your thumb.

Massaging the Nose-Throat Zone on the Top of the Foot

The zone of the nose-throat area runs on the top of the big toe along the base joint. This zone is best reached with the tip of the index finger. Massage point by point both lengthwise and crosswise.

Massaging the Lung Zone on the Top of the Foot

The lung zone on the top of the foot is massaged with the fingertips. Start close to the indentation near the top of the first two metatarsal bones, then massage lengthwise between the individual metatarsal bones point by point.

Massaging the Heart Zone on the Top of the Foot

The heart zone is located slightly below the base joint of the big toe and is slightly larger in the left foot than in the right. This zone, too, should be massaged lengthwise point by point with your fingertips.

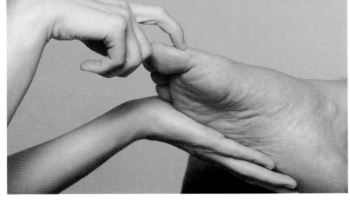

The zone of the nose-throat area is massaged both lengthwise and crosswise while your free hand supports the foot.

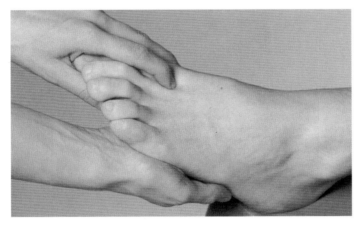

The gaps between the metatarsal bones are noticeable on the top of the foot.

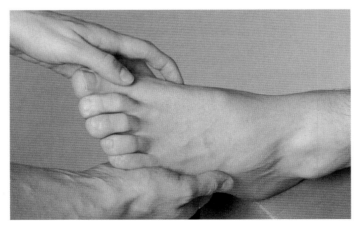

Far right: The zones of the nose-throat area, trachea, lungs, and heart are located on the top of the foot.

Massage the heart zone lengthwise with the tip of the index finger.

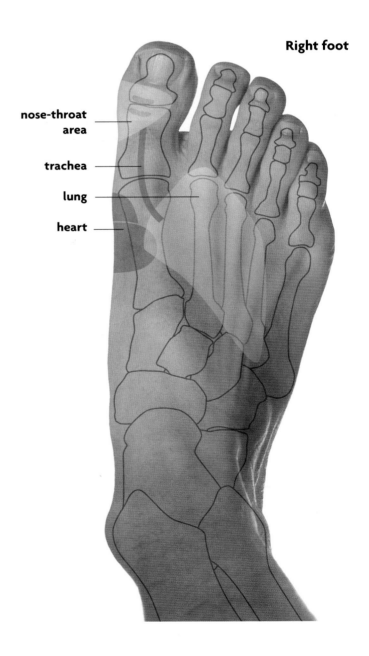

Right foot

nose-throat area

trachea

lung

heart

Massaging the Heart Zone on the Sole of the Foot

The heart zone extends from below the base joint of the big toe across two thirds of the length of the first metatarsal bone. This zone should be massaged point by point both lengthwise and crosswise with the tip of your thumb.

Massaging the Lung and Diaphragm Zones on the Sole of the Foot

Since they overlap, it is recommended that you massage the zones for diaphragm and lungs together. Starting at the base joint of the big toe and ending at the middle of the foot, massage point by point toward the heel. Carry out two or three lines of massage in this manner. When you have reached the space between the first and second metatarsal bones, shorter lines that extend from one third of the way down the metatarsal bones to the middle of the foot will suffice.

Follow this by massaging the zone of the lungs crosswise from top to bottom.

Massaging the Zone of the Solar Plexus

This zone is located at the point where the first metatarsal bone meets the medial cuneiform bone at the inside edge of the sole of the foot. Apply steady pressure at this spot with the tip of your thumb and hold this pressure for 1 to 2 minutes. You can do this on both feet at the same time.

Right foot

- trachea
- lung
- heart
- diaphragm
- solar plexus

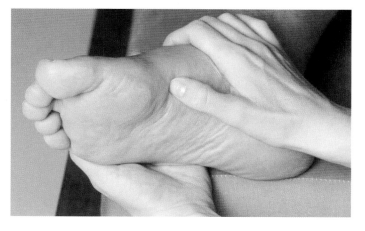

When massaging the heart zone, turn the foot slightly outward and support it with your free hand.

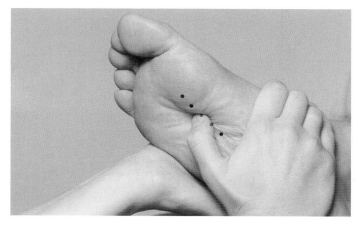

The muscle layer is much thicker on the sole of the foot, meaning that you can apply stronger pressure with your thumb here.

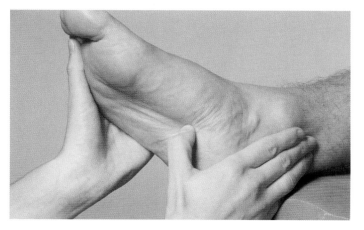

Far left: The zones of the organs of the rib cage are slightly larger on the sole of the foot than the corresponding zones on the top of the foot.

The solar plexus zone is massaged using steady pressure.

The Endocrine Glands

Many life processes are controlled through the hormones, which could be thought of as messenger substances. Hormones are secreted into the blood by endocrine glands. The word *endocrine* in this sense means "connected to internal secretion." Here we will discuss the function and location of three important kinds of endocrine glands: the thyroid, the pancreas, and the adrenal glands.

The thyroid is located in the neck, below the larynx and on either side of the trachea. It consists of two parts, called flaps, connected to each other. The most important hormones secreted by the thyroid are thyroxine and trijod-thyronine, whose functions, among others, are to increase the metabolism. Another thyroid hormone, calcitonin, regulates calcium levels in the blood and supports bone formation.

The pancreas is located near the top of the stomach, across the spine. Each day, the pancreas produces about 1.5 liters of liquid containing digestive enzymes that help break down food into its individual components. The pancreas also contains groups of cells (islets of Langerhans) that produce hormones that regulate blood sugar levels. The most well known of these substances is insulin, which lowers blood sugar levels. A lowered production or total absence of insulin leads to diabetes.

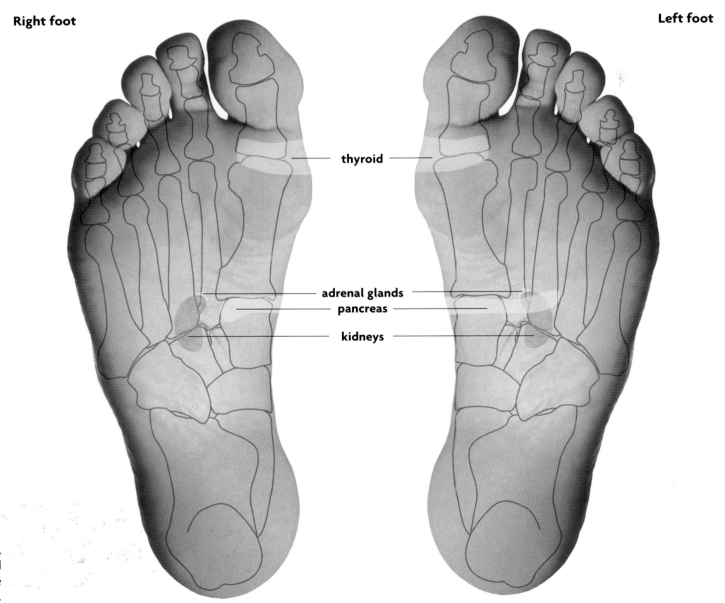

Right foot

Left foot

thyroid

adrenal glands
pancreas

kidneys

The pancreas, thyroid, and adrenal glands are endocrine glands.

The adrenal glands are small organs that sit like hats on the upper poles of the kidneys. Each consists of a cortex and a medulla. The adrenal cortex produces hormones that regulate levels of fluids and electrolytes, blood sugar levels, and the production of sexual hormones. These corticosteroids, as they're called, also have anti-inflammatory qualities. The adrenal medulla produces the important hormones adrenaline and noradrenaline. Adrenaline is known as a stress hormone because it is secreted in situations of stress, fear, and panic and enables the body to react quickly.

Massaging the Zones

Massage of the reflex zones of the thyroid, adrenal glands, and pancreas takes place on the soles of the feet.

Massaging the Thyroid Zone

The thyroid zone is located on the sole of the foot near the base joint of the big toe. Massage the area with the tip of your thumb point by point from top to bottom and then from left to right.

Massaging the Pancreas Zone

The zone of the pancreas extends in the right foot across the base of the first metatarsal bone and in the left foot from the first to the third metatarsal bone. Massage these zones point by point crosswise.

Massaging the Zone of the Adrenal Glands

This small zone is located at the base of the second and third metatarsal bones. Massage it point by point with the tip of your thumb, adjusting the pressure based on the sensitivity of your partner.

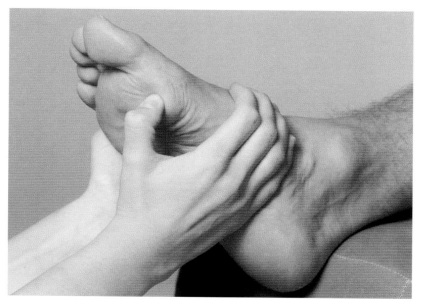

The zone of the thyroid is easiest to reach if you turn the foot slightly outward while supporting it with your free hand

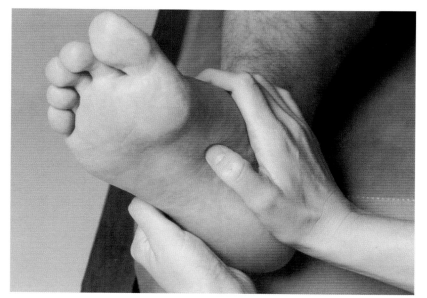

Massage the zone of the pancreas point by point in a horizontal line.

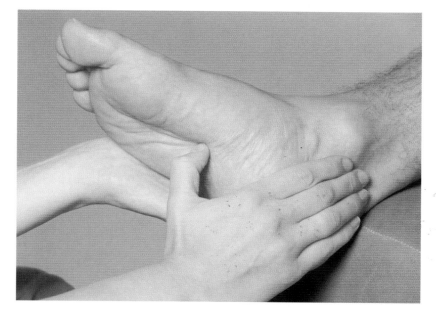

If you find a painful spot in the zone of the adrenal glands, use steady pressure followed by some strokes.

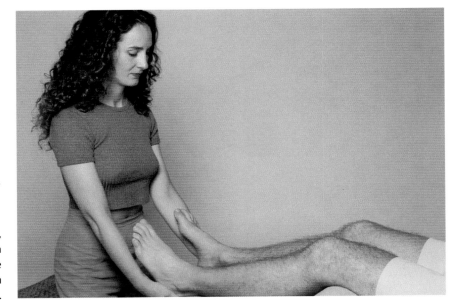

With the heel grip, you will deepen and harmonize the breathing rhythm of your partner.

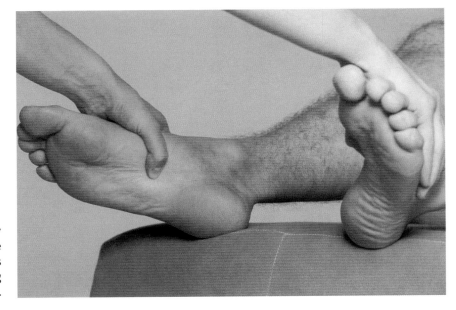

Using steady pressure on the solar plexus zones is relaxing and calming.

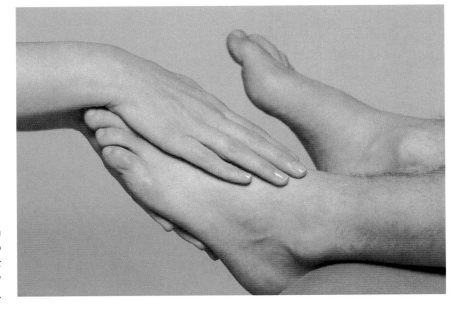

Strokes are an ideal way to conclude a foot reflexology massage.

Finishing the Reflexology Massage of the Foot

When you have massaged both feet, end the massage with soft strokes. There are a number of ways to do this. You can choose any one of them or combine them as you wish.

Stretching the Heels of Both Feet

Grasp the heels with your hands and then pull slightly on both heels. Note the breathing cycle of your partner and try to follow it: slightly increase the pull during exhalation and release the tension during inhalation.

Steady Pressure on the Zone of the Solar Plexus

Place one thumb on each of the two zones of the solar plexus. Apply light pressure and maintain it for 2 to 3 minutes.

Sandwich Strokes

Place one hand on the back of the foot at the level of the ankle joint and the other on the sole of the foot in the heel area. Glide both hands slowly toward the tips of your partner's toes.

Repeat this stroke on each foot two or three times.

Hands on the Soles of the Feet

To end, place the palms of your hands on the soles of your partner's feet. Rest your hands there for 1 to 2 minutes. Ideally, the feet will feel warm and relaxed after the massage.

Foot Reflexology at a Glance

Photocopy this page and hang it up in the space where you will administer foot reflexology massages.

Beginning a Foot Reflexology Massage

Concentrate on the energy of your hands. Make contact with your partner by touching the soles of his or her feet. Begin the massage with calm, gentle strokes. Gently stretch the heels.

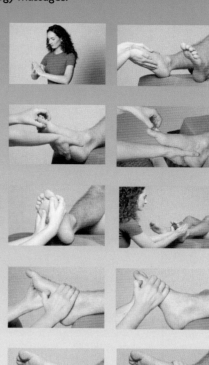

Massaging the Head Zones

The head zones are located in the area of the toes. Using the tweezers technique, massage all the toes from their base point by point. Start on the front (on the sole) of the toes and then massage their tops.

Massaging the Zones of the Neck, Shoulder Girdle, and Rib Cage

Massage the zones of the shoulder girdle and rib cage using the thumb walk on the sole of the foot and massage the zone of the upper arm using the caterpillar walk on the top of the foot. Then lightly shake the front of the foot to relax the shoulder girdle.

Massaging the Spine Zone

This zone is located on the inside edges of the feet. Massage it lengthwise using steady pressure. Note that the zone of the cervical spine is usually more sensitive than the other spine zones. Conclude with soft strokes.

Massaging the Zones of the Digestive Organs

Note that some zones extend across both feet. Massage the zones on the top of the foot with your index finger and those on the sole of the foot with your thumb. Work from the toes to the heels.

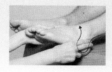
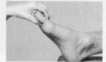

Massaging the Zones of the Lymphatic System

Massage the zones of the spleen, thymus, and armpit lymph nodes with your index finger and the zones of the head and throat lymphatic system with the tweezers technique. Finish massaging the zones of the lymphatic system with gentle strokes.

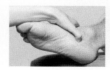
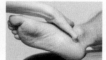

Massaging the Zones of the Urinary Tract and Pelvic Organs

Begin the massage in the kidney zone, then work via the zone of the ureter to the zones of the reproductive organs. Note the different location of the zones for the female and male reproductive organs.

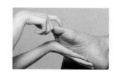
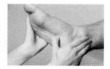

Massaging the Zones of the Solar Plexus and Organs of the Rib Cage

Massage the zones of the heart and breathing passages on the back of the foot with your index finger and on the sole of the foot with your thumb. Massage the zone of the solar plexus using steady pressure.

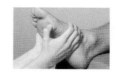
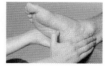

Massaging the Zones of the Endocrine Glands

Massage the zones of the thyroid and pancreas with your thumb and the zone of the adrenal glands with steady pressure on the sole of the foot. Note that the zone of the pancreas is larger on the left foot than on the right foot.

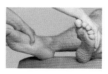
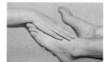

Concluding the Foot Reflexology Massage

Harmonize and deepen the breathing rhythm of your partner using the heel stretch. Sandwich strokes are the best way to conclude the massage. Let your hands rest for 1 to 2 minutes on the soles of your partner's feet after the massage.

Hand Reflexology Massage

In the same way that the human body can be projected onto our feet, it can be projected onto our hands. The individual zones on the hands correspond to the zones on the feet, although there are some anatomical differences. For example, the fingers, which like the toes represent the head zones, are significantly longer than the toes. The palm of the hand contains the zones for the internal organs, glands, and bones and muscles, but the palm of the hand is significantly shorter than the sole of the foot. When locating and massaging the reflex zones of the hand, you must adjust your massage to account for these anatomical differences.

Knowledge

How are hand reflex zones different from those of the foot? Especially for self-treatment, the reflex zones of the hand are more accessible. A hand reflexology massage can be carried out at any time and in any place. Hand massages are less effective than foot massages, however, and their effects wane more quickly. This is because the hands, as organs of touch, receive many more touch sensations than the feet, which makes the individual zones less sensitive. Nonetheless, a massage of the hands is a good alternative to a foot massage.

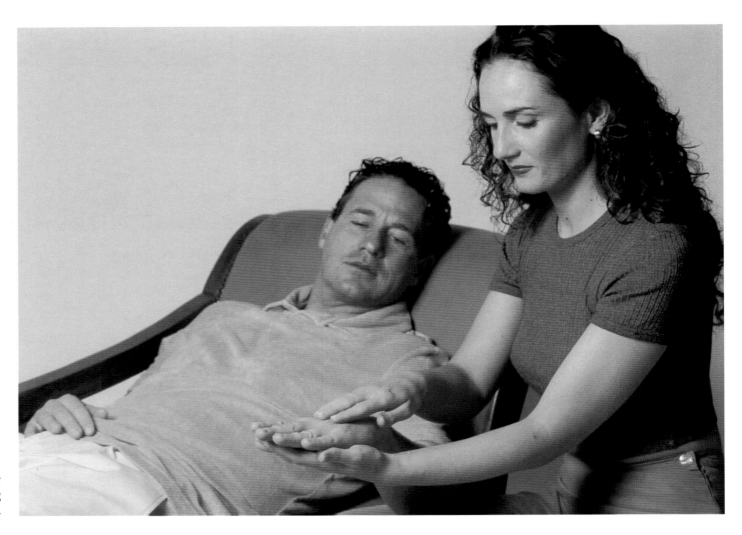

A hand reflexology massage is relaxing and soothing.

The Reflex Zones of the Hands

Fitzgerald's zone model, which divides the human body into ten zones, was presented on page 7 in the context of foot reflexology. This model can also be applied to the hands.

The Longitudinal Zones

The longitudinal zones run along the tracks of the fingers. Accordingly, the thumb is in the first longitudinal zone and the pinkie is in the fifth. The organs and structures in the middle of the body—the spine, heart, esophagus, mouth, and nose-throat area—are represented in the first zone.

The Latitudinal (Horizontal) Zones

Aside from the longitudinal zones, horizontal zones can be located on the hand as well. The fingers and thumb represent the head area; the metacarpal bones largely represent the chest and upper abdomen; and the heel of the hand, including the carpus (wrist bones), represents the lower abdomen and lower body.

Note: The division of zones into longitudinal and horizontal zones is done for the hand as it was for the foot. As such, the following descriptions will discuss the location of organs in the individual zones.

The First Horizontal Zone

The first horizontal zone includes the thumb and fingers and ends at their base joints. The head is represented on the insides of the fingers and thumb; this is where the zones for forehead, eyes, nose-throat area, mouth, and jaw are located. The back of the head is represented on the backs of the thumb and fingers. In addition, the tip of the thumb contains the zone of the pituitary gland, which can be described as the overarching steering element for the human body.

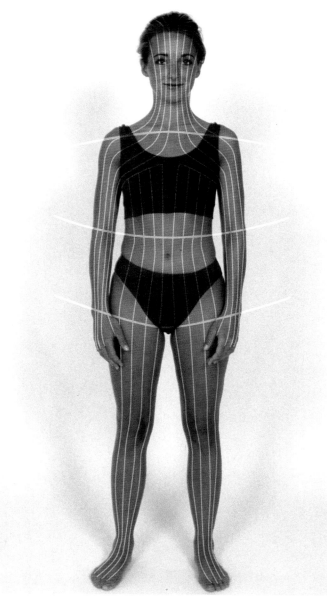

Left: The boundaries of the horizontal zones run along the base joints of the fingers and above and below the carpus.

Right: The longitudinal zones run from the head to the feet and from the shoulders to the hands.

The Second Horizontal Zone

The second horizontal zone extends from the base joints of the fingers to the base of the metacarpal joints and contains the zones of the organs of the rib cage such as the lungs and heart, as well as that of the aorta. The zones for the organs of the upper abdomen, such as the stomach, spleen, liver, and gallbladder, are also located here.

The Third Horizontal Zone

The third horizontal zone lies in the area of the carpus and contains the reflex zones for the lower abdomen and the lower body. This is where the intestines; the sexual organs, such as the uterus, fallopian tubes, and prostate; and the kidneys and bladder are represented. This area also contains the zones of the lumbar and sacrum region.

The Hand as a Tool

If you want to become proficient in hand reflexology massage, it helps to understand the structure of the hands. Our hands are very special tools. In contrast to the rather inflexible toes, our fingers and especially our thumbs have a wide range of motion. The thumbs can carry out circular motions and can touch every other finger. This high degree of mobility allows us to use our hands for a great variety of tasks. The spectrum of work that hands can do is immense, ranging from precise surgery and goldsmithing to activities that require less precision but more strength.

In addition, our hands are highly differentiated sensory organs. People who are born blind become familiar with large parts of the world using their hands. The sensitivity of the fingertips enables them to notice the slightest differences in surfaces. One example of this is Braille, a system of writing using raised dots that are read with the fingertips. The appearance of the hands can tell you much about the person they belong to. Well-shaped fingernails and smooth, well-cared-for hands are signs that the bearer pays attention to his or her hands and values his or her external appearance. Callused, muscular hands indicate that the bearer participates regularly in physical activity. The condition of the nails can also tell a lot about the moods of a person. Nervous people and those under a lot of stress tend to bite or pick at their nails, which can result in very short nails that don't extend to the tip of the finger. The nail bed in such cases can be torn or inflamed.

Left: The second horizontal zone encompasses the area of the metacarpal bones.

Right: The third horizontal zone is much smaller on the hand than the corresponding zone on the foot. The zones of the sacral bone and lumbar region as well as the organs of the lower abdomen are located here.

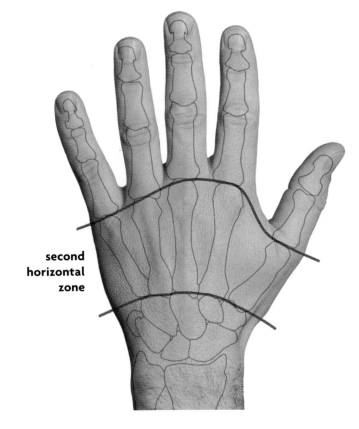

second horizontal zone

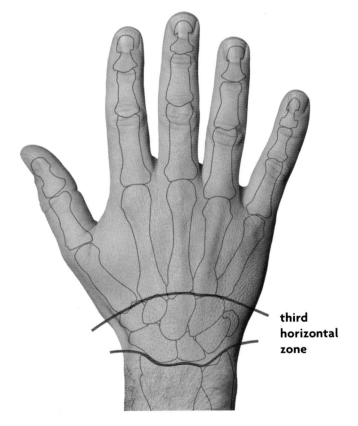

third horizontal zone

The Structure of the Hand

The functions of the hand are made possible by the special structure of its bones. Each hand is made up of a total of twenty-seven bones that are put together like a puzzle. The carpus, at the wrist, forms the base for free movement. Here, two rows of bones are connected to each other by strong tendons. Toward the arm are the navicular bone, lunate bone, and triquetral bone, along with the pisiform bone, which is located toward the outer edge. The four bones in the row above border the metacarpal bones. On the side of the thumb is the trapezium bone. The trapezoid bone is next to it, the capitate bone is in the middle, and the hamate bone is on the outside. The five metacarpal bones reach up to the finger joints. Each finger is made up of three bones (base, middle, and end), with the exception of the thumb, which has only a base and an end.

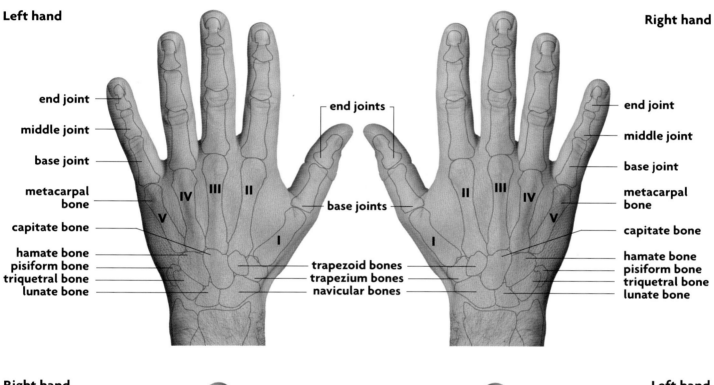

Left hand

Right hand

end joint

middle joint

base joint

metacarpal bone

capitate bone

hamate bone
pisiform bone
triquetral bone
lunate bone

end joints

base joints

trapezoid bones
trapezium bones
navicular bones

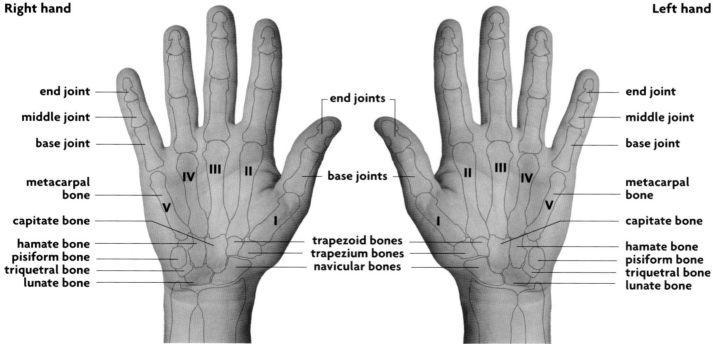

Right hand

Left hand

end joint

middle joint

base joint

metacarpal bone

capitate bone

hamate bone
pisiform bone
triquetral bone
lunate bone

end joints

base joints

trapezoid bones
trapezium bones
navicular bones

The hand is made up of twenty-seven bones.

Noteworthy Points for Carrying Out a Hand Reflexology Massage

As discussed, the human body is reflected in the reflex zones of the hand. These zones in turn can influence the body's organs. A reflexology massage of the hands can be carried out in much the same way as one of the feet. A thorough massage of the hand with the techniques shown here will be both harmonizing and relaxing. The advantage of hand massage is that it can be carried out at any time and in any place. Moreover, it is better suited for self-treatment than is foot massage. You can reach the indi-vidual zones more easily and carry out a massage under many different circumstances. If massaging someone else's hands, it is useful to keep a few things in mind. If possible, carry out the massage in a quiet, pleasant environment. The more relaxed your partner is during the massage, the more he or she will benefit from it.

Posture during the Massage

The reflex zones of the hand can be massaged while the recipient is sitting or lying down. Lying down has the advantage that it encourages relaxation. But if no suit-

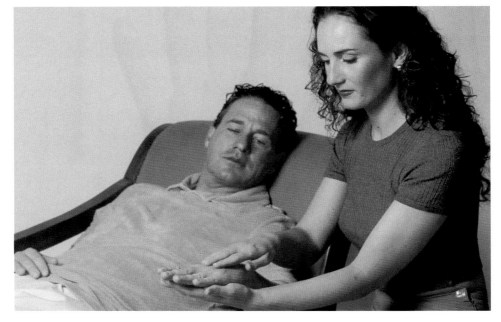

able location is available, you can carry out the massage while your partner is simply seated. In either case, pay attention to your own posture while administering the massage. Ideally, your shoulders are relaxed and you are sitting comfortably with your back straight. If you are in an uncomfortable position or are tense, you will experience fatigue more quickly and will not enjoy administering the massage.

Make sure that your upper body remains straight and your shoulders relaxed when you administer a massage.

Preparing the Hands

You will massage the individual zones with the tips of your thumbs and index fingers. Make sure that your fingernails do not extend beyond your fingertips, as this could make the massage unpleasant and could even cause injuries. The modalities of the massage are the same as for the foot massage. You can read in detail about the other things to pay attention to when administering a massage on pages 31–32.

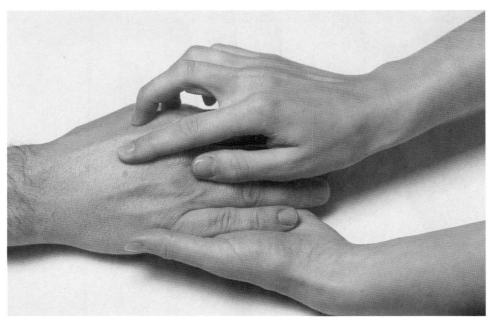

Hand reflexology massages have harmonizing and relaxing effects.

The Energy of the Hands

Carry out an "energy exercise" before administering a massage. Close your eyes and hold your hands in front of your body with your palms together. Concentrate on the palms of both hands. Feel the warmth that moves between your hands. Then move your hands apart, gradually increasing the distance between your hands, but only to the point where you can still feel the warmth and energy flow between them.

> **Tip: Loosening and Warming Up**
>
> Carry out the massage with warm hands.
>
> Loosen your hands by shaking them, lightly kneading them, or stretching them. To strengthen your hands, you can knead a small balloon filled with flour for about 2 minutes (see page 26 for instructions on how to make such a balloon). For a simple stretching exercise, place your hands together in front of your chest with your palms touching and hands pointing up. Move your hands down until you feel tension in the muscles of your fingers and lower arms. Keep up the tension for about 7 seconds, then release.
>
> Repeat this exercise two or three times.

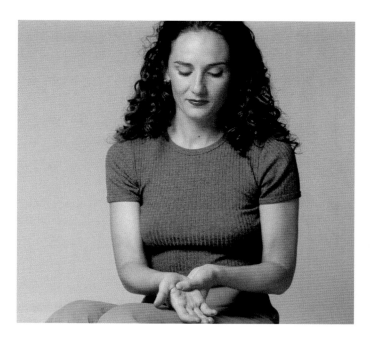

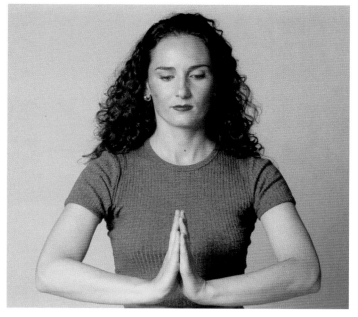

Left: Self-massage of your hands is best done while sitting down.

Right: Place your hands together in front of your chest. Move them down along the front of your body, keeping the palms together.

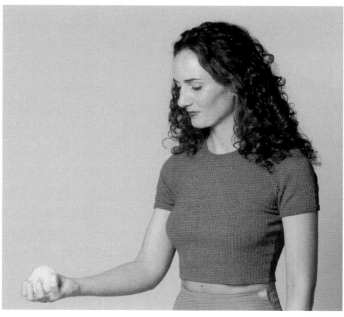

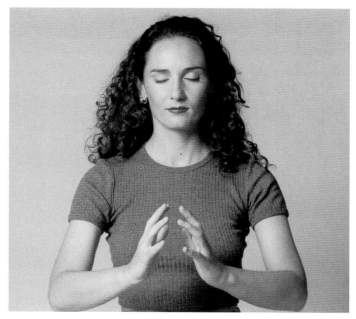

Left: Knead a balloon filled with flour for about 2 minutes with each hand. This strengthens and warms the hands.

Right: This perception exercise heightens the sensitivity of your hands.

What Painful Zones Mean

When you massage the hands of your partner with the following techniques, it is possible that you will encounter painful or extremely sensitive zones. These are often the result of energy imbalances.

Massage these areas especially gently, and respect the individual pain limits of your partner.

Dealing with Painful Zones

Usually, a painful zone can be alleviated by applying steady pressure. Place your thumb on the painful area and apply steady pressure for 1 to 2 minutes. The amount of pressure depends on your partner's tolerance. Usually this pressure will dissolve the painful zone. If the sensitivity of the zone

> **Tip**
>
> Your partner likely will want to know what part or organ of the body a painful zone corresponds to. Answer these questions with care. A painful zone on the hand does not necessarily indicate illness in the corresponding organ. Leave it to a doctor to make diagnoses, and remember that many painful spots will disappear during the course of a massage.

is not reduced, repeat this technique later on in the massage or at the end.

Reactions to the Massage

As is the case for foot reflexology massage (see page 30), your partner may have a number of possible reactions during or after the massage, aside from the painful zones.

These reactions can affect the whole body. A feeling of fatigue or sleepiness is common during or after the massage. Such a reaction is desirable because it shows a proper response from the body, signaling the switch from a tense to a relaxed mood.

During the massage, your partner may also experience "autonomic reactions." These include a lowered temperature in the hands and a feeling of cold all over the body. The hands may start to produce a cold sweat. You can deal with such situations by taking each hand of your partner between your own so that your hands cover your partner's. Apply light pressure to both the palm and the back of the hand.

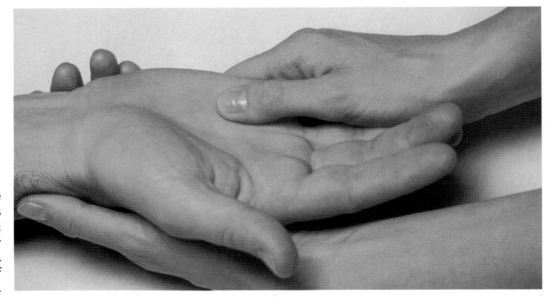

Steady pressure for 1 to 2 minutes dissolves painful tensions. To apply steady pressure, place the tip of your thumb flat . . .

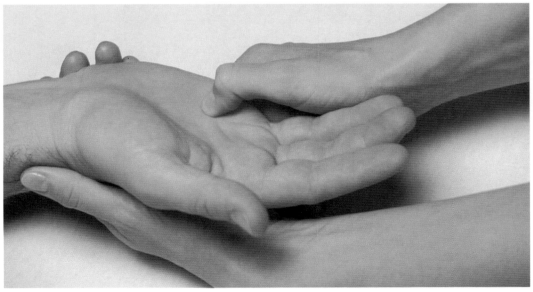

. . . and then roll it up on its tip, so that it is perpendicular to the affected spot.

The following simple techniques offer additional ways of dealing with such outbreaks during or after a massage.

Again, take the hand of your partner between your hands. Using both hands, stroke it, applying light pressure, from the heel of the hand along the palm toward the tips of the fingers. Repeat this stroke three to five times.

Also, inform your partner that existing ailments can sometimes worsen between massages. Such a reaction, however, is a positive effect since it indicates that the body of the recipient is responding to the reflexology massage. This initial worsening is only temporary.

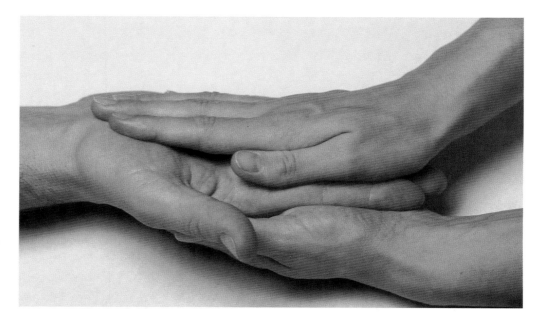

Covering the hands and applying slight pressure is a good way to counteract an autonomic reaction.

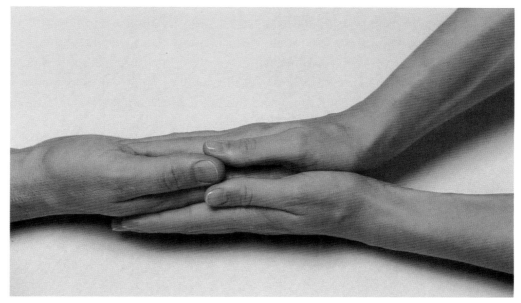

Take your partner's hand between your hands . . .

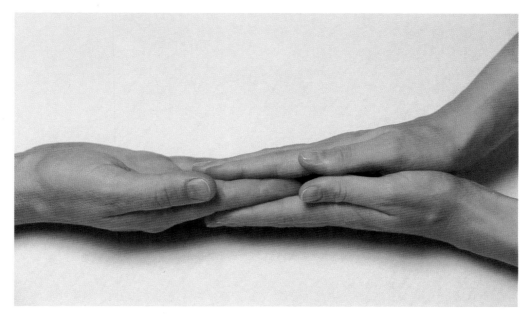

. . . and stroke it slowly and with gentle pressure in the direction of the fingertips.

Aids

You do not need any aids to carry out a relaxing hand reflexology massage. Neither massage sticks nor other tools are a match for the sensibility and touch of your own "instruments." Oils and lotions are also more of a hindrance than a help, as they may cause your fingers to slip from the areas you are massaging. However, if you want to, you may apply lotions and oils after the massage.

Duration and Frequency of the Massage

For a complete massage of both hands, you will need 30 to 45 minutes.

If the goal of the massage is to reduce tension and provide relaxation, daily sessions are best.

If the goal is to stabilize the recipient's energy and provide long-term positive effects for overall well-being, two or three massages per week is recommended.

If the goal is therapeutic treatment of a particular ailment or imbalance, you should administer the massage every two or three days.

Situations That Hand Massage Can Benefit

The situations for which hand reflexology massages can be of benefit are largely the same as for foot reflexology massages, as discussed in detail beginning on page 20. A regular massage is good prevention against ailments of all kinds and harmonizes the energy flows in your body.

Please note that reflexology massage is used for the treatment of functional disturbances and cannot be the sole treatment for illnesses. View hand reflexology massage as a complementary measure for the following conditions: sleeping problems, nervousness, feelings of stress and anxiety, hormonal disturbances, menstruation and pregnancy ailments, problems with the breathing passages, joint pains, skin problems, allergies, and ailments of the urinal tract or genitals. It also can serve as an accompanying therapy for severe illnesses.

Hand reflexology massages can also be combined with other natural-healing methods. Other reflex-zone therapies such as foot reflexology, acupressure, and acupuncture complement one another and even amplify each other's effects.

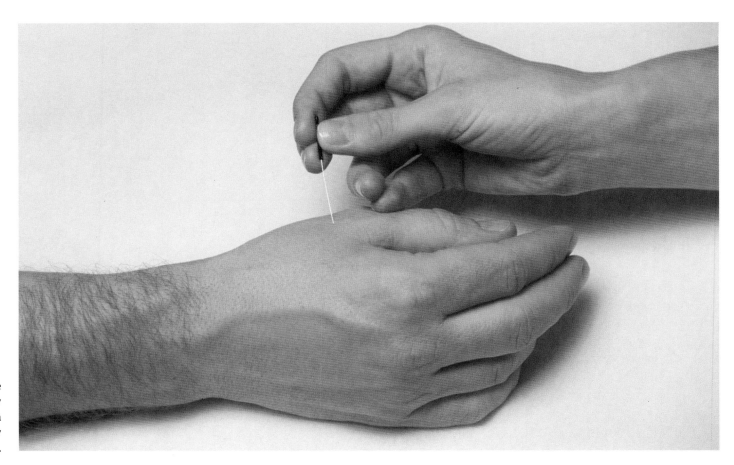

Acupuncture can amplify the effects of a reflexology massage.

Perfect Hands

The hands are usually the tools of our bodies that we use the most. Long-term mechanical uses can lead to ugly calluses and rough palms. Stress and nervousness can lead to dull, chewed-up nails and torn or inflamed nail beds. In the context of hand reflexology massage, it can be helpful to pay some attention to the state of your hands.

If your nails are painted, remove the nail polish, preferably with a remover that contains healing substances.

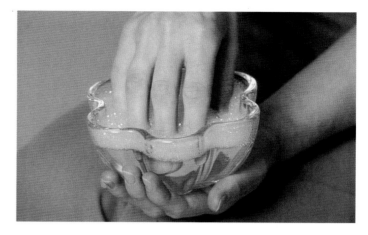

A handbath relaxes the hands and softens calluses.

A Handbath to Set the Mood

Bathe your hands in an appropriate-size bowl filled with warm water. You can add healing substances to the water. End the bath after 10 to 15 minutes and dry your hands thoroughly.

Calluses will now be softened and can be carefully scrubbed off using a pumice stone, which can be purchased in any drugstore. Wet the stone before use, and rinse and dry your hands well after removing the calluses.

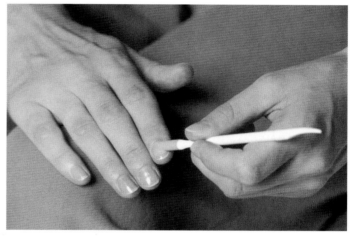

Carefully push back the cuticles with a stick designed for that purpose.

Nail Care

Now turn your attention to nail care. After the handbath, the cuticles will be soft and smooth. You can now carefully push them back with a stick designed for that purpose. You can remove excess skin around the nails with nail scissors, being sure not to cut the nail bed. Cut the nails themselves as straight across as possible, and round off the edges with a file. Your nails shouldn't be too long for administering reflexology massages.

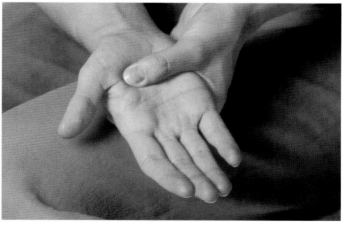

Massage the palm of the hand with circular movements.

Massaging and Putting Lotion on the Hands

After nail care, treat yourself to a hand massage. Start with either the right hand or the left. Begin by kneading the muscles of the palm with circular movements using your thumb, then move down to massage the base of the thumb and the edge of the hand. Then stroke the hand from the heel up to the fingers in several passes. Begin at the outer edge of the hand and end with the thumb. Finally, stroke each finger from its base to the tip. Massage the other hand in the same way. Afterward, apply lotion to your hands.

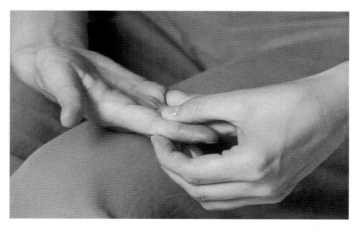

Then stroke each finger from its base to the tip.

Administering Hand Reflexology Massages

A hand reflexology massage relaxes and calms the recipient.

The main techniques do not differ significantly from those of the foot reflexology massage, which were thoroughly described beginning on page 36. The following summary offers a brief overview of the different techniques of a hand reflexology massage.

General Tips

The recipient of the hand reflexology massage can be either sitting or lying down. Lying down enables greater relaxation.

A space with a pleasant temperature and good ventilation is the optimal setting.

The hands of the recipient should be warm, since reflex zones react very little or not at all in cold hands. Ask the recipient to take off any jewelry, such as rings, before the start of the massage.

Start the massage with strokes of the whole hand before you focus on individual zones. Ask your partner how he or she is finding the massage. You can also get an idea of your partner's degree of relaxation by observing him or her, particularly the eyes. If you come upon sensitive zones, do

> **When Should You Not Massage?**
> Do not massage in the following situations:
> - There is an open wound in the hand area.
> - There is an acute injury in the hand area.
> - The hand has been resting for an extended period of time—for example, in a cast or after surgery.
> - The recipient has an acute or painful illness or one that requires surgery. In these cases, a massage may mask the symptoms and delay the beginning of necessary treatment.
>
> If in doubt, ask a doctor whether you can administer a hand reflexology massage.

not guess or offer diagnoses about possible illnesses those sensitivities may indicate.

For a thorough massage of both hands, plan on spending 30 to 45 minutes.

If your partner feels tired and wants to sleep after the massage, he or she should be allowed to do so.

The Massage Techniques

The techniques used on the hands are similar to those used in foot reflexology massages. Hand massages, too, use strokes as an introduction, to conclude the massage of individual zones, and for closure at the end of the massage. The techniques for the massage of individual zones are the same and include the application of point-by-point pressure using the tip of your thumb or index finger. The selection of techniques depends on what you want to achieve with your massage. For a simple hand massage designed to relax and harmonize the body, you should use primarily strokes. But if you want to target individual zones, you should use the more focused pressure techniques. The following sections introduce the individual techniques.

Practical Procedure for a Hand Massage

Begin with a few introductory strokes. Afterward, systematically massage all the zones. Note which zones are especially sensitive, and work on these more thoroughly

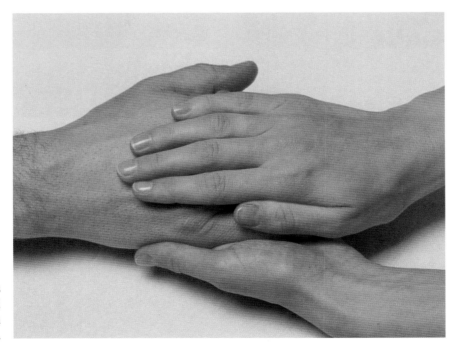

Sandwich strokes are an ideal introduction to a hand massage.

in a second round. If these zones remain sensitive after a second round of massage, repeat the massage after two or three days. Remember that a massage is supposed to be pleasant and relaxing, and make sure that you adjust your pressure based on the sensitivity of your partner.

On the back of the hand, bones and tendons are just under the skin and are easily felt. Massage these areas using only light pressure, and pay close attention to the reaction of your partner.

As is the case for foot reflexology massages, the various techniques for hand reflexology massages fall into different categories: either strokes and stretches or pointed-pressure exertions. For the introduction and closing of the massage, it is best to use strokes. The individual zones of the hand should be massaged with pointed pressure, exerted with your thumb or index finger.

Holding the Hands

Holding your partner's hands serves to initiate contact and relax your partner, allowing him or her to get ready for the massage to follow. Take one of your partner's hands between your own hands, which should be warm. Hold it there for a minute and focus your attention on your hands. Picture the energy flowing calmly between your hands and that of your partner. Feel the tension of your partner gradually decreasing as he or she prepares to receive a massage from you. Repeat with the other hand.

Strokes and Stretches

To begin and end the massage, use strokes. Strokes are also used during the massage to give closure to the massage of certain zones. Stretching the palms and fingers helps the massage recipient relax and get full benefit from the session.

Sandwich Strokes

Again, take your partner's hand into your own. Place one palm against your partner's palm and the other on its back.

Now, applying light pressure, slide your hands from the heel of your partner's hand up to the fingertips.

Repeat this stroke four or five times on both hands.

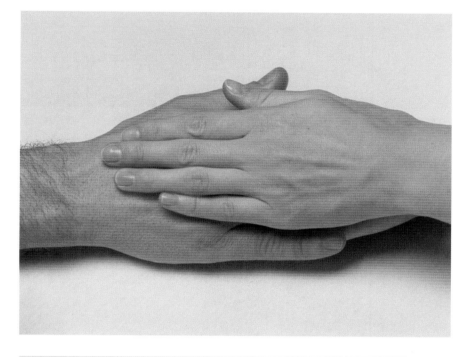

Take your partner's hand between your own. Applying light pressure, . . .

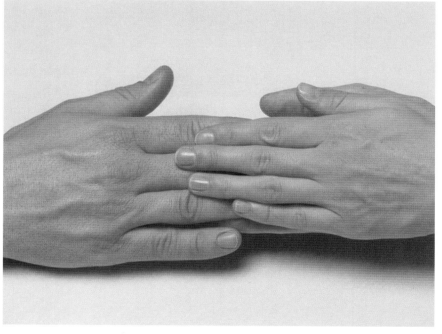

. . . stroke slowly over the hand up to the fingertips.

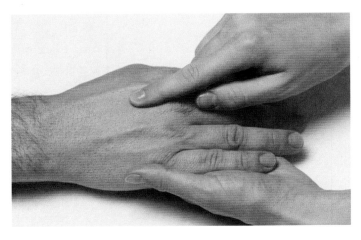

Find the space between two metacarpal bones near the carpus and glide the tip of your index finger in the space in toward the fingertips.

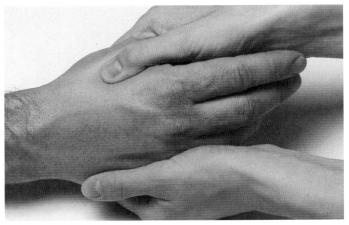

The first metacarpal space is much larger than the others because of the range of motion of the thumb, and it is easy to find. Stroke this space with your thumb tip.

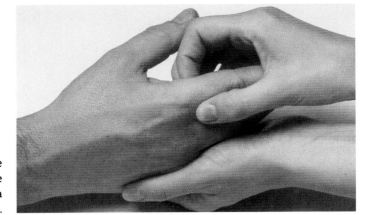

Using gentle pressure, stroke each finger a few times.

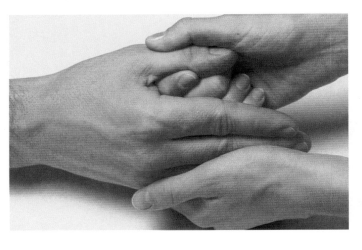

Left: The alternative finger-stroking technique makes it easier to stroke the thumb.

Right: The alternative finger-stroking technique can also be performed on the other fingers.

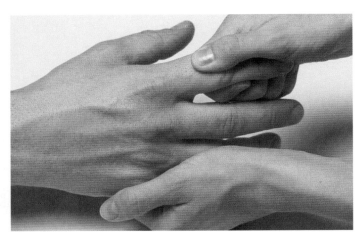

Stroking between the Metacarpal Bones

You can stroke the spaces between the metacarpal bones with your fingertip or thumb tip. The pipelike metacarpal bones are easily felt on the back of the hand. Locate one of these spaces near the carpus. Applying light pressure, run your index finger down the space toward the fingers. Repeat two or three times and then move on to the next space.

Stroking the Fingers

Stroking the fingers is also a very pleasant, relaxing technique. With light pressure, stroke each finger from its base joint to its tip using the tips of your index finger and thumb. Repeat this stroke two or three times on each finger.

An alternative version of this stroke can be done for the thumb. For this, stroke your partner's thumb with your thumb tip on the back of the thumb and with the side of your index finger on the inside of the thumb.

Stretching the Palms and Fingers

Because of the natural bent position of the fingers, the hand and finger flexion muscles are under constant tension. Stretching these muscles feels good and is a good way to begin the massage.

Taking your partner's hand with both your hands, put your thumbs next to each other on the palm and your fingertips on the back of your partner's hand. Straighten the fingers and carefully stretch the hand outward. Be sure that this stretch is not painful or unpleasant for the recipient. Keep up the tension for a few of your partner's breathing cycles.

The Pressure Techniques

You will massage the individual zones using pressure techniques. For these, you exert a focused pressure using your thumb or index finger. The pressure should be steady and stationary, moving forward in a zone point by point.

The Thumb Walk

The thumb walk is in many ways the most basic technique. It is used mainly on the palm of the hand, where the bones are well protected by a thick layer of muscles. You exert pressure with your thumb by rolling it from the tip so that the top joint is upright, perpendicular to the palm. You will be able to feel tense tissues with your thumb tip and will apply pressure to them. Then release the pressure and "walk" your thumb to the next spot, only a few millimeters away. By alternating pressure and release, you can work through the zones point by point.

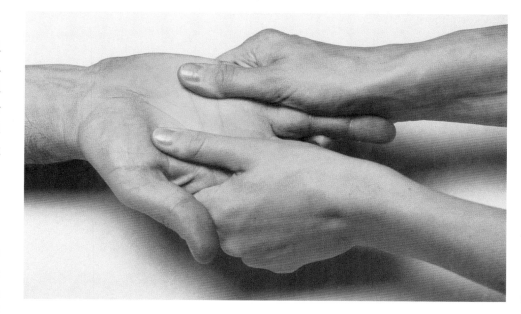

Gently stretching the finger muscles is a pleasant introduction to hand reflexology massage.

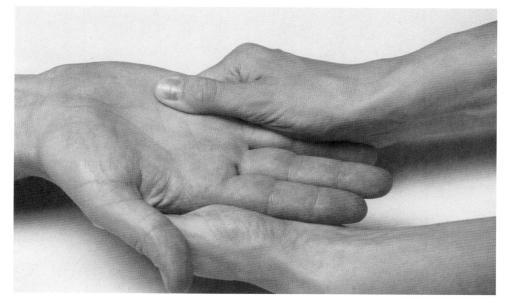

For the first phase of the thumb walk, place the tip of your thumb on the area to be massaged without applying any pressure.

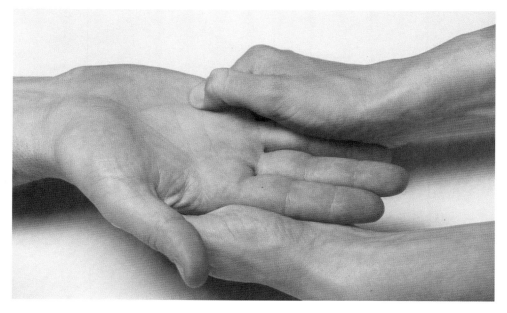

In the second phase, bend your thumb and apply pressure with the tip on the area below it.

The Technique of Steady Pressure—the "Anti-Pain" Technique

If you encounter a sensitive or painful zone during the course of your massage, try to resolve deep-seated tensions using the steady-pressure, or "anti-pain," technique.

Apply steady pressure to the painful zone using the tip of your thumb. The pressure should be only as strong as your partner tolerates. Keep up the pressure for 1 to 2 minutes.

Often this technique will simply dissolve the painful zone. If, however, the sensitivity to pain is not reduced, repeat this massage in a later cycle. Always be sure, though, to adjust the pressure to the pain tolerance of your partner.

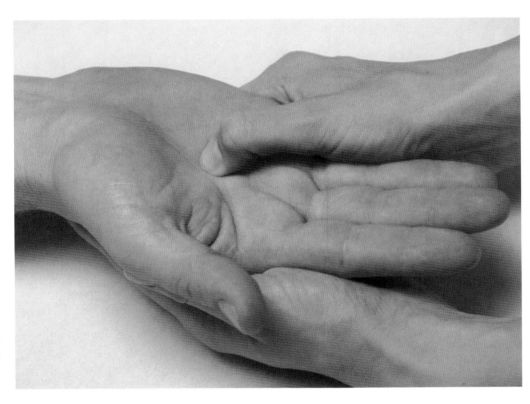

Painful zones can often be resolved using the technique of steady pressure.

The Caterpillar Walk with Your Index Finger

Perform the caterpillar-walk technique with your index finger, rather than your thumb, on those zones that cannot tolerate strong pressure—for example, on the spaces between the metacarpal bones on the backs of the hands. Place your finger berry (pad) lightly on the zone to be massaged and roll from it up to your fingertip.

Apply only as much pressure as your partner can tolerate. Keep up the pressure for a few seconds and then gradually release.

Now move your index finger to the next spot in line and repeat the application of pressure with your finger berry.

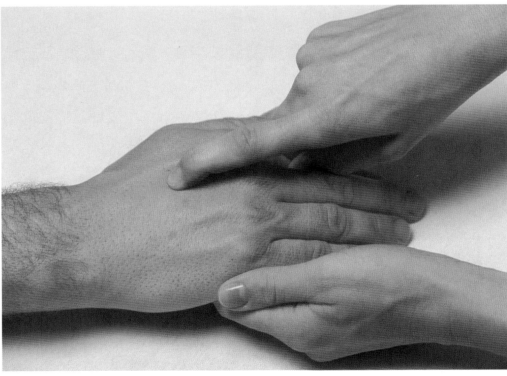

Massage the area between the metacarpal bones millimeter by millimeter using the top of your index finger.

The Tweezers Grip

With the tweezers grip, you use your index finger and the top of your thumb to apply pressure to individual zones. For example, you can take the webbed skin between the fingers between the berries of your thumb and index finger and give it a light, comfortable tug. You can also use this grip to massage the individual fingers point by point.

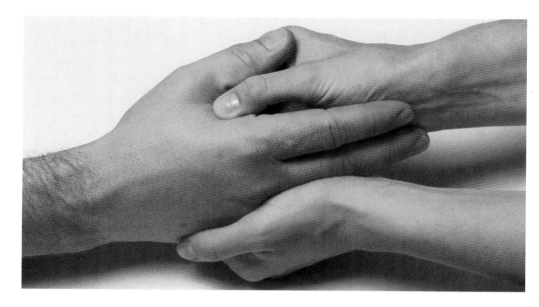

Grip the webbed skin between the fingers between the top joints of your thumb and index finger using the tweezers technique.

Techniques at a Glance

STROKES AND STRETCHES

Holding the Hands
Close your eyes and take deep breaths. Focus your attention on your hands and feel the energy collecting in them.

Sandwich Strokes
Place your hands over the hand of your partner. Slowly glide from the carpus to the fingertips and beyond.

Stroking the Metacarpal Bones
Stroke the spaces between the fingers along the back of the hand with the tip of your index finger or thumb.

Stroking the Fingers
Slowly stroke a single finger from its base joint to its tip and beyond. Repeat for each of the other fingers.

Stretching the Palm and Fingers
Place the tips of your thumbs on your partner's palm and the fingertips on the back of the hand. Applying steady pressure, gently stretch the palm toward both outer edges.

PRESSURE TECHNIQUES

Thumb Walk
Use the tip of your thumb to apply pressure on the palm of the hand point by point. Picture the points like pearls on a necklace, lying immediately adjacent to one another.

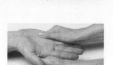

Steady Pressure
For painful areas, place the top joint of the thumb perpendicular to the area and apply steady pressure.

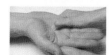

Caterpillar Walk with the Index Finger
Place the top joint of the index finger flat on the hand. Bend your finger in the middle joint and apply pressure with your fingertip. Release the pressure and roll the fingertip forward to the next point.

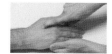

Tweezers Grip
Use the top joints of your thumb and index finger to stretch the webbed skin between the fingers. You can also massage fingers point by point using this technique.

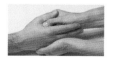

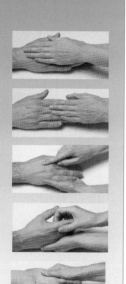

The Location and Massage of Individual Zones

The following will discuss the location of the individual zones on the hand and how they should be massaged. It will be easier to orient yourself and find the zones if you recall the zone model of Fitzgerald, with its division of the body into ten longitudinal zones. The zones of the middle of the body are projected onto the thumbs; zones two, three, four, and five appear on the index, middle, ring, and pinkie fingers, respectively. Using the zone model, you can fairly clearly and easily assign the body's organs and other parts—head, brain, mouth, nose-throat area, heart, spine, et cetera—to the individual parts of the hand and the fingers. The massage described below should be performed on both hands.

The Head and Throat Zones

The head and throat zones are represented on the thumb and fingers. The zones of the front of the body lie on the back of the hand and the zones of the back parts of the body on the palm. The teeth zones are set above and below the middle joints of the fingers, and the jaw zone is at the joint of the thumb.

Locating the Zones on the Back of the Hand

The zone of the forehead area is located on the tip of the thumb. Below it, around the base joint of the thumb, is the zone of the nose-throat area. The zone of the face is set over the thumbnail area. The eye zone is on the middle joints of index and middle fingers, while the ear zone is on the backs of the fourth and fifth fingers.

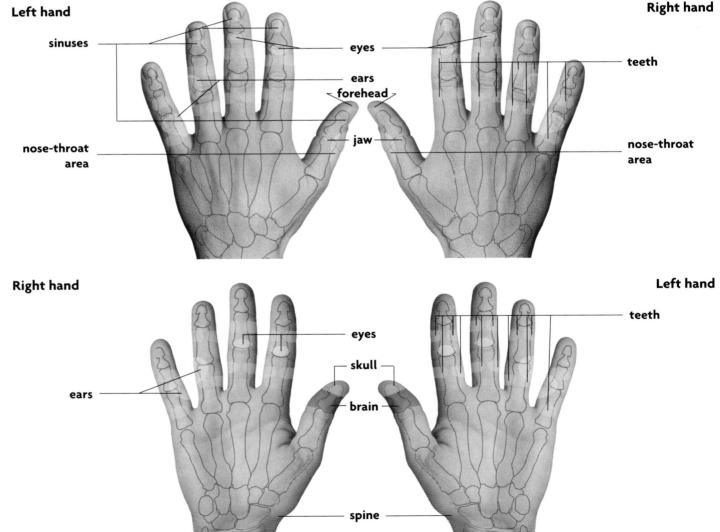

The zones of the forehead, nose-throat area, eyes, ears, jaw, and teeth are located on the backs of the hands.

The zones of the skull, the brain, and again the eyes, ears, jaw, and teeth are on the palms of the hands.

Locating the Zones on the Palm of the Hand

The inner side of the thumb tip represents the zone of the skull, while the zone of the brain is located at the tip of the thumb. The zone of the neck muscles is on the inner side of the thumb's base joint. The eye zone is represented on the index and middle fingers and the ear zone on the ring finger and pinkie.

Massaging the Head and Throat Zones

Carry out a few strokes as an introduction. Take your partner's hand into both of your own and stroke gently with light pressure from the carpus up to the fingertips (see also sandwich strokes, page 38).

Massaging the Jaw and Teeth Zones

The zones of the jaw and teeth extend to both sides of each finger on the base and the middle joints. These zones should be massaged point by point using the tweezers grip.

Begin the massage with the base joint of the thumb. Take the front and back sides of the thumb between your thumb and index finger like they were a pair of tweezers and apply light pressure.

Release the pressure, move your fingers up to the next point, and apply pressure again. Repeat as necessary until you have massaged the entirety of the zones on all the fingers.

Massaging the Zones of Forehead, Neck, and Brain

Massage these zones point by point using your thumb. Begin with the zone of the forehead at the tip of the thumb and massage point by point through the brain zone and neck zone (down the length of the base joint; see the diagram on page 96) to the bottom of the base joint.

Use this technique to massage the other fingers as well.

Massaging the Zones of Ears and Eyes

The eye zone is on both sides of the hand on the second and third fingers. The ear zone is also on both sides of the hand but on the fourth and fifth fingers. Massage these zones on the palm side of the hand point by point using the thumb walk. Apply only light pressure, and be sure to adjust it to your partner's sensitivity.

The zones on the backs of the fingers are best massaged with the tip of the index finger.

After you have massaged all the zones, carry out a few strokes to transition to the next phase of the massage.

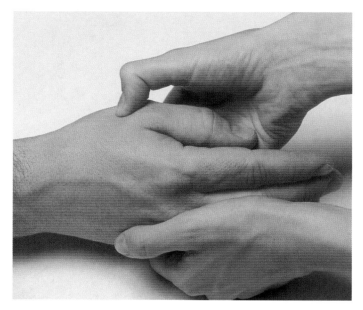

Use the tweezers technique to massage the fingers point by point from the base joints to the tips.

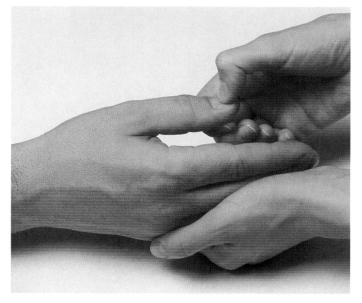

Use the thumb walk to massage the zones of the forehead, brain, and neck.

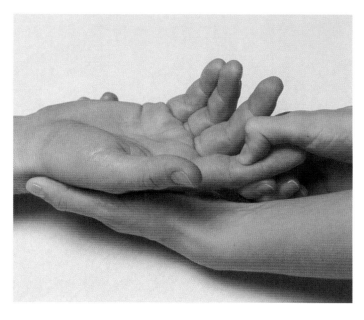

The eye and ear zones should be massaged using only light pressure.

The Zones of the Neck, Shoulder Girdle, and Rib Cage

The zones of the neck, shoulder girdle, and rib cage are in the area of the metacarpal bones. This is a rather long area that makes up the upper two thirds of the hand.

Locating the Zones on the Palm of the Hand

You will find the neck zone at the base joint of the thumb. The shoulder girdle zone—composed of the shoulder muscle, shoulder blade, and shoulder joint—extends crosswise across the base joints of the other four fingers and extends to the metacarpal bone of the pinkie. On the fifth metacarpal bone you will find the shoulder joint at the top, near the base joint; the upper arm in the middle; and the elbow joint at the bottom, near the carpus.

Locating the Zones on the Back of the Hand

The zone of the rib cage lies over the metacarpal bones. The sternum zone is located over the metacarpal bone of the thumb; the collarbone zone runs crosswise across the base joints.

Right hand   **Left hand**

The zones of the shoulder muscles, shoulder blades, upper arms, shoulder joints, neck, and rib cage are located on the palms.

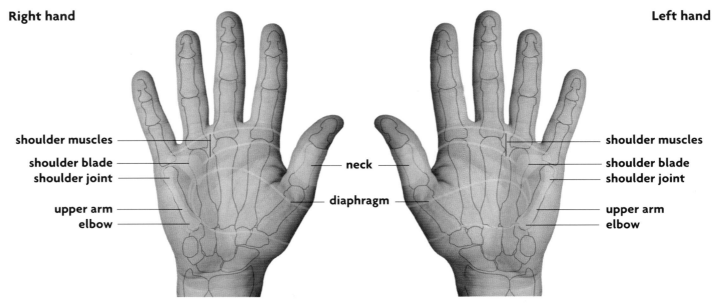

Left hand   **Right hand**

The zones of the sternum, ribs, collarbone, and upper arms are located on the backs of the hands.

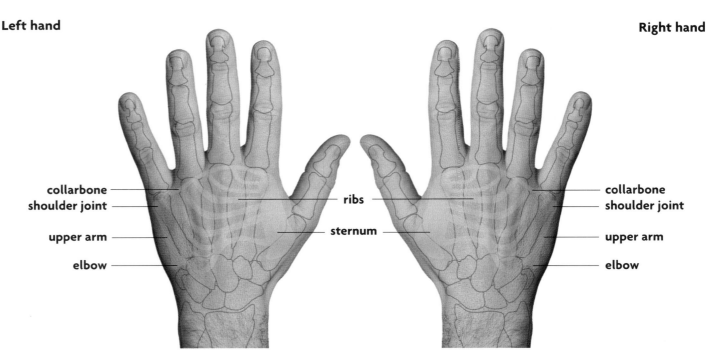

Massaging the Zones

The palm of the hand is best massaged point by point with the tip of the thumb. On the back of the hand, the bones are covered by only a very thin layer of skin. This area, including the spaces between the metatarsal bones, are best massaged with the tip of the index finger.

Loosening the Shoulder Girdle Zone

To begin massaging the neck and shoulder zones, loosen the zone of the shoulder girdle by moving the metacarpal bones. Gently holding the last four metacarpal bones steady with one hand, carefully move the metacarpal bone of the thumb up and down. Then hold metacarpal bones three to five while carefully moving the metacarpal bone of the index finger up and down. Continue in this manner until you have loosened all the metacarpal bones.

Massaging the Zones of the Neck and Shoulder Girdle

The zones of the neck and shoulder girdle are best massaged point by point with the tip of the thumb. Massage each zone, following the lengths of the metacarpal bones one by one. This way you will cover all areas. The zone of the muscles of the shoulder girdle is in the area of the finger base joints. Massage this zone from left to right and right to left in several paths. Then turn your attention to the neck zone, which extends along the base joint of the thumb.

Massaging the Zones of the Upper Arm and Rib Cage

The zone of the upper arm is slightly to the side of the metacarpal bone of the pinkie. This zone is best massaged point by point with the tip of the index finger, starting at the base joint and moving toward the carpus. Afterward, use the tip of the index finger to massage the zone of the rib cage. Although the zone of the rib cage runs in paths across the back of the hand, massage in vertical lines along the spaces between the metacarpal bones from the base joints to the carpus. Do not massage directly on the bones.

Finish the massage of these zones with a few strokes.

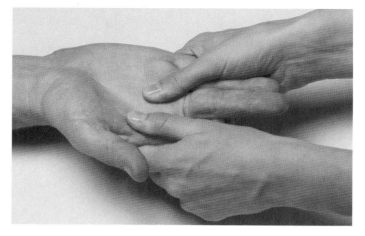

Moving the metacarpal bones helps loosen the zone of the shoulder girdle.

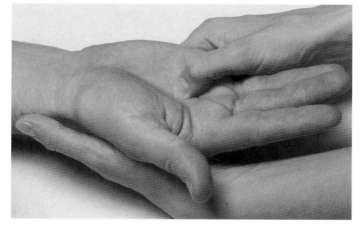

Massage the zones located on the palm in paths that run both lengthwise and crosswise.

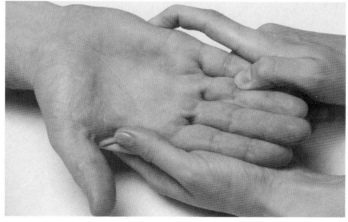

The upper-arm zone is located slightly at the edge of the hand. It is best massaged with the tip of the index finger.

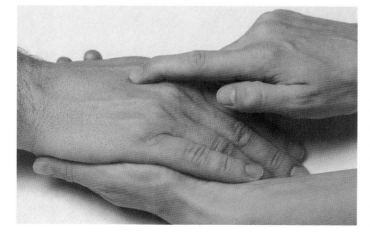

Massage the zone of the rib cage on the back of the hand using the tip of your index finger. Do not massage directly on the bones.

The Zones of the Spine, Pelvis, and Thighs

The spine runs right along the middle axis of the body. It consists of several parts: cervical spine, thoracic spine, lumbar spine, sacrum, and coccyx. The sacrum anchors the spine in the pelvic circle. According to the theory of Fitzgerald's zone model (see page 7), the spine is located in the first longitudinal zone, which in the case of the hand is the thumb.

Locating the Zones on the Palm of the Hand

The zones of the different parts of the spine run along the side of the thumb. The zone of the cervical spine is located to the side of the upper base joint. The zone of the thoracic spine runs alongside the first metacarpal bone. The zone of the lumbar spine is in the area of the carpus. The sacrum and pelvis zones extend across the wrist.

Locating the Zones on the Back of the Hand

The pelvis zone extends across the entire wrist. The zones of the thigh and hip start at the border of the carpus with the ulna (i.e., on the lower part of the forearm closest to the pinkie finger).

The zones of the cervical spine, thoracic spine, lumbar spine, sacral bone, and pelvis are located on the palms of the hands.

The zones of the pelvis and tailbone are also located on the back of the hands. The zone of the hip and thigh is here as well.

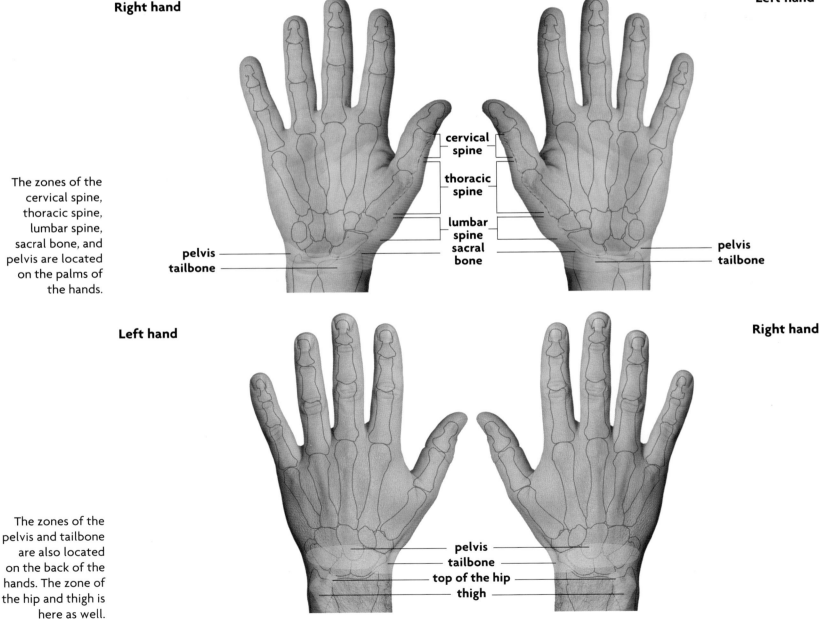

Right hand   Left hand

cervical spine
thoracic spine
lumbar spine
sacral bone
pelvis
tailbone
pelvis
tailbone

Left hand   Right hand

pelvis
tailbone
top of the hip
thigh

Massaging the Zones

Massage the zones of the spine and sacrum on the outer edge of the thumb with the palms of your partner facing up. To begin, start with a few strokes of the hand.

Massaging the Zones of the Cervical and Thoracic Spines

Begin the massage directly below the base joint of the thumb in the zone of the cervical vertebrae. Work point by point toward the carpus. Since the bones in this area are located very close to the surface, be sure to apply only a very light amount of pressure.

Massaging the Zones of the Lumbar Spine, Sacrum, and Pelvis

The zone of the lumbar spine begins below the metacarpal bone of the thumb in the area of the carpus. This zone is usually very sensitive to pressure, since it contains tendons of the thumb and finger muscles as well as large blood vessels. For this reason, massage the area only very lightly with your index finger, moving point by point. Starting from the end of the lumbar spine zone, massage across and toward the wrist, which will cover the zones of the sacrum and pelvis.

Massaging the Zones of the Hip and Thigh

These zones, too, are massaged on the palm side of the hand. Begin above the carpus in the zone of the sacrum and massage across the wrist until you feel the lower end of the ulna. The zone of the hip is in this area.

Follow the ulna and massage the zone of the thigh.

In this area, too, the bones and tendons are covered by only a thin layer of skin and are sensitive to the touch. Work with a very light amount of pressure and adjust the pressure based on the sensitivity of your partner.

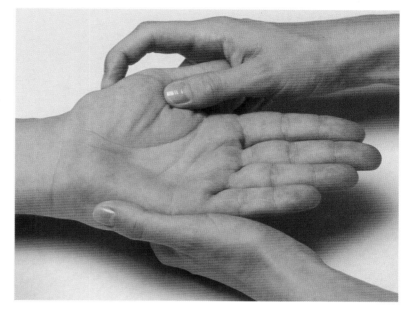

Massage the zones of the cervical spine and thoracic spine using the tip of your index finger.

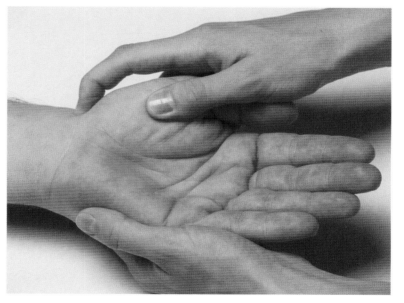

The zone of the lumbar spine ends in the zone of the sacral bone, which runs across the wrist.

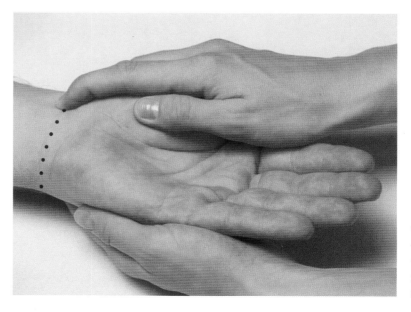

Working across the carpus, you will massage the zones of the hip and thigh.

The Zones of the Digestive Tract

The zones of the digestive system are located at the transition area between the metacarpal bones and the carpus, as well as in the area of the carpus. Since the carpus is very small, the zones in it blend into one another, especially on the inside of the hand, and are difficult to separate.

Locating the Zones on the Palm of the Hand

The zone of the large intestine, or colon, begins in the right palm. It extends across the palms of both hands and in the left hand drops down, beneath the fourth metacarpal bone, before turning back across the wrist, ending in the zone of the rectum.

The liver zone is found crosswise in the area of the first four metacarpal bones on the right palm. The zone of the stomach is on the left palm, crossing the first metatarsal bone. Below it are the zones of the small intestine and the pancreas.

Locating the Zones on the Back of the Hand

The zone of the mouth cavity is on the back of both hands, on the sides of the thumbs at the level of the base joints. It extends downward into the zone of the esophagus. The zone of the gallbladder is on the right hand, in the area where the fourth metacarpal bone transitions to the carpus.

Right hand

Left hand

The zones of the esophagus, large intestine, liver, and stomach are located on the palms of the hands.

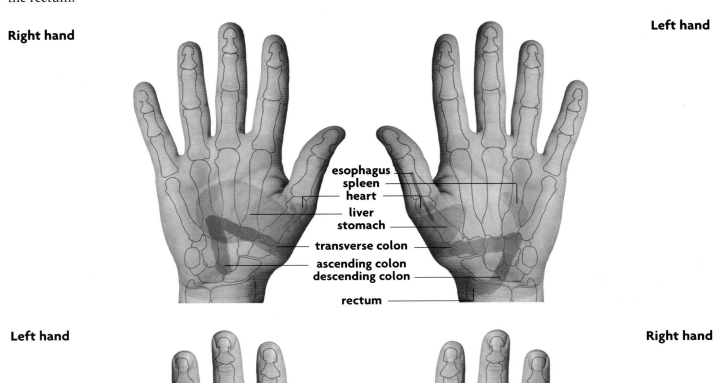

esophagus
spleen
heart
liver
stomach
transverse colon
ascending colon
descending colon
rectum

Left hand

Right hand

The zones of the mouth, esophagus, and gallbladder are located on the backs of the hands.

mouth
esophagus
gallbladder

Massaging the Zones

Because many of these zones overlap, the zones of the organs of the upper abdomen can be massaged only as a whole.

The zone of the esophagus is an exception, as it runs along the thumb before ending in the area where the zones of the upper abdominal organs are located.

Massaging the Zone of the Esophagus

The zone of the esophagus is best massaged point by point with the tip of the thumb, working in several paths.

Start each path on the side of the thumb and work lengthwise past the carpus region to the outer side.

Now massage the zone in several horizontal lines from top to bottom.

Massaging the Zones of the Mouth Cavity and Gallbladder

Massage the zones of the mouth cavity and gallbladder on the back of the hand using your index finger. The zones are located on the bones themselves and should thus be massaged only very lightly. You can find the zone of the gallbladder by touching the space between the third and fourth metacarpal bones and following it down to the carpus.

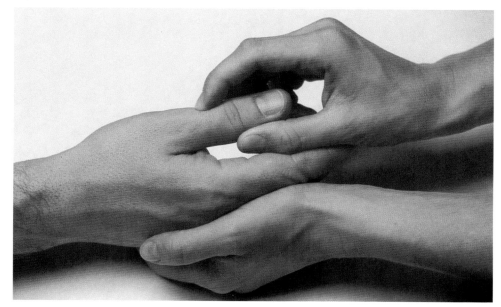

The zone of the esophagus ends in the zone of the organs of the upper abdomen.

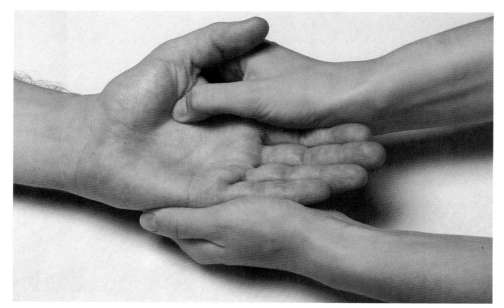

The zones of the organs of the upper abdomen should be massaged with the thumb tip in several paths running lengthwise and crosswise.

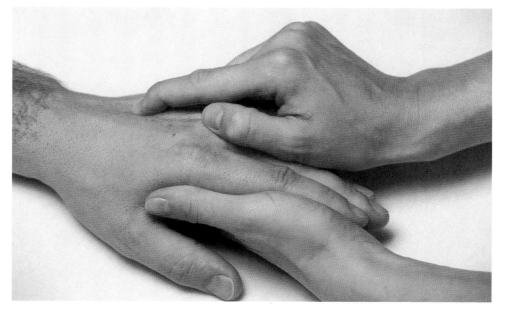

The zone of the gallbladder is located at the end of the space between the third and fourth metacarpal bones.

The Zones of the Lymphatic System

These are a number of different zones that are spread out over the hands. The zone of the lymph drainage area of the lower body begins above the carpus, while the zone of the head's lymphatic system is located on the webbed skin between the fingers.

Locating the Zones on the Palm of the Hand

Lengthwise, striplike zones on both hands below the carpus represent the lymph drainage system of the lower body. The zone of the armpit lymphatic system is located below the base joints of the fourth and fifth fingers, in the space between the metacarpal bones, on both hands. The zone of the lymphatic system of the head and throat is located in the webbed skin between the fingers. The zone of the spleen is located in the lower third of the fourth metacarpal bone in the left hand.

Locating the Zones on the Back of the Hand

The lymph drainage system of the thigh is represented on both hands in a horizontal strip that crosses the the wrist below the carpus. The zones of the armpit lymphatic system and the spleen are in the same position as on the palms of the hands.

The zones of different lymphatic areas are located on the palms of the hands . . .

. . . as well as on the backs of the hands. The spleen is represented only on the left hand.

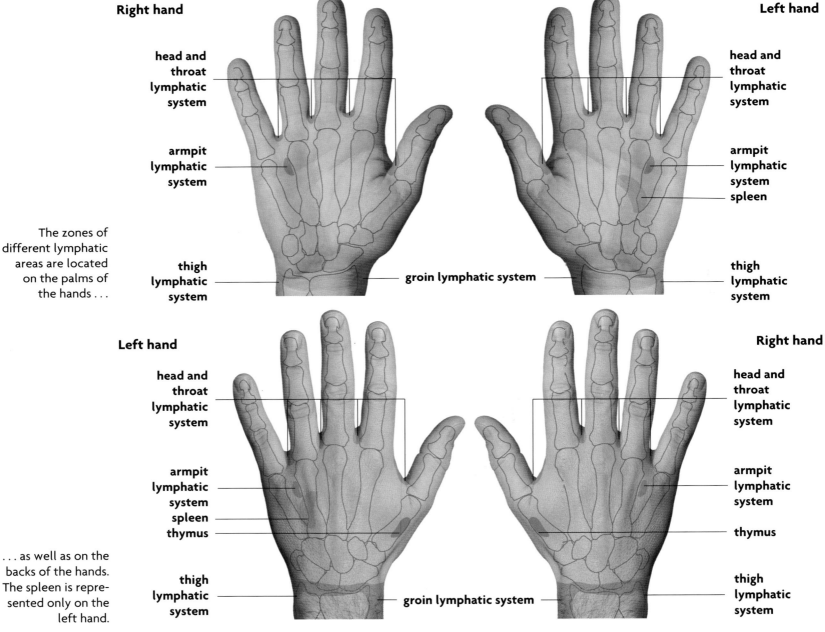

Right hand

head and throat lymphatic system

armpit lymphatic system

thigh lymphatic system

Left hand

head and throat lymphatic system

armpit lymphatic system
spleen

thigh lymphatic system

groin lymphatic system

Left hand

head and throat lymphatic system

armpit lymphatic system
spleen
thymus

thigh lymphatic system

Right hand

head and throat lymphatic system

armpit lymphatic system

thymus

thigh lymphatic system

groin lymphatic system

The zone of the tonsils is found on the front of the thumb, at the height of the base joint. The tonsils aid in the body's early defense against substances that enter the body via the mouth or breathing passages. The zone of the thymus is found in the middle of the first metacarpal bone.

Massaging the Zones of the Lymphatic System

Massage the zones of the lymphatic system in the following order: zones of the lower body and groin, zones of head and throat, then the zones of the individual organs.

Massaging the Zone of the Lower-Body and Groin Lymphatic Systems

With one hand, hold your partner's hand with the back of the hand facing up. With your other hand, stroke the pinkie side of the hand with the sides of your thumb and index finger, gliding from the carpus toward the fingertips and applying light pressure. Perform this stroke three or four times. Then rearrange your grip so that you can stroke the thumb side of the hand, again moving toward the fingertips and applying light pressure. Repeat this stroke three or four times.

Now turn your partner's hand so that the palm faces up. Stroke the outer edge of the lower arm, from about one hand width above the wrist up to the fingertips, using the sides of your thumb and index finger and applying light pressure. Repeat this stroke three or four times.

With these strokes, you have massaged the zones of the lymphatic systems of the lower body and groin.

On the palms, the following zones remain to be massaged: the zones of the lymphatic system of the head and throat, of the armpit, and of the spleen.

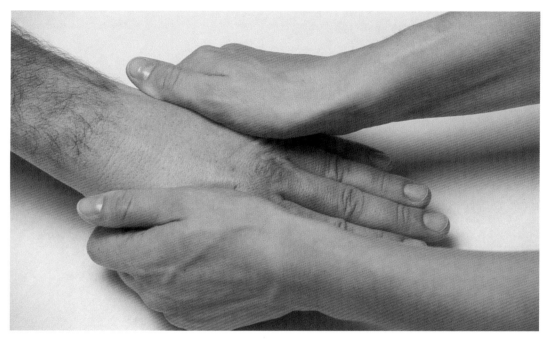

Use your thumb and index finger to stroke the pinkie side of the hand from the wrist to the fingertips.

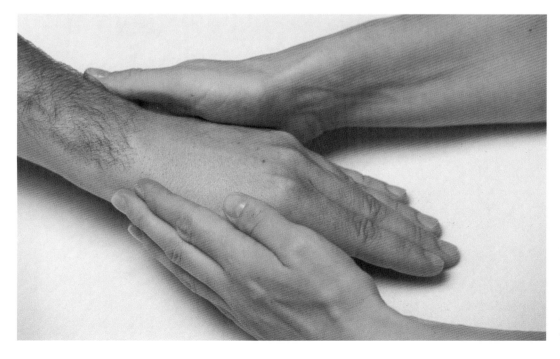

Massage the zones of the lymphatic systems of the middle thigh and pelvis on the thumb side of the hand.

Massaging the Zones of the Head and Throat Lymphatic System

These zones are located on the skin between the fingers. This region is best massaged with the berries of your thumb and index finger. Begin in the space between the thumb and index finger. Place your fingers slightly above the first and second metacarpal bones and then close your fingers over the skin between the thumb and index figner, so that the webbed skin is grasped between your two fingertips. Lightly tug at the skin, maintaining the tension for 4 or 5 seconds. Repeat three times, then repeat this massage for the webbed skin between all the other fingers in turn.

Massaging the Zones of the Armpit Lymph Nodes and the Spleen on the Palms

Hold your partner's hand with its palm facing up. Find the metacarpal bone of the pinkie finger and place the tip of your thumb in the space between it and the fourth metacarpal bone. From here, use your thumb tip to massage point by point in the metacarpal space from the carpus up to the base joint in several paths. Repeat three or four times. With this massage, you are covering the zones of the spleen and the lymph nodes of the armpit. These zones also appear on the back of the hand.

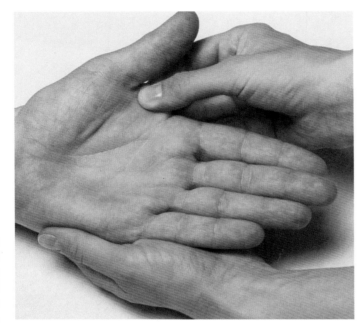

Use your thumb and index finger to massage the zones of the head and throat lymphatic system.

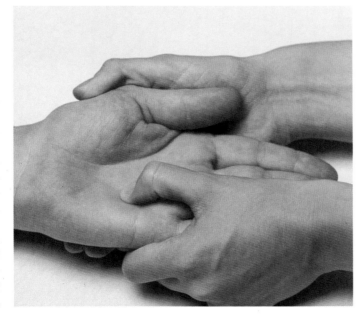

Far right: The zones of the lymphatic systems of the armpit, the head and throat, and the spleen are massaged on the palm of the hand.

Massage the zones of the spleen and the armpit lymphatic system using your thumb.

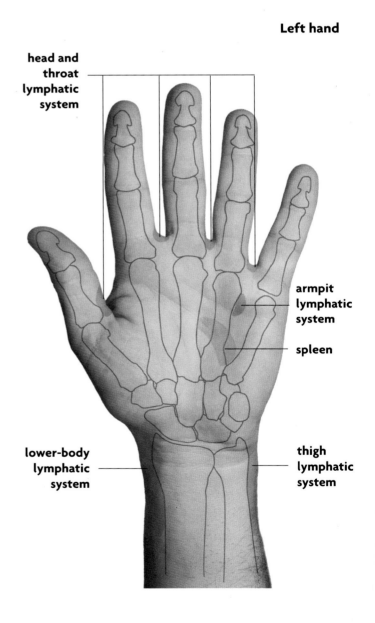

Left hand

head and throat lymphatic system

armpit lymphatic system

spleen

lower-body lymphatic system

thigh lymphatic system

On the back of the hand, the following zones remain to be massaged: the zones of the lymphatic system of the armpits, the tonsils, the thymus, and the spleen.

Massaging the Zones of the Arm Lymphatic System and the Spleen on the Back of the Hand

Hold your partner's hand with its back facing up. Find the space between the metacarpal bones of the pinkie and ring fingers. Place the tip of your index finger on this space near the carpus and massage point by point up toward the fingertips. Repeat three or four times. With this massage, you are also treating the zones of the spleen and of the drainage region of the lymph vessels of the arms. Note that the

zones of the armpit lymphatic system and the spleen also appear on the palms (see page 106).

Massaging the Zones of the Tonsils and the Thymus

Turn the hand of your partner so that the side of the thumb faces up. Massage the base joint of the thumb with the tip of your index finger in several paths, moving from top to bottom. Apply only light pressure, as the bone is directly under the skin here and is very sensitive. Afterward, massage the upper third of the first metacarpal bone with the tip of your index finger.

This also covers the zone of the thymus.

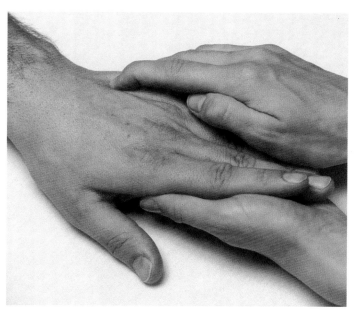

Massage the space between the metacarpal bones of the fourth and fifth fingers.

Left hand

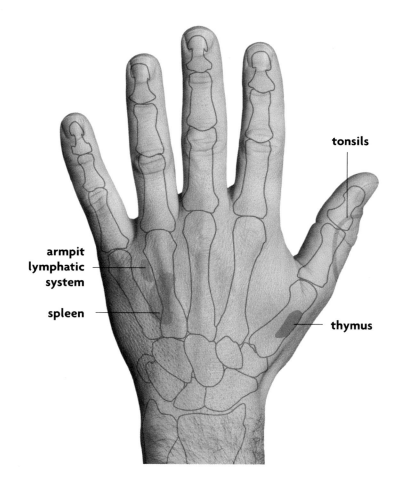

tonsils

armpit
lymphatic
system

spleen

thymus

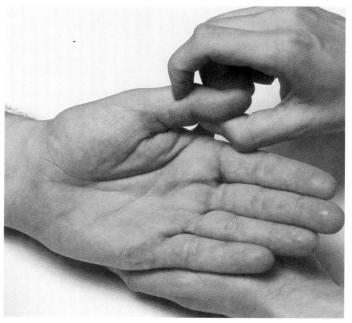

Far left: The zones of the tonsils, thymus, spleen, and armpit lymphatic system are located on the back of the hand.

The zones of the tonsils and thymus are located on the outside edge of the thumb.

The Zones of the Pelvic Organs and the Urinary Tract

The bladder and genitals are located in the middle axis of the body, or the first longitudinal zone, which is the zone represented on the thumb.

Locating the Zones on the Palm of the Hand

The zone of the kidney is in the palm of the hand, near the carpus between the second and third metacarpal bones. From here, a thin band runs diagonally across the carpus toward the base of the thumb on the side of the hand. This is the ureter zone, which connects to the zone of the bladder.

Locating the Zones on the Back of the Hand

Because the kidneys are located deep inside the body, they and the ureter are not projected onto the back of the hands. Only the zone of the genitals area can be found here, on the side of the lower arm at the end of the radius. At the wrist joint both the radius and ulna join with the most proximal carpal bones.

The zones of the kidneys, ureter, and bladder are located on the palms of the hands.

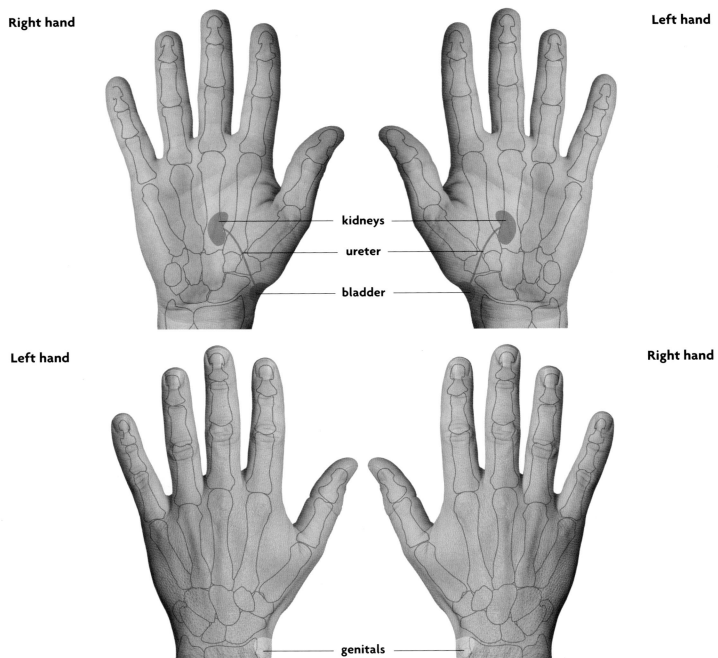

Right hand

Left hand

kidneys

ureter

bladder

Left hand

Right hand

The genitals zone is located on the backs of the hands.

genitals

Massaging the Zones

You'll massage the zones of the kidneys, ureter, and bladder on the palms of the hands. You'll massage the zone of the genitals on the backs of the hands.

Massaging the Kidney Zone

Hold your partner's hand with its palm facing up. Locate the zone of the kidney by finding the space between the metacarpal bones of the index and middle fingers. Follow this space down to the carpus. The place where your thumb stops is exactly the zone of the kidney.

This zone is often somewhat sensitive to the touch. Massage this small area point by point, staying parallel to the two metacarpal bones, with the tip of your thumb.

Massaging the Zones of the Ureter and Bladder

Starting from the kidney zone, you can now massage point by point across the carpus and the thumb joint to the outer edge of the hand. The movement takes you from the kidney zone to the bladder zone, following the natural direction of urine in our bodies.

Massaging the Genitals Zone

Now turn your partner's hand so that the back faces up. Supporting the hand with one of your own, use the tip of your index finger to massage the genitals zone, which lies to the side of the radius bone, point by point. Be careful in this area, as the bones here are covered by only a thin layer of skin and are very sensitive to the touch.

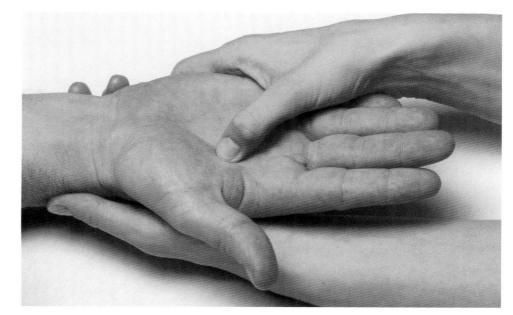

The kidney zone is in the place where the metacarpal bones of the index and middle fingers join to form a V.

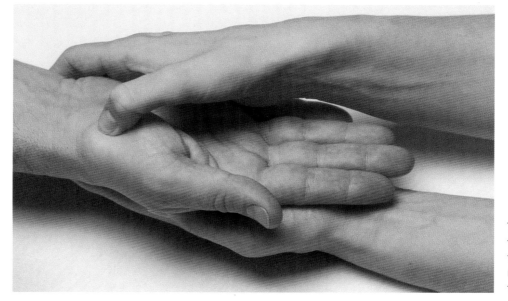

The thin zone of the ureter ends in the bladder zone near the edge of the hand.

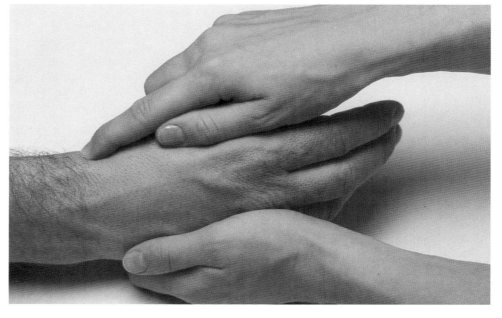

Be careful when massaging the small zone of the genitals in the wrist joint area of the radius and carpus.

The Zones of the Organs of the Rib Cage and the Solar Plexus

The zones of the rib cage, including the lungs and heart as well as the large blood vessels, cover nearly the entire middle of the palms. The zone of the front part of the rib cage is located on the back of the hands, while the zones of the chest organs and the large blood vessels found in back of the rib cage are located on the palms.

Locating the Zones on the Palm of the Hand

The zone of the lungs covers the area from the first to the fourth metacarpal bone. The line between the metacarpal bones and the carpus, running horizontally, represents the zone of the most important breathing muscle, the diaphragm.

The heart zone is located on the side of the first metacarpal bone. It is slightly larger on the left hand than on the right, which corresponds to the natural shape and location of the heart. The zone of the solar plexus (see page 72) is on the base of the first and second metacarpal bones.

Locating the Zones on the Back of the Hand

The zone of the front part of the rib cage is located on the back of the hand. You can find this zone across the second to fourth metacarpal bones (see page 98). A small, narrow zone around the base joint of the thumb represents the nose-throat area. The thin zone of the trachea connects the two areas.

Right hand

Left hand

The zones of the trachea, lungs, heart, diaphragm, and solar plexus are located on the palms of the hands.

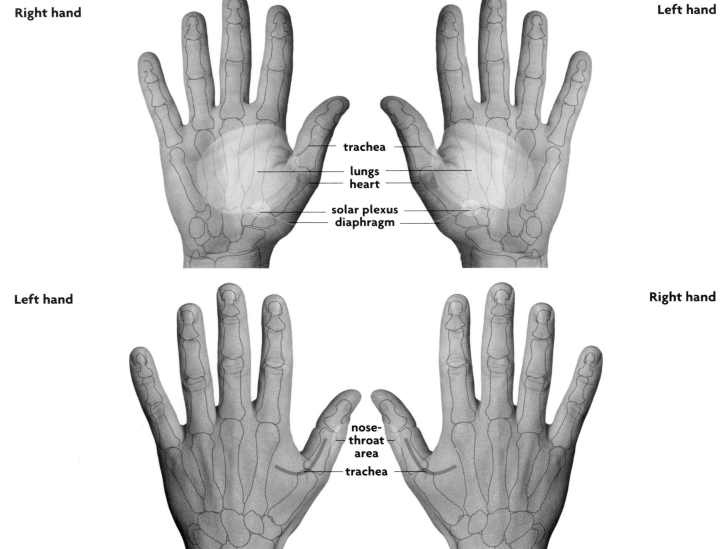

trachea
lungs
heart
solar plexus
diaphragm

Left hand

Right hand

The zones of the nose-throat area and the trachea are located on the backs of the hands.

nose-throat area
trachea

Massaging the Zones on the Palm of the Hand

Begin by massaging the zones on the inside of the hand.

Massaging the Zone of the Heart and Lung

Massage the spaces between the metacarpal bones with the tip of your thumb. Starting on the side of the thumb, move point by point from the base joint toward the carpus. Repeat for each of the other metacarpal spaces. Conclude by massaging the horizontal zone of the diaphragm at the base of the metacarpal bones. Work from left to right and vice versa.

Massaging the Zone of the Solar Plexus

This zone can be found at the inside edge of the base of the first metacarpal bone. Apply steady pressure to this spot, adjusting the pressure to suit your partner. Maintain this pressure for 1 to 2 minutes.

Massaging the Zones on the Back of the Hand

Now massage the back of the hand.

Massaging the Zones of the Nose-Throat Area and Trachea

Starting at the top of the base joint of the thumb, use your index finger to massage point by point the small area around the base joint. Then massage along the inside of the thumb until you reach the gap between the first and second metacarpal bones. Now move lengthwise toward the carpus. Turn the hand so that the back faces up and massage the space between the first and second metacarpal bones from the base joints to the carpus.

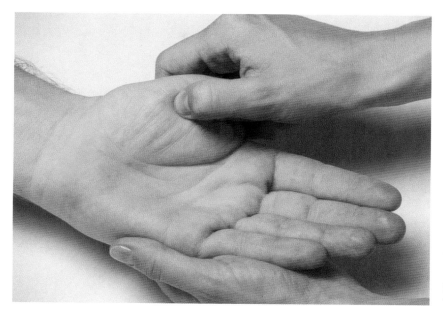

Massage the zones of the heart and lungs using your thumb, working in lengthwise paths toward the carpus.

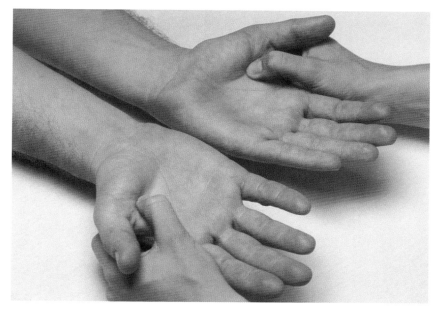

You can apply steady pressure to both hands at the same time.

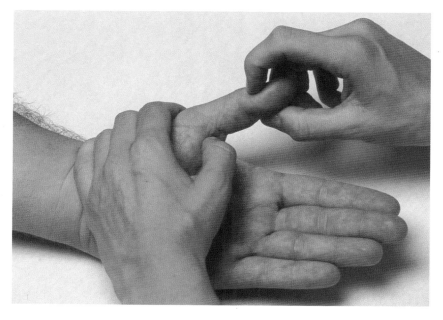

Use the index finger to massage the zone of the nose-throat area.

The Zones of the Endocrine Glands

The zones of the endocrine glands, including the thyroid, adrenal glands, and pancreas, are spread out across the palms and backs of the hands.

Locating the Zones on the Palm of the Hand

The thyroid zone is located in the area of the thumb base joint. The very small zone of the adrenal glands can be found by locating the gap between the second and third metacarpal bones and following it down to the carpus. The adrenal glands zone is located slightly above the V formation of the two bones.

You'll find the pancreas zone in the area of the thumb metacarpal bone and the carpus. It runs horizontally and is slightly wider on the left hand, which corresponds to the actual size and location of the pancreas in the abdomen.

Locating the Zones on the Back of the Hand

The only zone on the back of the hand is that of the thyroid. It runs in a tongue shape across the base joint of the thumb.

Right hand

Left hand

The zones of the thyroid, adrenal glands, and pancreas are located on the insides of the hands.

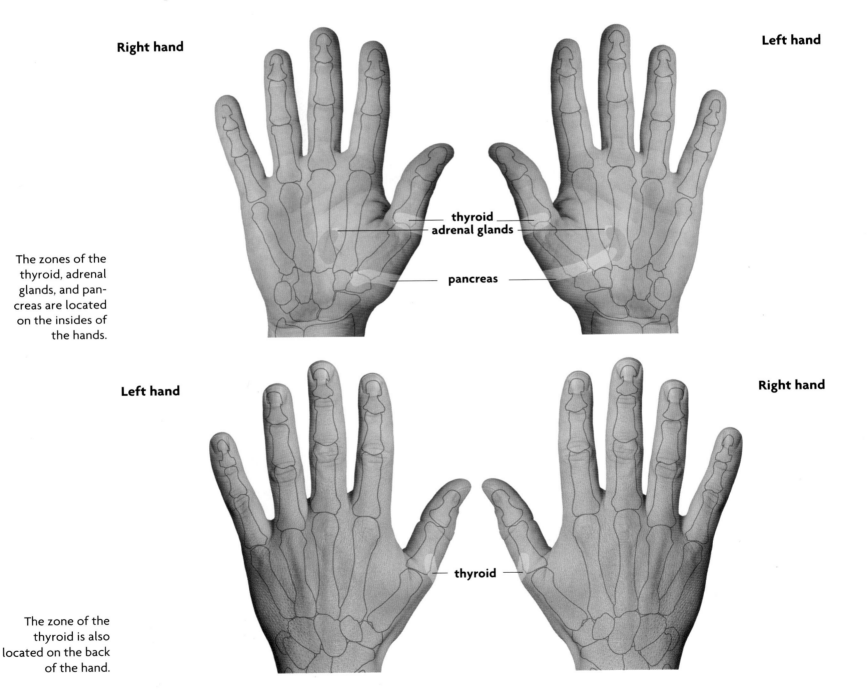

thyroid
adrenal glands

pancreas

Left hand

Right hand

The zone of the thyroid is also located on the back of the hand.

thyroid

Massaging the Zones

Begin by massaging the zone of
the thyroid on the back of the
hand. Turn your partner's hand
so that the back of the hand
faces up.

Massaging the Zone of
the Thyroid

Place the tip of your index finger slightly above the base joint
of the thumb and massage this
zone point by point in paths
that run both lengthwise and
horizontally. Then turn over
the hand so that the palm faces
up and massage the zone on the
front of the thumb's base joint.

Massaging the Zone of the
Adrenal Glands

Find the second and third
metacarpal bones with your
thumb and index finger. Follow
the gap between them toward
the carpus.

    The zone of the adrenal
gland is located in the V or
angle that these two bones create. Massage this small zone
with the tip of your thumb.

Massaging the Zone of the
Pancreas

Locate the metacarpal bone of
the thumb and trace it back to
the carpus. At its end, at the
level of the wrist wrinkle, is
the horizontal zone of the pancreas. Massage this zone with
the tip of your thumb in several
paths from left to right and vice
versa.

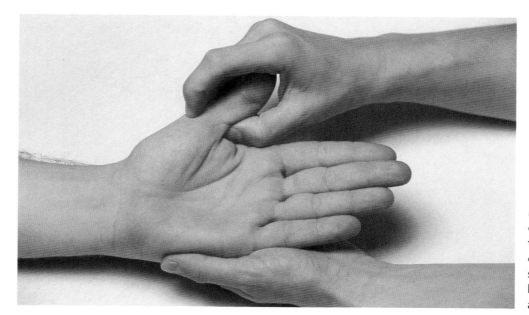

Massage the zone
of the thyroid on
the front and back
of the thumb in
several paths going
both lengthwise
and crosswise.

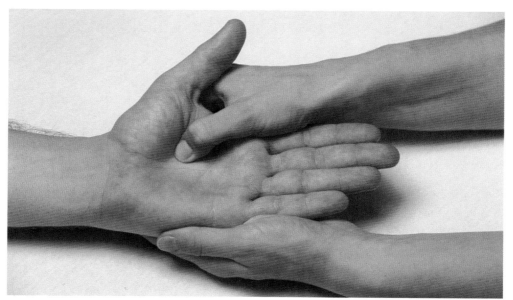

Use your thumb
to massage the
zone of the
adrenal glands
on the palm.

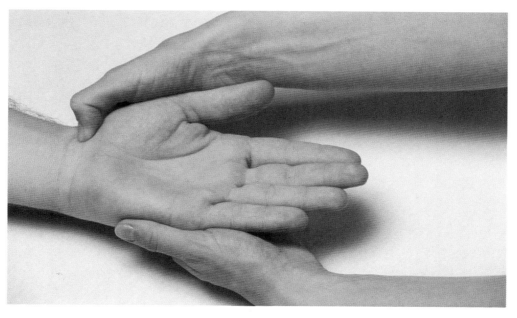

Use your thumb to
massage the zone
of the pancreas.

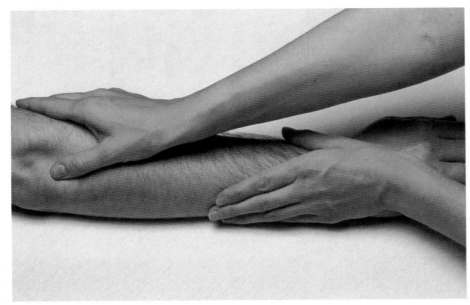

First place your right hand flat on the lower arm.

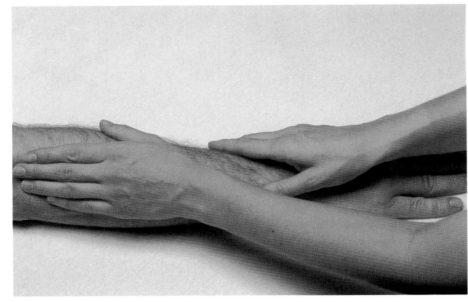

While the right hand slides down, place your left hand above the right so that they follow one another. Repeat this cycle.

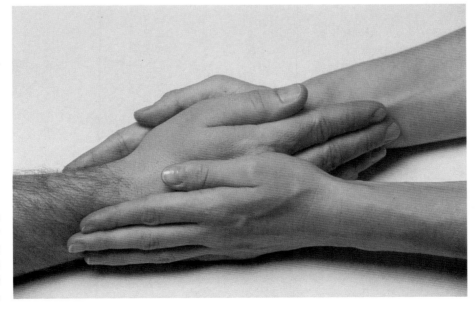

Take your partner's hand between your own and apply light pressure while gliding to the fingertips.

Concluding the Hand Massage

After you have systematically massaged the zones discussed here, conclude with a few strokes. Include the lower arms in these strokes. First stroke the outsides (pinkie sides) and then the insides (thumb sides) of the lower arms and hands. Then make a few circular strokes on the inside and outside of the arms, in rhythm with your partner's breathing. Make similar strokes on the palms and backs of the hands. Use sandwich strokes to conclude the massage.

Stroking Hand over Hand

Have your partner's hand and lower arm lying flat with the back of the hand facing up. Place your right hand on the lower arm and glide down with soft but increasing pressure in the direction of the fingertips. While the right hand is moving downward, place your left hand in the spot where it started. The left hand now follows the right. When the right hand reaches the fingertips, place it above the left and continue. This creates a circular, rhythmically repeating and very relaxing movement.

Carry out this stroke on the outside and inside of both arms and hands.

Sandwich Strokes

Take the hand of your partner between your own. Applying light pressure with both your hands, pull your hands across the carpus, middle hand, and fingertips and beyond.

Repeat this stroke three or four times on each hand.

Hand Reflexology Massage at a Glance

Photocopy this page and hang it up in the space where you administer hand reflexology massages.

Beginning the Hand Reflexology Massage

Take your partner's hands between your warm hands and rest them there for a moment. Carry out a few strokes as an introduction to the massage. Sandwich strokes are especially well suited for this.

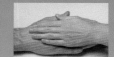 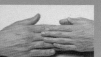

Massaging the Head and Throat zones

Massage the zones of the forehead and the nose-throat area on the back of the hand using the thumb walk. Massage the eye and ear zones with the tip of your index finger and the zones of the jaw and teeth with the tweezers technique.

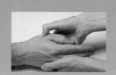 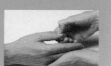

Massaging the Zones of the Neck, Shoulder Girdle, and Rib Cage

Loosen the zones by moving the metacarpal bones. Massage the zones of the neck and shoulder girdle on the palms of the hands with the tip of your thumb and the zone of the rib cage on the backs of the hands with the tip of your index finger.

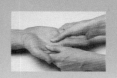 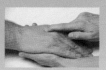

Massaging the Zones of the Spine, Pelvis, and Thighs

Start by massaging the zones of the cervical spine and thoracic spine, working point by point toward the carpus. On the backs of the hands, use your index finger to massage the zones of the sacral bone, pelvis, and thighs.

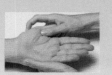 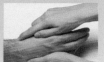

Massaging the Zones of the Digestive Tract

Massage the zones of the esophagus and gallbladder point by point using the tip of your index finger. Massage the zones of the abdominal organs in horizontal and vertical lines using the tip of your thumb.

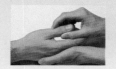 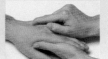

Massaging the Zones of the Lymphatic System

Stroke the lymphatic zones of the lower body to the fingertips. Massage the head lymphatic-system zones in the webbed skin between the fingers, then massage the zones of the spleen and armpit lymphatic system between the fourth and fifth metacarpal bones.

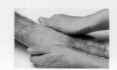 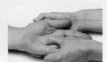

Massaging the Zones of the Urinary Tract and Pelvic Organs

Massage the very small kidney zone with the tip of your thumb. From here, work the zone of the ureter up to the zone of the bladder on the outer edge of the hands. Note that the zone of the genitals is sensitive to pressure.

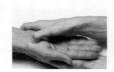 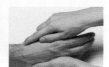

Massaging the Zone of the Solar Plexus and Organs of the Rib Cage

Massage the zones of the heart and lungs using the tip of your thumb, massaging toward the carpus. Massage the zone of the solar plexus using steady pressure. Massage the zone of the nose-throat area along the first metacarpal bone.

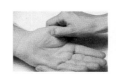 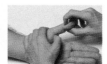

Massaging the Zones of the Endocrine Glands

Massage the zones of the adrenal glands and pancreas on the palm of the hand with the tip of your thumb. Massage the zone of the thyroid on both the palms and the backs of the hands in horizontal and vertical lines.

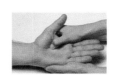 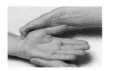

Concluding the Hand Reflexology Massage

Carry out a few circular strokes on the inside and outside of the arms in rhythm with your partner's breathing. Carry out similar strokes on the palms and backs of the hands. Use sandwich strokes to conclude the massage.

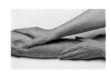 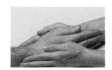

Ear Reflexology Massage

It is possible to project the human body not only onto the foot and hand, but also onto the ear. Systematic research and description of the represented zones have led to a map of the reflexology zones on the auricle (outer ear). As a variant of ear acupuncture, ear reflexology massage is a great way to treat yourself or a partner.

Knowledge

As discussed in the introduction, the body can be represented in its entirety on some of its parts. This principle is manifested in one example in our cerebral cortex. Measurements have shown that individual body parts and regions are represented in specific zones of the cerebral cortex. The size of their zones in the cerebral cortex derives from the number of receptors they have. Lips and fingertips, for instance, have a high number of receptors that allow them to record temperature, touch, pressure, and vibrations, and

they have a much larger zone in the cerebral cortex than, for example, the legs and elbows. Examining the assignations of the individual body parts zones in the cerebral cortex leads to a picture—distorted though it may be—of the body.

Similarly, the reflex zones of the ear correspond to certain parts of the body. Thus, disturbances in certain parts of the body can express themselves as sensitive zones or points on the auricle. Conversely, certain areas of the auricle can be stimulated to produce effects on the corresponding body parts, much like a reflex.

Milestones of Ear Massage

About one hundred years before the Julian calendar was instituted, a classic textbook of traditional Chinese medicine, *Huang Di Nei Jing*, outlined in basic terms the relationship between the auricle and other body regions. Beginning around 400 B.C., the teachings of the Greek physician Hippocrates influenced medicine in many parts of the Western world. Many reports from this time describe the treatment of back pain by the application of tiny burns to certain zones of the auricle. From 618 to 907 A.D., during the time of the Tang dynasty, twenty therapeutic points on the front and back of the auricle were described in China. Eventually, ear acupuncture was spread over land and sea to India and Africa. In 1637, the Portuguese physician Zaratus Lusitanus published a case study about the treatment of a painful back problem by applying targeted small burns to a zone on the auricle.

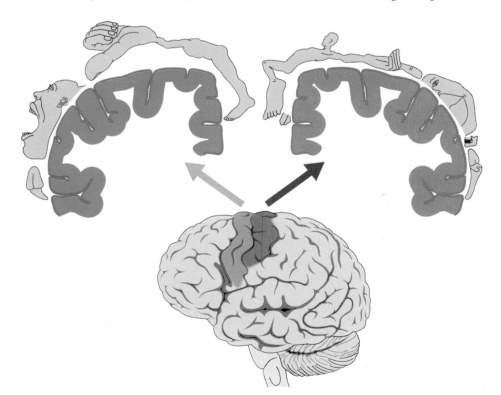

The cerebral cortex reflects a distorted picture of the human body, with the lips and fingers taking up more space than, for example, the legs.

In the 1950s, the French physician Paul Nogier observed small burn zones on certain areas of the ear among some of his patients who had previously seen a folk healer for back pain. Through systematic examination, Nogier worked out the reflex cartography of the ear. In this work, he compared the shape of the auricle with that of an upside-down embryo (page 6). He presented his findings at a symposium in 1956 under the term *auricle therapy*. In the 1970s and 1980s, ear acupuncture was used increasingly in medical clinics for its painkilling properties.

The Construction of the Ear

The basic construction of the auricle consists of elastic cartilage tissue that gives the ear its characteristic shape. The auricle is bordered by a rim of such tissue called the helix. The helix is subdivided into the helix root (sometimes called the crura of the helix), the helix body, the tuberculum darwini (a small bump on the helix), and the helix tail, which ends in the earlobe. Inside the helix is the anthelix, which divides into two branches on its upper end, the superior anthelix crus and the inferior anthelix crus. These two branches enclose a triangular indentation called the fossa triangularis. On its lower end, the anthelix ends in a larger bump called the antitragus. Below the helix root is the tragus, an extended, canoe-shaped prominence. The position of the helix root marks the division of the auricle into an upper part and a lower part. The inner auricle is divided into two parts, the cymba concha above the helix root and the cavum concha below the helix root. The auditory canal ends in the cavum concha.

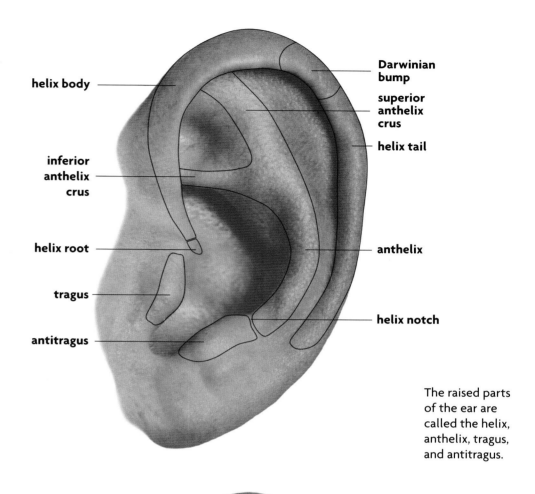

The raised parts of the ear are called the helix, anthelix, tragus, and antitragus.

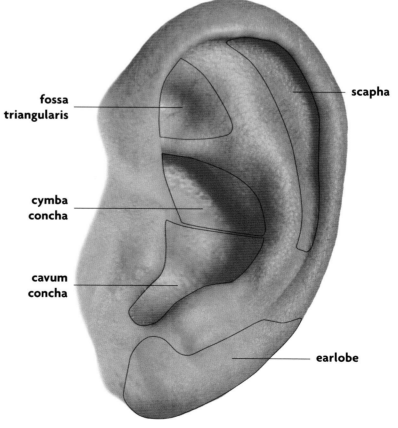

The indented parts of the ear are the inner auricle, which is divided between the cymba concha and the cavum concha, and the fossa triangularis.

The Ear as a Picture of the Body

Assigning reflex zones of individual body parts to the auricle goes back to the work of Nogier. The image of the upside-down embryo, which Nogier developed, can help you remember how the body areas relate to the regions of the ear. The head is depicted in the area of the earlobe. The zone of the spine extends along the helix up to the anthelix. The leg and the pelvis are in the fossa triangularis in the upper part of the ear. The zones of the arm and hand extend along the helix. Around the helix root are the zones of the internal organs. The zones of the heart and lung are located in the cavum concha, while the stomach and liver zones are grouped around the helix root. The intestines zone and the zones of the organs of the lower abdomen (kidneys, bladder, and ureter) are located in the cymba concha in the upper half of the auricle.

How Body Zones Relate to the Individual Parts of the Auricle

The embryo model is a good mnemonic device for remembering the approximate location of the zones. However, the individual zones can be located even more precisely. The zone of the spinal vertebrae is a ribbon on the tip of the anthelix. The disks that serve as buffers between the individual vertebrae and reduce the impact of shocks on the spine are represented in a second ribbon, immediately adjacent to the zone of the vertebrae. The zones of the endocrine glands (pituitary, thyroid, pancreas, adrenal gland cortex, and others) make up a third ribbon. A fourth ribbon-shaped zone on the inside the anthelix represents the autonomic nerves that run along the spine.

The spine consists of several parts: the cervical spine, thoracic spine, and lumbar spine as well as the sacrum and coccyx. These four zones in their different shapes are

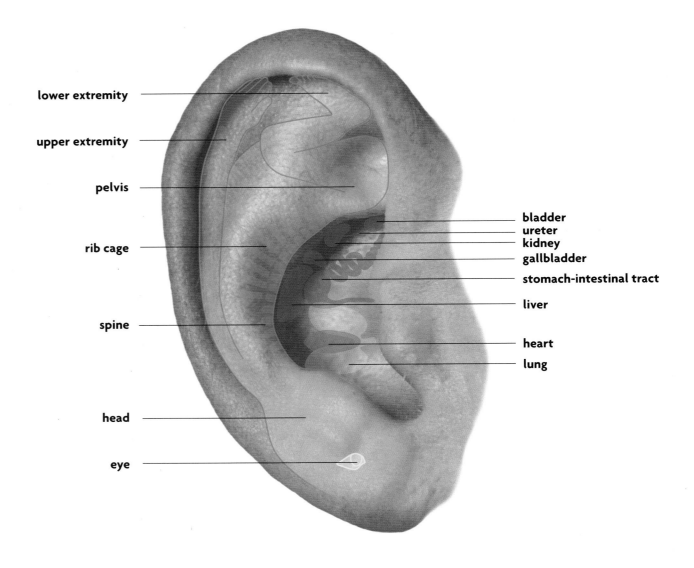

lower extremity

upper extremity

pelvis

rib cage

spine

head

eye

bladder
ureter
kidney
gallbladder
stomach-intestinal tract
liver
heart
lung

Based on the embryo model, the body zones can be transferred to the auricle.

grouped around the bend of the anthelix. The zone of the cervical spine is in the lower part, while the bend itself represents the zones of the thoracic and lumbar spines. The sacrum and coccyx zone is located in the upper part of the anthelix.

The spine forms the central column of a system of muscles and tendons that ultimately makes our upright posture possible. The zone of these tendons and muscles is represented as a broad band that takes up the upper part of the helix. The zone of the upper body is in the area of the canoelike indentation between the helix and the anthelix. The zone of the lower body area is located in the area of the fossa triangularis and the bordering branches of the anthelix. The zones of the sensory organs and the head are located on the earlobe.

The zones of the stomach and intestinal tract surround the helix root. The zones of the kidneys and the urinary tract are in the cymba concha. The zones of the liver and pancreas are located opposite the helix root. The zones of the organs of the rib cage—for example, the heart and lungs—are in the cavum concha.

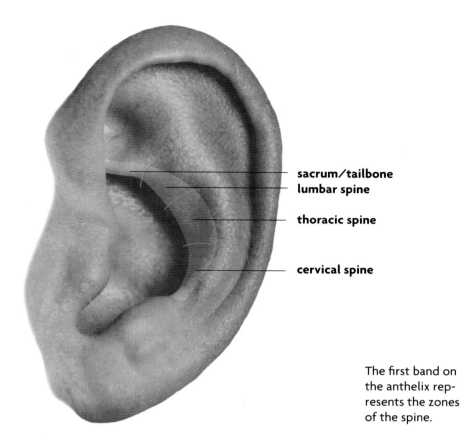

sacrum/tailbone
lumbar spine

thoracic spine

cervical spine

The first band on the anthelix represents the zones of the spine.

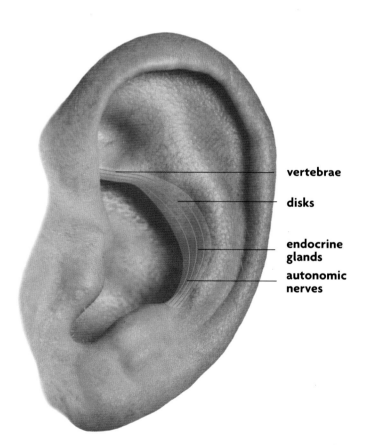

vertebrae

disks

endocrine glands

autonomic nerves

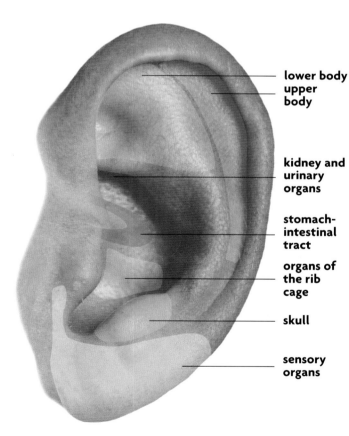

lower body
upper body

kidney and urinary organs

stomach-intestinal tract

organs of the rib cage

skull

sensory organs

Left: The second, third, and fourth bands on the anthelix represent the zones of the disks, endocrine glands, and autonomic nerves.

Right: The zones of the internal organs are represented in the cymba concha and the cavum concha.

Administering Ear Reflexology Massages

Ear reflexology massage is both very effective and easy to master. It is well suited for treating yourself or a partner.

Useful Knowledge for Administering Ear Massages

The following basic concepts and tips will give you the necessary information to make a good entry into administering ear reflexology massages.

Possibilities and Limits of Ear Reflexology Massage

Ear reflexology massage can be helpful in the treatment of many different ailments. Pain of a variety of causes, such as back pain, toothache, or headache, can be cured especially well. Generally, all functional ailments—those for which no physiological problem can be shown to be the cause—can be treated by reflexology. Reflexology massage can also be used as a complementary measure to other therapeutic treatments. However, acute pain should be addressed by a medical doctor before you proceed with a massage. If you are unsure whether you can apply reflexology massages, discuss your concerns with a physician. Do not carry out ear massages if the skin of the ear is infected or injured. Finally, in the case of severe illnesses accompanied by fever or those that require surgical intervention, do not carry out reflexology massages.

Duration and Frequency of the Massage

The duration and frequency of the ear massage depend on the physical condition of your partner and your goal. In the case of acute pain, you can administer massages more frequently—for example, daily or every two days. An overall harmonizing massage can be administered at any time. For such a massage you will need 10 to 15 minutes.

Generally, you will always massage both ears, even in cases in which the symptoms are occurring on only one side of the body. In those cases, however, start your mas-

Situations for which Ear Reflexology Will Not Work

There are situations in which an ear reflexology massage doesn't work, despite a good setting. Possible reasons for this are:
- A general weakness of the body—for example, from fasting
- Ingestion of certain medication used to treat anxiety, sleeping disorders, or depression
- Consumption of drugs or alcohol
- After surgery on the auricle

sage with the ear on the side where the symptoms are occurring.

Preparation and Administration of the Massage

For the following section, much will depend on whether your goal is to have a more general, relaxing massage or to alleviate existing ailments. Moreover, you will need to differentiate between treating yourself and treating a partner. If you are massaging yourself, you can massage both ears at the same time, while either sitting or lying down. If you are massaging a partner, you should—when possible—administer the massage with your partner lying down. Lying down makes it easier for your partner to relax, and it allows you to rest your hands on a surface, which is easier for your back. An added benefit is that a recipient who is already lying down will easily be able to give in to any feelings of sleepiness that might follow the massage.

The Ear Massage Step-by-Step

When massaging a partner, the following steps will help you structure your massage.

Step One

Ask your partner to remove any ear jewelry.

Step Two

Carefully examine the individual zones of the ear. The location of any small red dots, flakes, swellings, and noticeable vessels and scars could offer clues to disturbances in the corresponding body zones or organs. However, do not make a premature diagnosis, and be sure not to frighten your partner with premature comments.

Step Three

Systematically touch the auricle to identify any sensitive zones. Use the tip of your thumb or index finger to do this, and make sure that your fingernails do not extend past your fingertips, as you might otherwise cause injury to the auricle.

Step Four

Carry out the massage using the techniques described on the following pages (stroking, shaking, circling, pressing points). Depending on what your goal is for the massage, you can administer either a general harmonizing and relaxing massage or one that is focused on a specific ailment.

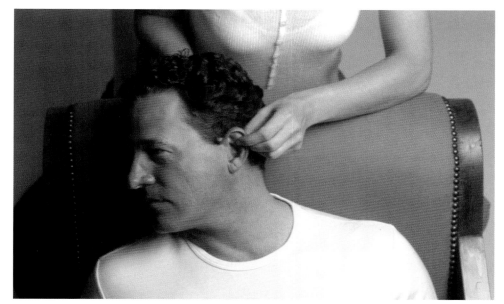

When massaging a partner, massage one ear after the other.

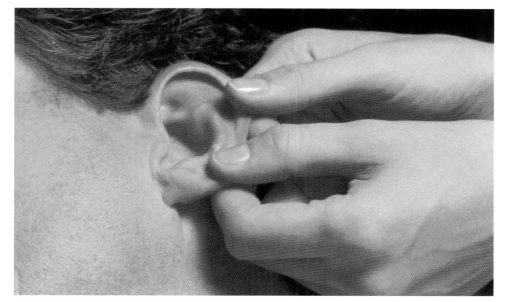

Take care with scars or skin irritations, such as red spots

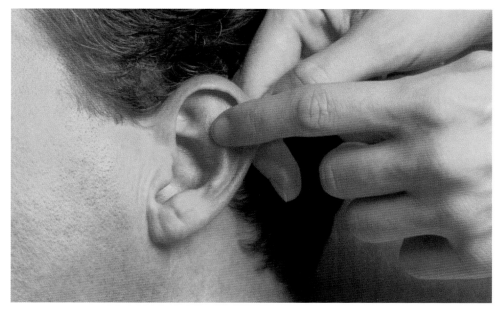

Carefully touch the auricle to locate any sensitive zones.

Basics of Ear Massage

You can use the following techniques when massaging a partner or on yourself. Taken together, they form a basic program that can be used to treat specific ailments, as well as to give a relaxing and harmonizing massage.

Massage Techniques

You can carry out an ear massage with four simple, basic techniques. With these techniques you will stroke, circle, or press the individual points or shake sections of the auricle. Be sure to administer a massage only with warm hands. If necessary, warm your hands before giving a massage.

During or after the massage, the recipient will generally experience a warm sensation in the massaged ear. This is a desirable feeling and shows the positive effects of the massage. The feeling of warmth or reddening of the ear may remain for a few minutes after the massage.

On many parts of the ear, the skin is very thin and is accordingly sensitive. Be sure to start with light pressure and to increase it only very gradually.

Always watch your partner's face. This will allow you to register even small changes in his or her expression, which signal pain or discomfort.

Right ear

Left ear

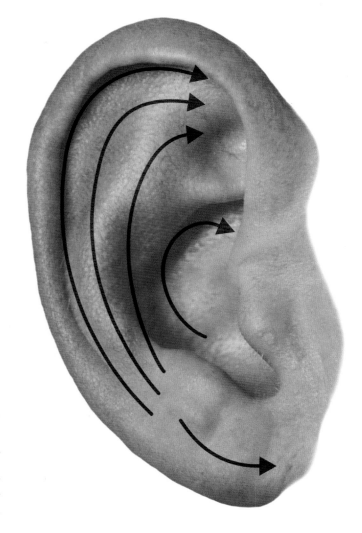
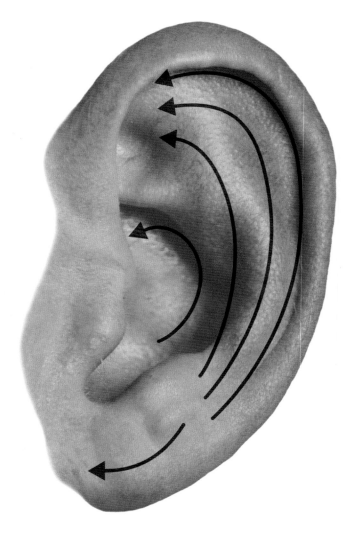

The strokes are made in several paths, beginning at the helix tail and ending at the inside wall of the inner auricle.

Stroking

Stroke the upper part of the ear with the thumb berry. Start on the inside of the helix and follow its course up to the top of the ear. Then start again on the inside of the helix and stroke again, this time slightly inside the first path, up to the top of the ear. Finally, stroke with the tip of your thumb along the top part of the inside auricle. This type of stroke is good for self-massage, too. Afterward, stroke the earlobe with the thumb, with the index finger of the same hand providing the counterpoint. Finish by massaging the earlobe with the thumb.

Shaking

Grasp the outside of the ear in the area of the helix using the tip of your thumb and bent index finger. Carry out gentle shaking motions. These movements loosen and relax the muscles that surround the auricle. They can also have a relaxing effect on the neighboring muscles of the head.

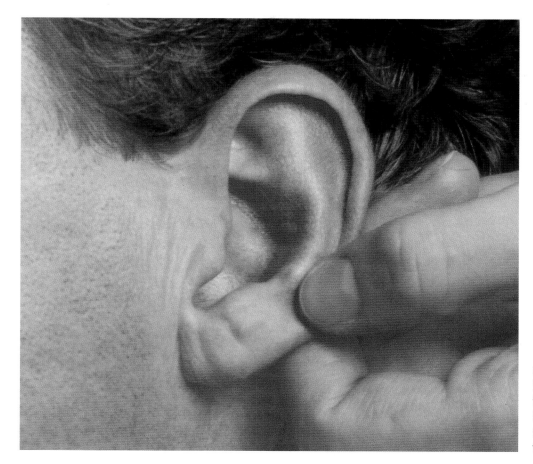

Stroke the ear in several paths from top to bottom, gradually moving toward the inner auricle.

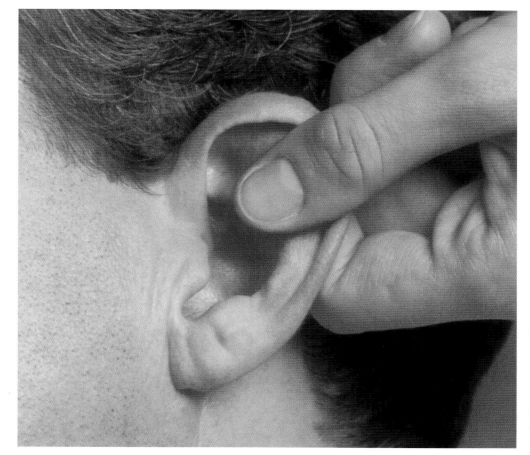

Lightly shaking the ear relaxes the muscles around it.

Circling

Use the tip of your index finger to move the skin on the auricle in small circles. Carry out these movements in the area of the indentation between the helix and the anthelix. Begin in the area of the earlobe and massage in this way up to the top of the ear. Now massage the area of the cavum concha with the tip of your index finger, making small circling movements around the helix root.

Pressing

For this phase of the massage, you will apply pointed pressure in several paths that run along the helix. The pointed pressure is administered with the tip of the index finger. Place the tip of the index finger on the ear and apply a strong, steady pressure—but only as strong as is still pleasant for your partner. This pressing technique is especially good for treating sensitive zones. Keep up the pressure for

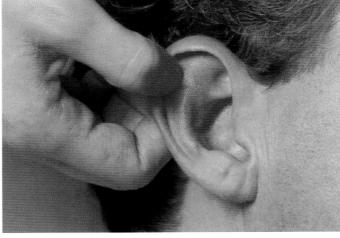

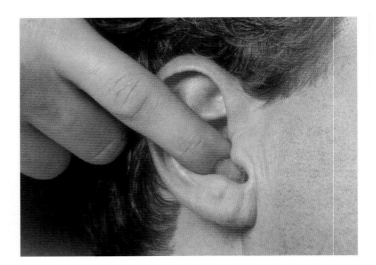

Left: Circular movements cover the whole ear.

Right: The zones of the inner auricle are best massaged with the index finger.

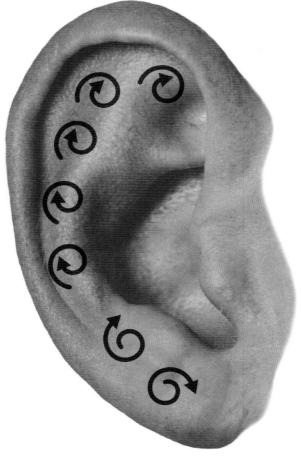

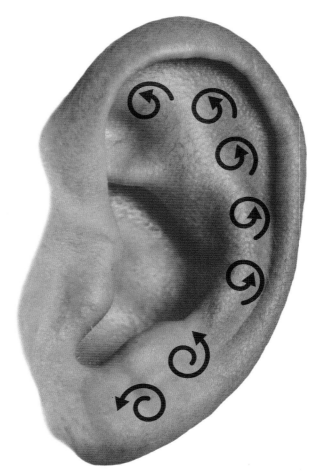

Carry out small circular movements along the helix up to the tip of the ear.

2 to 4 seconds. Start above the earlobe between the helix and the anthelix and massage point by point along the groove up to the top of the ear. The next treatment path begins above the earlobe on the tip of the anthelix and follows the anthelix to the upper edge of the ear. The third treatment path begins in the lower auricle and runs along the inner auricle wall up to the upper edge of the ear. Use several pressure points in the area of the fossa triangularis. Then massage the area around the helix root point by point.

Afterward, take the earlobe between your thumb and

> **Note**
>
> Many people have a point in the fossa triangularis that is sensitive to pressure. This point has a large spectrum of effectiveness: it alleviates pain, stops infection, and calms the person.

index finger and apply pressure in several crosswise lines.

Conclude with some lengthwise strokes of the ear. A reddening or intensive feeling of warmth in the massaged ears after the massage is normal and shows that the body is responding to the massage.

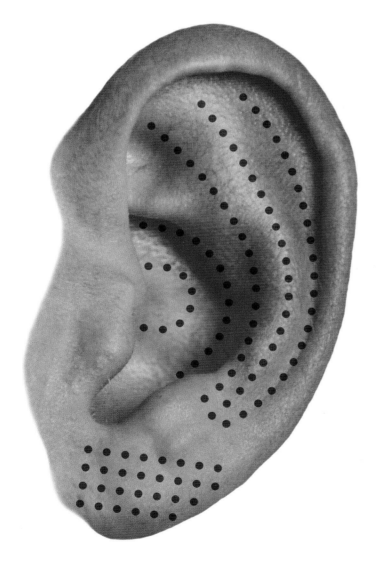

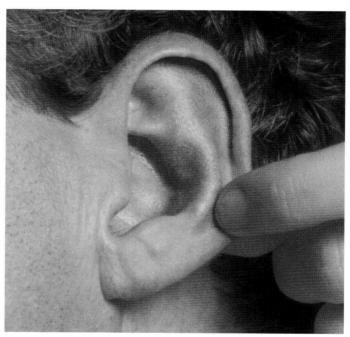

Apply pressure along the helix using your index finger.

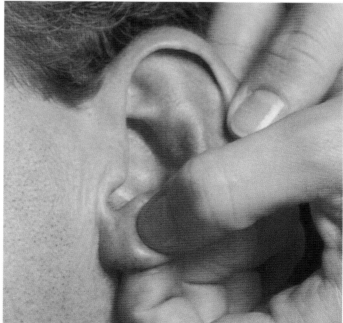

Far left: Administer the pressure-point technique along several paths.

After massaging the helix and the inner auricle, press the earlobe in horizontal lines.

The Individual Zones

This section will introduce you to the individual zones and points of the ear.

Note: In general, the reflex zones of the ear are very small, and in the following text they will be referred to as points. Keep in mind that there are likely to be several points under your fingertip at any one time during the massage.

The Points in the Head Zone

The head zone is represented in the earlobe. Certain points in this area can be massaged to alleviate pain or other problems.

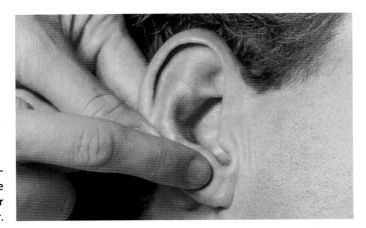

Apply point-by-point pressure using your index finger.

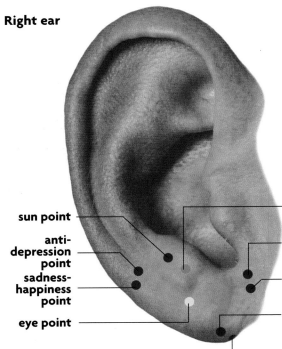

Right ear

sun point
anti-depression point
sadness-happiness point
eye point

forehead point
anti-aggression point
worry-fear point
main omega point
analgesia point

The points of the head zone are massaged to relieve pain and psychological problems.

The Antiaggression point

This point has psychological effects. It calms the recipient, especially in the case of an aggressive mood that appears as a result of a chronic illness.

It is also used as a complementary therapy in the treatment of addiction.

The Fear-Worry Point

This point affects real and imagined fears.

The Antidepression Point

Massage of the antidepression point can relieve psychological problems like depression and melancholy.

The Sadness-Happiness Point

This point should be massaged if a person is sad or lacks energy.

The Analgesia (Alleviating) Point

This point, as its name implies, alleviates pain and can be massaged in the case of severe pain.

The Forehead Point

Massage the forehead point to treat headache in the frontal forehead or in the case of illness of the sinuses, nerve pains in the facial area, dizziness, or insomnia.

The Eye Point

The eye point is exactly in the middle of the earlobe. It can be massaged to relieve problems with the eyes, migraines, and headaches.

The Main Omega Point

This point has a regulating effect on psychological well-being, leading, for example, to the release of psychological tension resulting from prolonged illness.

Note about the Massage

Massage the earlobe with the tip of your thumb or index finger either lengthwise or crosswise. Place the pressure points close to one another to treat all sensitive points.

Locating the Zones of the Shoulder Girdle, Neck, and Chest Area

The zones of the spine, which can be broken down into the cervical, thoracic, and lumbar spine, extend along the top of the anthelix.

Small strips that run parallel to the anthelix represent the structures of the spine, including the zones of the vertebrae, the disks, and the autonomic nerves.

The zone of the muscles and tendons in the spine run along the broad indentation between the helix and the anthelix. The zones of the shoulder girdle and the neck and chest area are located close to it, and thus all can be massaged together.

Locating the Shoulder Joint Point

The point representing the shoulder joint is in the indentation between the helix and the anthelix.

Locating the Zone of the Neck and Chest Area

This zone extends between the helix and the inner auricle in a broad area opposite the helix root. It begins at the helix notch and extends one third of the distance to the point where the anthelix branches.

Note about the Massage

The massage of these zones occurs along lines that run closely parallel. Be sure to place your points close to one another to cover all the zones.

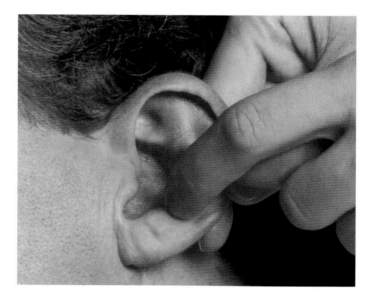

Massage the zones of the neck, shoulder, and thoracic spine in close parallel lines.

Left ear

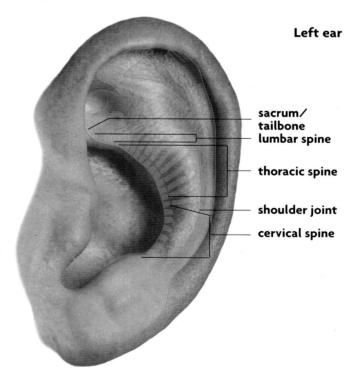

- sacrum/ tailbone
- vertebrae/ disk zone
- lumbar spine
- thoracic spine
- shoulder joint
- cervical spine
- autonomic nerves

Left ear

- sacrum/ tailbone
- lumbar spine
- thoracic spine
- shoulder joint
- cervical spine

Keep reminding yourself of the embryo model—it will make it easier to locate zones on the ear.

Right ear

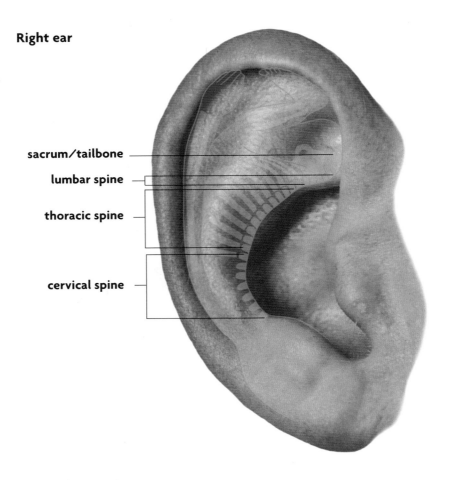

sacrum/tailbone
lumbar spine
thoracic spine
cervical spine

The Spine

The bend of the spine in the human body is reflected in the pronounced shape of the anthelix. It is easy to see the location of the spine by recalling once again the embryo model.

Locating the Reflex Zones

If you follow the spine in this picture, you will recognize its individual parts.

In the first part is the zone of the seven cervical vertebrae. It is followed by the zone of the thoracic spine, which, with its twelve vertebrae, is the longest part of the spine. Horizontal to this are the zones of the lumbar spine and the sacrum and coccyx. The width of the spine zone extends from the indentation between the helix and the anthelix over to the inner auricle wall.

Locating the Zone of the Cervical Spine

This zone begins at the tip of the anthelix diagonally opposite the helix root. The lower third of the inner wall of the anthelix is the zone of the related muscles and tendons, and below it on the inside of the auricle in the cavum concha is the zone of the disks.

Locating the Zone of the Thoracic Spine

The zone of the thoracic spine connects directly to that of the cervical spine. It runs along the rising and upper part of the anthelix.

Locating the Zone of the Lumbar Spine

The zone of the lumbar spine extends from the zone of the thoracic spine in the upper and horizontal part of the anthelix. The zone ends in the area of the sacrum.

Right ear

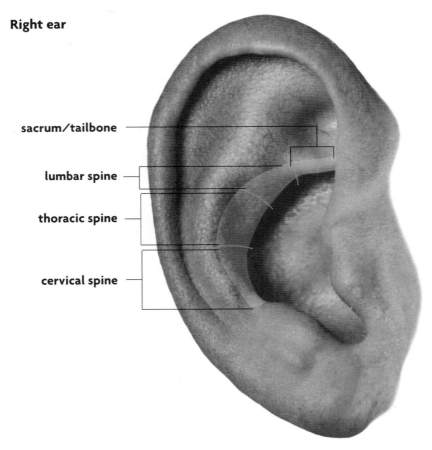

sacrum/tailbone
lumbar spine
thoracic spine
cervical spine

Compare the location of the zones with the embryo model.

Massaging the Zones of the Spine

The spine zones as a whole form a broad ribbon. Often, several points of this zone are sensitive to pressure, but any sensitivity usually lessens or disappears altogether over the course of the massage.

Massaging the Zone of the Cervical Spine

The zone of the cervical vertebrae begins immediately behind the bulge of the earlobe. Carry out the massage in closely parallel paths from the helix to the inside edge of the anthelix. Place the points close to one another. Afterward, massage the zone inside the inner auricle wall with the tip of your index finger.

Massaging the Zone of the Thoracic Spine

Support the earlobe with your free hand and massage point by point from the helix in lines toward the inside edge of the anthelix. Then massage the zone inside the inner auricle wall both lengthwise and horizontally.

Massaging the Zones of the Lumbar Spine, Sacrum, and Tailbone

Massage the zones of the lumbar spine, sacrum, and tailbone in lengthwise paths that run close to one another. First work the zone from the anthelix to the inner auricle wall with the tip of your thumb, then massage inside the inner auricle wall with the tip of your index finger.

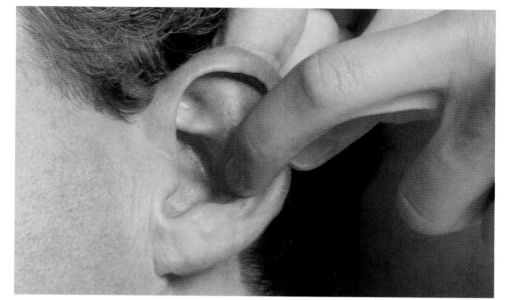

Massage the zone of the cervical spine inside the inner auricle wall in several paths running close together, both lengthwise and crosswise.

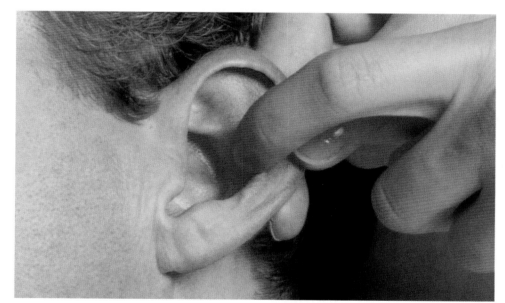

Massage the zone of the thoracic spine from the helix to the anthelix.

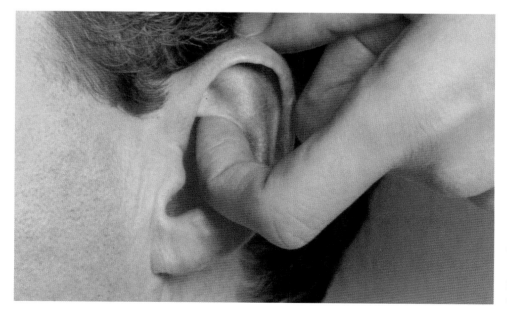

The zone of the lumbar spine is best reached with the tip of the index finger.

Locating the Zones and Points of the Organs of the Rib Cage

The rib cage houses the lungs and the heart. Next to these organs are the large vessels of the aorta as well as the trachea and esophagus. These organs are represented in the ear by relatively large zones, which may be painful if there are problems with the corresponding organ. On the other hand, these organs are also represented by very specific, small points. Both the zone and the point are described for the lungs. Because the lung zone is larger than the lung point and the lung point is within the lung zone, you will massage the whole zone, which will cover the individual point.

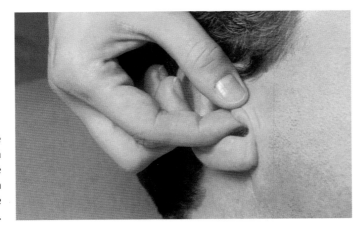

The inner nose point is hidden on the back edge of the skin in front of the auditory canal.

Right ear

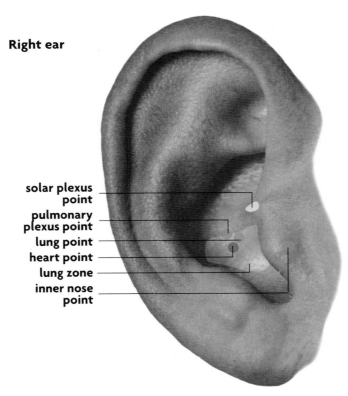

solar plexus point
pulmonary plexus point
lung point
heart point
lung zone
inner nose point

You will find the points and zones of the rib cage in the cavum concha, the lower part of the inner auricle.

The Lung Zone

The lung zone covers the upper half of the cavum concha. In the case of illness of the breathing organs, this zone will be more sensitive than the rest of the ear.

The Lung Point

The lung point is located in the middle of the lung zone. This point, too, becomes sensitive in case of lung problems. It can also be massaged as part of the treatment of nicotine addiction.

The Pulmonary Plexus Point

This point can be stimulated in the case of illness of the breathing passages along with cramps, as is the case with asthma, for example.

The Heart Point

The heart point is located at the deepest indentation of the inner auricle. Massage the heart point in cases of nervousness, insomnia, rapid heartbeat, and all other heart problems caused by internal unrest.

The Solar Plexus Point

This point is located on the helix root. Massage of this point can be helpful in cases of nervous problems such as anxiety before exams.

This point can also be stimulated to treat problems in the upper abdomen.

The Inner Nose Point

The inner nose point is located in a somewhat hidden spot, on the inside of the bump of the earlobe. It is useful in dealing with infections of the nasal mucous membranes or the sinuses.

Notes about the Massage

Masage the zones and points of the organs of the rib cage point by point with the tip of your index finger. Work the cavum concha with several treatment paths running parallel to one another. The inner nose point is best massaged with the tweezers grip: Carefully press the small bump in front of the auditory canal between the tips of your thumb and index finger.

Locating the Zones and Points of the Digestive Organs

The zones and points of the digestive organs are located around the helix root.

The Stomach Zone

The zone of the stomach circles the helix root in a U shape. Massage of this area can be helpful in the case of nausea, stomach problems, or eating disorders.

The Liver-Gallbladder Zone

This area is located opposite the stomach zone and reacts to illnesses of the liver and the gallbladder.

The Liver Point

The liver point is used to treat general upper abdominal problems. Interestingly, this point can also be used to treat eye problems and to support the treatment of addiction.

The Zone of the Small Intestine

The slightly elongated zone of the small intestine follows the zone of the stomach and is located above the helix root. Massage this zone in the case of illness of the small intestine or upper abdomen.

The Stomach-Cardiac Point

Massage of the stomach-cardiac point can be beneficial in the treatment of a sensitive stomach, upper abdominal problems linked to nerve problems, and sensations of discomfort caused by overeating.

The Spleen Point

Massage the spleen point in the case of digestive problems or functional disturbances in the upper abdomen.

Notes about the Massage

Massage the zone of the digestive organs using your index finger, working around the helix root point by point in a semicircle. Enlarge this circle in several paths until it includes the zones of the liver, gallbladder, and spleen.

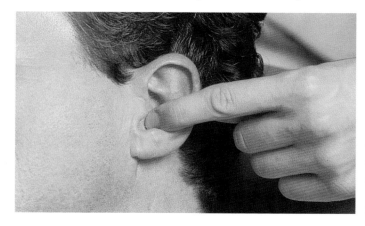

Use your index finger to massage the zones of the digestive organs in the area of the upper auricle.

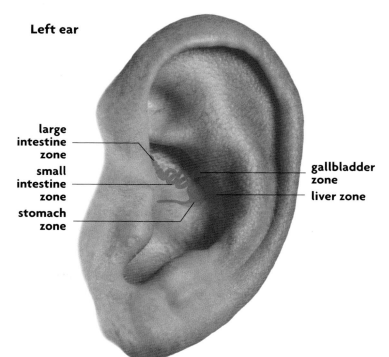

Left ear

large intestine zone
small intestine zone
stomach zone

gallbladder zone
liver zone

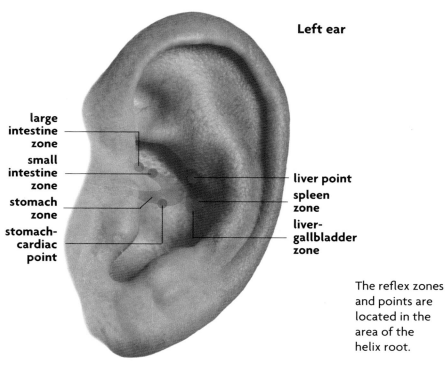

Left ear

large intestine zone
small intestine zone
stomach zone
stomach-cardiac point

liver point
spleen zone
liver-gallbladder zone

The reflex zones and points are located in the area of the helix root.

The Zones and Points of the Pelvic Organs and Urinary Tract

The points and zones of the pelvic organs and urinary tract are located in the cymba concha, the upper part of the auricle. Two exceptions are the points of the uterus and ovaries. They are located on the fossa triangularis and the earlobe, respectively.

The kidney-bladder zone is elongated, in contrast to the kidney point, which is small and lies inside the kidney-bladder zone.

The Kidney-Bladder Zone

The kidney-bladder zone is an elongated, slightly oval zone in the upper part of the inner auricle wall. It is located immediately below the end of the fossa triangularis.

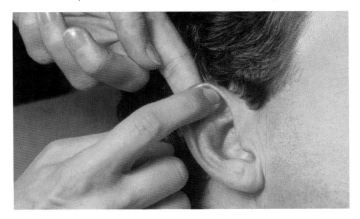

Massage the uterus point at the upper edge of the fossa triangularis.

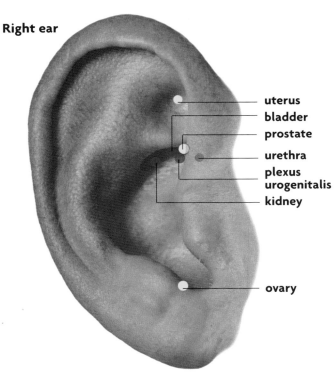

Right ear

uterus
bladder
prostate
urethra
plexus urogenitalis
kidney

ovary

The location of the zones of the pelvic organs deviates from the theme: some zones are located far apart from each other.

The Kidney Point

This point is located inside the kidney-bladder zone. It is often sensitive in the case of pain, weakness, or illness of the kidneys.

The Urethra Point

This point is located just to the side of the helix edge, above the helix root, and becomes noticeable in the case of pain or infection of the urethra.

The Prostate Point

This point is located very close to the urethra point. It can be sensitive when the prostate is infected, as well as in the case of unspecific pain in the lower body.

The Plexus Urogenitalis Point

This point corresponds to the web of nerves that surrounds the reproductive organs. It can be massaged to relieve cramplike pains in the abdomen.

The Uterus Point

This point is located slightly away from the preceding points. It is found at the upper edge of the fossa triangularis, below the helix. It is effective for gynecological problems.

The Ovaries Point

The point of the ovaries is also outside the zone of the pelvic organs and urinary tract. It is located at the edge of the indentation above the earlobe and can be of benefit when massaged in the case of a number of hormonal illnesses as well as in the case of infertility.

Notes about the Massage

Massage this area in several paths using the tip of your index finger. Start with the zone of the urethra, then massage the uterus point on the upper edge of the fossa triangularis. Massage the point of the ovaries with the tip of your thumb using the tweezers grip. Of course, if the massage recipient is a man, the points for the uterus and ovaries should be skipped.

Begin at the lower edge of the indentation and massage along the indentation point by point, slowly moving upward.

Special Points

The following points cannot be assigned to specific organs or systems. They have a holistic effect and usually have a range of applications.

The Allergy Point

The allergy point is located at the upper tip of the ear. It is massaged with the tweezers grip, between the thumb and index finger, to treat allergies.

The *Shen Men* Point

Shen men roughly translates from the Chinese as "gate of the gods." This point has calming and anti-inflammatory effects and is one of the most important points of ear reflexology. It is located in the fossa triangularis and should be massaged with the tip of the index finger. To locate the shen men point, divide the fossa traingularis into four equal quadrants (see dotted lines on illustration). The shen men will fall in the lower right-hand quadrant on the left ear and in the lower left-hand quadrant on the right.

The Omega-1 Point

The omega-1 point is located at the upper edge of the rising helix body. It can be massaged to treat nerve-based stomach and intestinal problems.

The Omega-2 Point

The omega-2 point is located on the helix. It has psychologically balancing effects.

The Sympathetic Point

The sympathetic point is below the helix in the extension of the inferior anthelix crus, the lower branch of the anthelix that encloses the fossa triangularis. It has relaxing, balancing effects and is viewed as a point for muscle relaxation.

The Excitation Point

The excitation point is located on the inside wall of the antitragus. This point is effective for illnesses that come from imbalances in the autonomic nervous system. It also fights infection and relieves pain, calms, and contributes to restoring psychological balance.

The Frustration Point

The frustration point is located where the helix transitions to the skin of the face. It can be massaged in the case of severe psychological stress that requires a high degree of willpower, for example, to achieve weight loss or quit smoking.

The Polster Point

The polster point is massaged to treat pain at the back of the head, dizziness, or low blood pressure. It has a calming and pain-relieving effect as well.

The Jerome Point

The jerome point is at the end of the helix tail. Massage of this point relaxes hardened muscles, contributes to balance in the autonomic nervous system, and has positive psychological effects.

The Point of Desire

This point is located on the outer edge of the helix at the level of the jerome point. It can be of benefit when massaged in the case of those getting treatment for addiction, quitting smoking, or trying to lose weight.

The Adrenal Glands Point

The adrenal glands point is located at the edge of the tragus, toward the nose. It is effective in cases of joint pain and rheumatism and also in the case of hay fever, allergic skin problems, or chronic fatigue.

The Thyroid Point

The thyroid point is located on the deepest part of the indentation in the earlobe area. It is massaged to treat functional disturbances of the thyroid, such as hyper- or depressed functioning, in tandem with medical treatment.

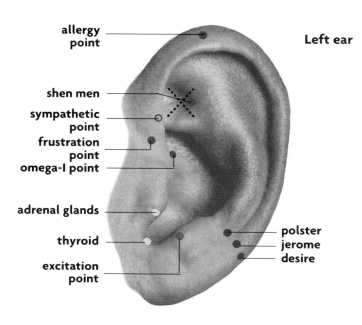

allergy point — shen men — sympathetic point — frustration point — omega-1 point — adrenal glands — thyroid — excitation point — polster — jerome — desire

Left ear

The special points are frequently used in acupuncture. Using them in reflexology massage requires some experience.

Head Reflexology

Reflexology massage of the head is another way to influence certain organs or systems of the body. The reflex zones of the head are located on the temples and forehead.

Knowledge

The practice of head reflexology massage has evolved from scalp acupuncture. Scalp acupuncture is a highly effective method of treating a variety of pains as well as functional disturbances (see page 18) and illnesses of the nervous system. Reflexology massage is nearly as effective: Massaging the points and zones with the techniques described here will allow you to effectively treat specific ailments. The respective points and zones are in the area of the hairline on the forehead and temples and are thus easily accessible for a massage.

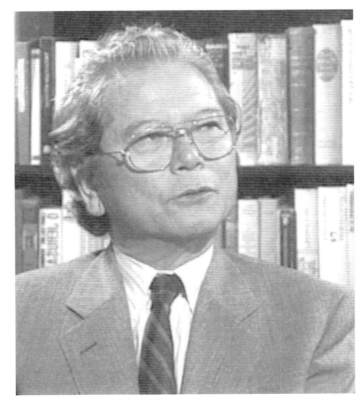

Dr. Toshikatsu Yamamoto is considered the founder of new scalp acupuncture.

Historical Background

Dr. Toshikatsu Yamamoto, the founder of today's scalp acupuncture, was born in Japan. He went to medical school in Japan, Germany, and the United States and was trained in surgery, gynecology, and anesthesia. He eventually returned to Japan and opened his own practice in Nichinan. He later expanded this practice to a private clinic; today it has become a large clinic and rehabilitation center. In the early years of his practice, Yamamoto by accident discovered a point on the scalp that in the true sense of the word became the starting point of his method. He then started to search for other points that could be used successfully in the treatment of the various illnesses of his many patients. He systematically evaluated his experiences and found that the points he described formed a microsystem, a reflection of the body on itself. The reflex system Yamamoto discovered is especially well suited for treating specific and chronic disturbances of the musculoskeletal system. His scalp acupuncture method is easy to learn and apply, and it is a very effective form of acupuncture with few side effects. It can easily be combined with other biological and medical treatment methods. The head reflexology massage described here is a special type of acupressure, or the pressing of a selection of acupuncture points, in this case those described by Dr. Yamamoto. This massage can be done either as a self-massage or on a partner.

The New Scalp Acupuncture

The reflexology massage of the head presented here is based on the findings of the Japanese physician Toshikatsu Yamamoto. In the 1960s, he developed a new acupuncture system called "Yamamoto's New Scalp Acupuncture" (abbreviated YNSA). The therapeutic results were so impressive that his method quickly spread beyond Japan to Europe and the United States.

The Reflex Zones

The following sections will introduce you to the individual reflex zones of the head. It is necessary to know the precise location of the zones and their effects in order to carry out an effective massage.

An Overview

The basic principle underlying the massage of the points on the head is that here we are able to locate zones that correspond to certain parts of the musculoskeletal system, the sensory organs, and parts of the nervous system. The points on the front of the head are located in a symmetrical pattern that corresponds to the two body halves, and they are repeated on the back of the head. There are also points both in front of and behind the ears. Note that we will describe only a selection of a wide range of possible points.

In case of illness or disturbance of the musculoskeletal system, sensory organs, or nervous system, the corresponding zones on the head become sensitive. This is usually expressed as a sensitivity to pressure, which makes the zones easy to find and massage.

Especially problems with a sudden onset can be quickly alleviated by massaging the corresponding points on the head. Alleviation of the symptoms can begin even during the massage.

Because the points are easy to locate and sensitive to the touch in the case of disturbance, head reflexology massages are a good entry point for reflexology in general.

The A and B Zones

Yamamoto named zones based on the sequence of their discovery in an alphabetical manner. The A zones are located about 0.5 centimeter from the middle axis at the hairline. They are each about 2 centimeters long and 2 to 4 millimeters wide. These zones represent the head and the cervical vertebrae. In the case of ailments like headache, migraine, neck pain, and dizziness, they become sensitive. The A zones can be subdivided into smaller parts from the top to the bottom. The zone for the first cervical vertebra is at the top and that of the seventh vertebra is at the bottom.

The B zones are located just outside the A zones and are of the same size as the A zones. They represent the cervical vertebrae, the neck, and the shoulders and become sensitive in the case of pain in or injury to these areas.

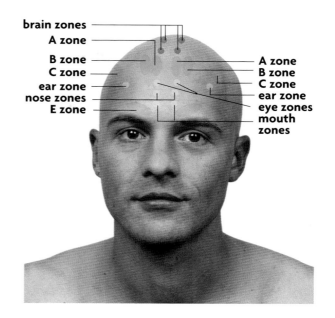

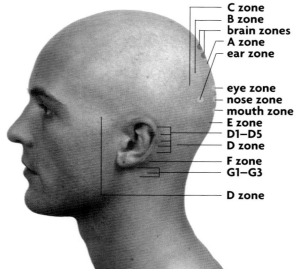

Top and center: The reflex zones on the front of the head are repeated on the back of the head.

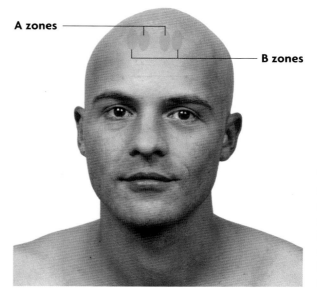

The A and B zones are located symmetrically on either side of the middle axis and represent the head and shoulder area.

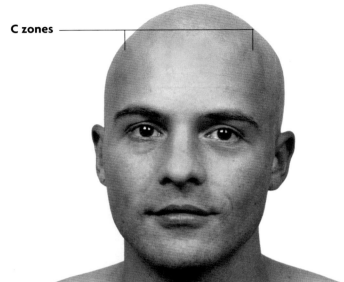

C zones

The C zones are located in the area of the receding part of the hairline and are divided from top to bottom into the areas of the shoulder joints, elbows, and hands.

The C Zones

The C zones are located in the area of the "receding" part of the hairline. They are about 2 centimeters long and 2 to 4 millimeters wide. The C zones correspond to the shoulders, the upper and lower arms, and the hands. They will have a heightened sensitivity to pressure in the case of pain following injury or surgery, aching shoulder joints, rheumatic ailments, tennis elbow, or other pain in the area of the shoulders, arms, and hands. The C zones can be divided into the separate joints from top to bottom: the shoulder joints are at the top of the C zones, the elbow joints are in the middle, and the hands are at the bottom.

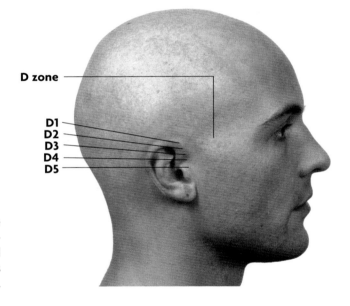

D zone

D1
D2
D3
D4
D5

There is a difference between the elongated D zones and the row of D points bordering the ear.

The D Zones and D Points

The D zones and D points refer to two different areas. The D zones are horizontal zones about 2 centimeters wide and 0.5 to 1 centimeter high. They are easily located above the cheekbones, at the hairline on the temples. These zones represent the lumbar spine, the pelvis, and the lower body. The D points 1 through 5 are found in front of each ear. From top to bottom they are lined up like a chain of pearls. Each point has a diameter of 3 to 4 millimeters. Each point represents one of the vertebrae of the lumbar spine.

The D zones and points are sensitive in the case of lower back pain or pain in the hip, knee, or foot.

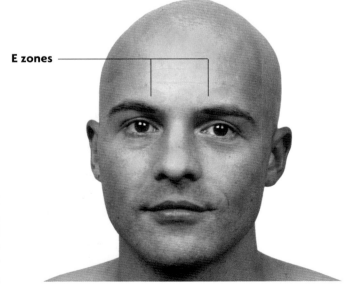

E zones

The E zones extend diagonally across the eyebrows and can be divided into twelve smaller zones.

The E Zones

The E zones run diagonally from the inside edges of the eyebrows upward. They are about 2 centimeters long and 2 to 4 millimeters wide. The E zones represent the rib cage, the thoracic spine, and the stomach.

Pain in the rib cage—for example, because of shingles, asthma, or another problem of the breathing passages—can cause these zones to become sensitive.

The E zone can be further subdivided into twelve segments that represent the twelve vertebrae of the thoracic spine.

The Zones of the Sensory Organs (Eyes, Nose, Mouth, and Ears)

The eye zones are about 0.5 centimeter away from the middle axis, just below the A zones (see page 135).

The zones for nose and mouth are directly below the eye zones. The ear zones are slightly below the C zones (see page 135). These zones represent the sensory organs they are named after.

The zones of the sensory organs (eyes, nose, mouth, ear) have a heightened sensitivity in the case of illness of ears, nose, sinuses, mouth cavity, teeth, gums, or ears.

The F Zones and G1 through G3 Points (Points of the Knee Joints)

The F zones are located on the highest points of the mastoid processes, which are the easy-to-feel bony bumps behind the earlobes, toward the back of the head. The F zones represent the area innervated by one of the main nerves of the legs, the sciatic nerve. This nerve runs along the backs of the thighs and divides into several branches. If the supply area of this nerve is injured, the corresponding F zone becomes sensitive.

Each of the G zones consists of three points that are grouped around the bony part of the mastoid process. All three points relate to the region of the knee joint and become sensitive when this joint is injured.

The Zones of the Brain

The zones of the brain are located in the scalp area above the A zones. They are subdivided into many different zones, but these subdivisions are of little importance in the context of reflexology massage.

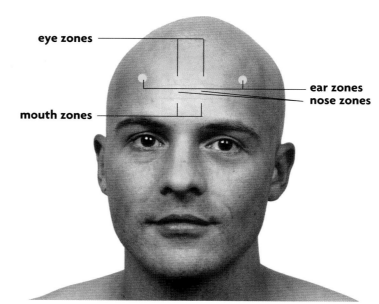

The zones of the eyes, nose, and mouth are located on a line below the A zone. The ear zone is located in the extension of the C zone.

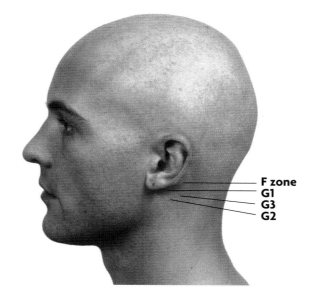

The F zone and the G points are located on and around the mastoid process, which can be felt behind the ear lobe.

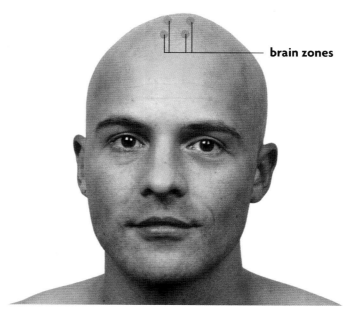

The zones of the brain are located on both sides of the middle axis, an extension of the A zone in the scalp area.

Administering Head Reflexology Massages

Head reflexology massages are easy to administer and can be used to treat acute pain from a great variety of causes.

Noteworthy Knowledge for Administering Head Massages

The following will give you some information about the application spectrum and prerequisites for a successful massage.

Use and Limits of Head Massage

Head reflexology massages can be used for many different purposes. Acute or chronic pain from a range of causes can quickly be alleviated using head reflexology massages. However, if the intended recipient has acute pain that necessitates surgery, a life-threatening illness, a severe infection such as pneumonia or tuberculosis, or an infection of the skin on the head, do not administer a massage. Please be extremely careful when the recipient suffers from pain of unknown origin or is in a state of exhaustion or weakness—for example, after fasting or physical exertion. You should also not administer head reflexology massages during pregnancy because of the heightened fragility of the body's circulation during that time. If you are unsure whether one of these exceptions exists, consult with a physician.

Possible Reactions

Since it is a highly effective type of massage, head reflexology massage can cause unexpected reactions. However, they are easily managed.

The Initial Worsening

Ailment symptoms may temporarily worsen after the massage. This phenomenon is of short duration, however, and indicates that the massage was done properly and was successful. Make sure you explain this to the recipient.

Reactions of the Circulation

The massage can lead to dizziness, light-headedness, and even fainting for sensitive people. To prevent this, always carry out a head reflexology massage with your partner lying down.

Therapy Obstacles

If the desired treatment effect does not materialize, a cause may be that the right points were not targeted or that the massage was not carried out correctly. Psychological and physical states of exhaustion can also have a negative effect on the success of the massage.

Duration and Frequency of the Massage

In case of acute problems, the massage should be carried out frequently, ideally twice a day for 2 to 10 minutes, and its strength (the pressure you apply) should be intensive and strong. In the case of chronic ailment or pain, one or two massages per week will suffice, and the pressure should be lighter and the massage longer.

Preparation and Execution

Explain to your partner that the massage could be unpleasant or even somewhat painful, and that feelings of sleepiness are possible after the treatment. Ideally, allow for a rest period of 30 minutes after the massage. Administer massages only with your partner lying down.

Planning the Massage

In contrast to the other types of reflexology, there is no overall harmonizing type of basic treatment for the head massage. Treatment is based on existing problems. For example, if your partner suffers from acute lower back pain, locate the D zone and D points 1 through 5 and treat them as long as the pain remains. Usually, pressure, tension, and pain in this zone will dissolve during or after the massage. The ailments in the corresponding body region will improve at the same time.

Massaging the Zones

For head reflexology massages, treat only those zones that require attention due to painful sensitivity to touch or pressure. Such sensitivity implies the existence of specific ailments.

Basic Techniques

Three basic techniques are used for head reflexology massages: touching, rubbing/circling, and pressing.

Touching

Precisely locating painful or sensitive zones is a prerequisite for the success of your massage. Touch all the zones from top to bottom with the tip of your thumb or index finger in circling or stroking motions. Note the muscle or bone structures under the skin and any small, tough knots. If you encounter one of these knots, your partner will clearly voice pain from the pressure of your touch.

Rubbing/Circling

As soon as you have located a sensitive point, you can massage it in the following way: Place the tip of your thumb on the *punctum maximum,* or the area on the point that is most painful. Apply pressure and make small, circling movements on the painful zone. The tip of your thumb must not move across the skin in these circling motions, as this would irritate the skin. Imagine that you are grinding sugar with your thumb.

Pressing

The rubbing or circling on a painful point as described above is a very intense and at times unpleasant treatment. If your partner cannot tolerate it, you can instead massage the painful point with pointed pressure. To do this, again locate the punctum maximum with the tip of your thumb. Bend the thumb so that its tip is perpendicular to the painful spot. Apply steady, stationary pressure to that point for 1 to 2 minutes. Adjust your pressure based on the sensitivity of your partner.

When you have finished treating the painful point, resume touching the remainder of the zones to see if any other sensitive points are present. If you find more sensitive points, treat them as above.

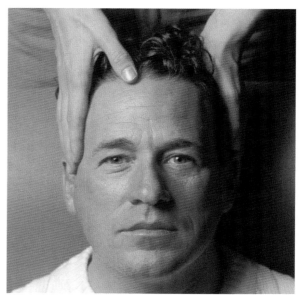

Locate the sensitive zones.

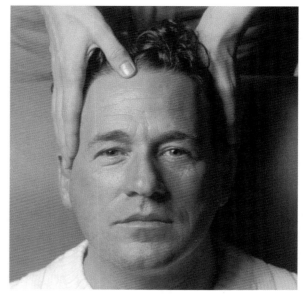

In the circular movement, the thumb and the skin move together above the point.

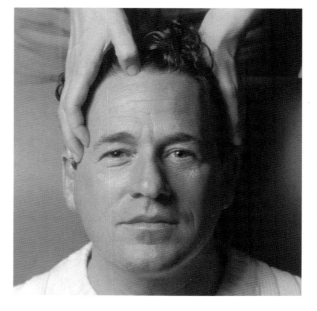

If the circular movement is too painful, apply steady, stationary pressure for 1 to 2 minutes, with the thumb perpendicular to the area being treated.

Special Massage Techniques

The following will demonstrate how to massage individual zones in a pointed manner.

The steps to be followed are always the same: First touch the zone, then locate the most sensitive point, and then massage it with either circling or stationary pressure.

Massaging the A and B Zones

The A and B zones are massaged in the same way. Touch each zone from the bottom up to the top, then put the tip of your thumb directly on the punctum maximum. Carry out circling motions until the pain in the massaged area recedes or disappears.

Massaging the C Zones

The C zones run diagonally in the area of the "receding" corners of the hairline. First touch each zone, following its diagonal shape. Then locate the punctum maximum and carry out circling motions.

Massaging the D Zones

The D zones are elongated, slightly oval zones along the hairline on the temples. To find one, set your thumb on the horizontal edge of the cheekbone, then move it above this edge to the hairline. Touch the D zone from left to right, then place the tip of your thumb on the most sensitive point and carry out circling motions.

Massaging Points D1 through D5

The points D1 through D5 run vertically like a chain of pearls along the front edge of the ear. Among this row, locate the most sensitive point and carry out circling motions. It is possible that several points will be sensitive.

Left: In this picture, the thumb is in the middle of the B zone, on the punctum maximum.

Right: The C zone runs diagonally in the area of the receding hairline. Follow this diagonal line when touching the zone.

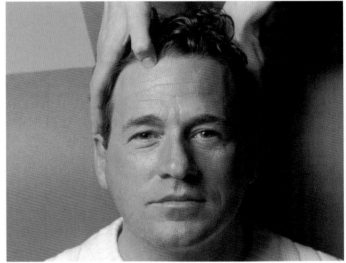

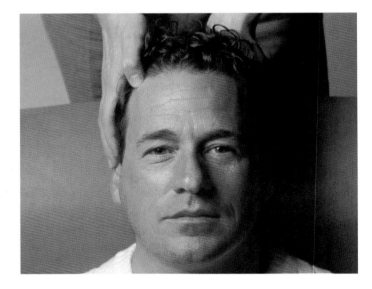

Left: The D zone is located above the cheekbone, at the hairline.

Right: Points D1 through D5 are located vertically along the front of the auricle.

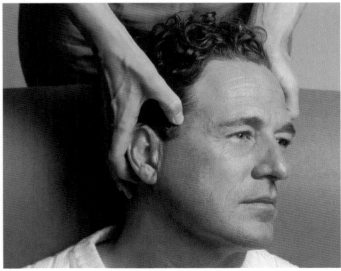

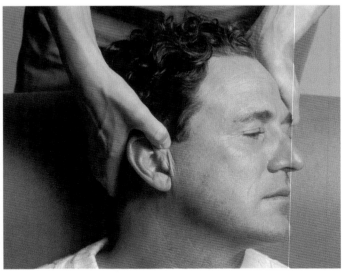

Massaging the E Zones and the Zones of the Sensory Organs

The E zones run diagonally across the eyebrows and are subdivided into twelve individual segments representing the twelve vertebrae of the thoracic spine. Touch each zone from the inside out. When you have located the most sensitive point, place the tip of your thumb on it and carry out small circling motions. Do the same for the zones of the eyes, nose, mouth, and ears, which are also located on the forehead.

Massaging the F Zone

Find the mastoid process behind each ear. On the highest point of these bones you will find the F zones. Place the tip of your thumb on the most sensitive point of each zone and carry out circling motions.

Massaging Points G1 through G3

The points G1 through G3 are located very close to the F zones, at the front, bottom, and back edge of the mastoid process. Touch the points with your thumb and massage the most painful point with circling movements. In some cases, the points that represent the knee joint will all be sensitive. In that case, massage all the points.

Massaging the Brain Zones

The brain zones are in line with the A zones in the scalp area. Touch the zones both lengthwise and crosswise and massage the most painful points with circling movements.

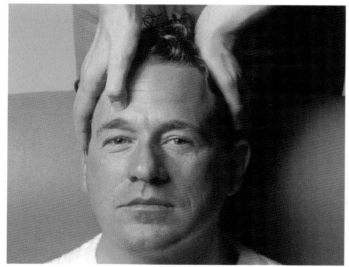

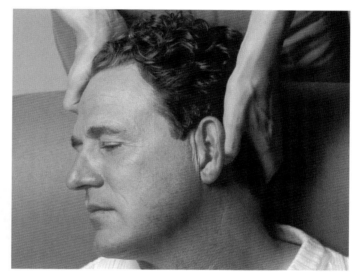

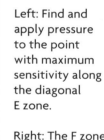

Left: Find and apply pressure to the point with maximum sensitivity along the diagonal E zone.

Right: The F zone is located at the highest part of the mastoid process.

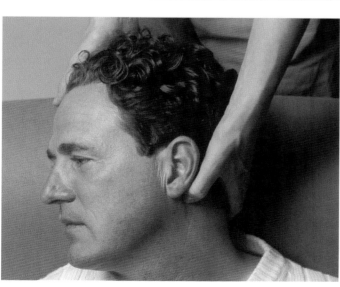

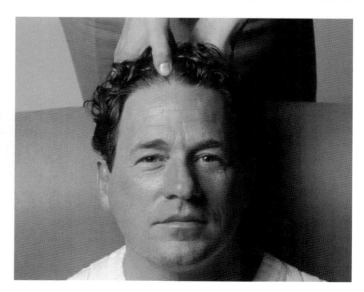

Left: Locate the most sensitive G point around the edges of the mastoid process.

Right: The zone of the brain is located in line with the A zone in the scalp area.

Shiatsu

In contrast to foot, hand, ear, and head reflexology, with their well-defined reflex zones, shiatsu deals with the whole body and is a complex and holistic system. To understand shiatsu, it helps to understand the differences between Western and Eastern medicine.

Knowledge

In our Western world, medicine is largely symptom based, meaning that medical treatment is usually focused on ailments of or injuries to individual body parts. In contrast, Eastern medicine principally looks at the human body as a whole. In that sense, health is based not on the functioning of individual body parts but rather on the harmonic distribution and uninterrupted flow of life energy throughout the body. Illness is a result of an imbalance in energy distribution. Recognizing and treating energy imbalances in the body is the most important principle of Eastern medicine. The means that are applied toward this end can be divided into several groups: acupressure, shiatsu, and other types of body massage; nutrition; therapy with primarily plant-based medicine; acupuncture; breathing therapy; and meditation.

You have to experience shiatsu on your own body to understand it. The treatment is presented here in such a way that it is accessible to Westerners who have no significant previous knowledge of the field. You will learn simple techniques with which you can administer a relaxing massage of the whole body.

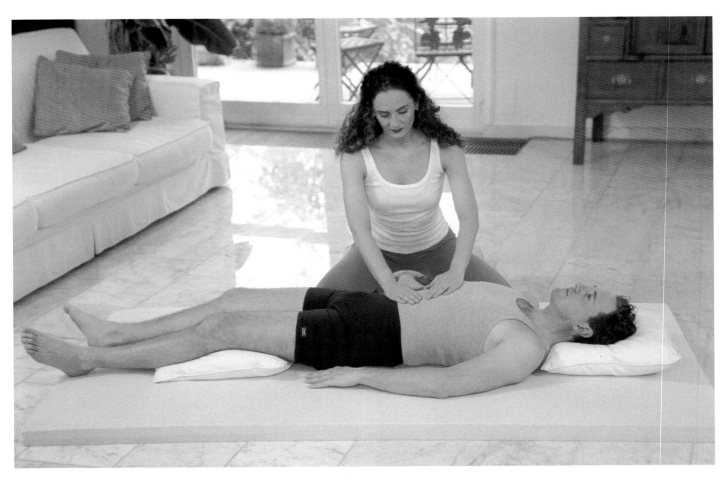

A shiatsu massage should always encompass the whole body.

What Is Shiatsu?

Shiatsu is a holistic body therapy or healing massage that originated in the Far East. In Japanese, *shi* means "finger," and *atsu* means "pressure." Freely translated, *shiatsu* thus means "pressure with the finger."

The Historical Background of Shiatsu

The roots of this type of therapy can be traced back all the way to the time of the legendary Yellow Emperor (about 2000 B.C.) in China. The Yellow Emperor Huang Ti was known for his intense interest in different medical questions. He held long medical debates with his advisers, Chi Po and Lei Gong, which were later written down in the famous work *Huang Ti Nei Jing* (The Yellow Emperor's Classic of Internal Medicine).

It is believed that Buddhist monks brought this knowledge from China to Japan about a thousand years ago. In Japan, many strokes and techniques were developed further and adapted to the different cultural circumstances. However, shiatsu was officially recognized as a healing massage only in the middle of the twentieth century in Japan. In the meantime, different styles had developed, with different focuses. News of this healing massage in the 1970s reached the West, first the United States, then Australia, and finally Europe.

The Basic Philosophic Principles

Shiatsu can be summarized in the simple principle of treating each person "holistically." However, this basic principle obscures the complex philosophical structure of ancient Eastern medicine. This philosophy views the universe with all its creatures and components as one big unit. Each creature is a small depiction of this larger whole. This philosophy can be illustrated with a simple example: Compare your body to a mechanical clockwork. Such a clockwork consists of many big and small wheels and levers. In their harmonious and precise interaction, these components drive forward the second, minute, and hour hands. A spring, which you compress by winding the clock, delivers the energy that drives the clockwork. If even a single lever or wheel gets stuck, the whole system stops working and the clock stops. The clockmaker now has to find out which part is responsible for the problem and repair the damage. Only once all parts resume working together can the clock run again.

Now transfer this example to the human body. All parts of the body work together like a clockwork. If one organ fails—for example, the heart—the body dies unless it receives outside help.

But what energy drives our bodies? In our example, the clock is driven by a spring that is powered by an outside force. Once the spring has unwound completely, the energy is used up and the clock stops. The energy that drives the human body, that flows through it and keeps it alive, is life energy. This energy is called *chi* (in Japan and China) or *prana* (in India).

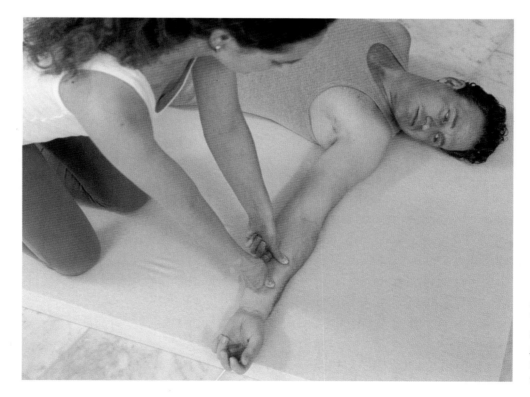

Shiatsu means "finger pressure" and refers to a Japanese healing massage technique.

How Does Shiatsu Work?

In a simplified explanation, the techniques used in shiatsu balance and harmonize chi. Shiatsu removes blockages to chi, which result in a lack of chi in associated parts of the body, and thus leads to well-being.

Chi—Life Energy

From the viewpoint of Far Eastern philosophy, at birth each person receives a certain amount of life energy, called inherited or original energy. Once this energy is used up—much like in a battery—life ends and the person dies. This life energy is stored in the abdomen, called the *hara*. From here, the life energy or chi courses through the body. When the body is evenly supplied with life energy, it is in perfect health. When this is not the case, illness may result. This is the starting point for shiatsu. When applied properly, it allows the practitioner to recognize and remedy energy imbalances and leads to well-being. In this way, shiatsu is well suited to preventing illnesses.

The Hara

In the view of Far Eastern medicine, the hara is the center of the body and the source of life energy. Freely translated, *hara* means "lower abdomen." But it also has a deeper meaning signifying the center of life. The hara is the place of physical balance, of emotional and spiritual energy. From a physical point of view—for example, when looking at the weight distribution of the human body—the area between the navel and the pubic bone is the central point of the body. The lower the center of gravity lies, the greater the stability and balance of the body. Conversely, the higher the center of gravity, the more fragile and insecure the body's balance. Take a simple example: Picture a smooth bowl with a rounded bottom. If you place a marble inside it, the marble will first roll around a bit and then come to rest in the center of the bottom of the bowl. If you turn the bowl over and place the marble on the high point of its bottom, its balance will be very fragile, and it will soon roll down one of the sides. It is interesting to note that all Eastern martial arts as well as dance, music, painting, and, of course, shiatsu come "from the gut," namely the hara.

Note

The life energy, or chi, is concentrated in a very small point about three finger-widths below the navel. This point is called the *tan tien*, and it is from here that life energy originates and to this point that it returns.

The Movement Comes from the Abdomen

A shiatsu session begins with concentrating on your own hara. When done correctly, all movements originate directly from your hara. For this to be the case, your hara has to be open. The following exercise helps you get in touch with and open your hara.

Perception Exercise for Your Hara

You can carry out this exercise sitting on the ground or on a chair. What is important is to sit upright. Place your hands together in your lap with your palms facing up. Ideally, your arms will form a circle, such that energy can circle your hara without disruption. Next, focus your attention on your breathing. With each breath, try to inhale more deeply into your abdomen, until you are breathing only with your abdomen. Place your hands on your abdomen and breathe "into" your hands. While doing this, take note of how your abdomen rises and falls.

Now imagine that you are breathing in and out of your *tan tien*, the center of your life energy. Feel how, with each breath, the energy in this point is becoming increasingly concentrated. From here, the warmth spreads throughout your hara. As soon as you feel this warmth spread, begin the next step: Feel your hara opening and energy flowing from it into your body. You may feel this as your hara releasing a warm light that spreads throughout your body. Your thoughts may wander during this exercise. This is normal. Try to calmly lead your thoughts back to the exercise. If you are unable to do this, do not feel pressured to continue the exercise. Instead, end it here and repeat it at a later point. The more often and regularly you do this exercise, the stronger your feeling for your hara will be. Try to do this exercise daily.

The Hands

Aside from the hara, shiatsu massage also assigns a special importance to the hands. Your hands should be warm and smooth. Your nails should not extend past the fingertips, since many massage techniques are done directly with the fingertips and long nails would injure your partner. Take off any jewelry such as rings, bracelets, and watches before the massage. For a thorough massage, your hands not only should be smooth but also should have the necessary strength and stamina to last 30 to 45 minutes. To this end, carry out regular stretching and strengthening exercises, especially immediately before giving a massage.

The Energy of the Hands

In the same way in which you increase your perception of the hara, you can increase your perception of your hands. For this, do the following simple perception exercise after you have finished warming up and stretching your hands.

Perception Exercise for the Energy of the Hands

Take up a comfortable position. Breathe in and out regularly and calmly. Throughout the exercise, keep your shoulders relaxed at your sides. Lifting only your hands, hold your palms in front of your body facing each other but not touching. Focus your attention on your palms. Feel the warmth that emanates from each palm to the other. Only once you are sure you are feeling this warmth should you take the next step. Then imagine this warmth to be an energy flow between your hands and start to play with it: Begin with small, slow circles in opposite directions, then increase the distance between your hands as far as you can while still feeling the energy or warmth between them. Now imagine that you will transfer this warmth and energy to your partner in the following massage. In the beginning, you may find it hard to perceive the warmth and energy flow between your hands. Remember that your hands have to be warm for the exercise. The more you do this exercise, the more honed your perceptiveness will be.

Summary

Shiatsu should not be used:
- In the first trimester of pregnancy
- After a heavy meal
- In the case of infection or illness accompanied by fever
- In the case of high blood pressure

Possibilities and Limits of Shiatsu

Shiatsu serves to balance the body's energy and thus improve well-being. The techniques introduced here have a preventive function. Before you carry out a shiatsu massage, find out whether the intended recipient manifests any counterindications. For elderly people and children, you should use only gentle techniques and carry out the massage with only very light pressure. Body areas with localized problems, such as open wounds, infections, varicose veins, and rheumatic ailments, should not be massaged.

Also, do not carry out a massage if your partner has just eaten a heavy meal, has an illness accompanied by a fever, or has very high blood pressure. Pregnant women should not have a shiatsu massage in the first trimester, and in the second and third trimesters, many techniques should be applied only in a limited manner, if at all. Such counterindications are marked by special notes in the text. People with a serious health problem, such as a weak heart, cancer, or osteoporosis, should be treated only by an experienced shiatsu practitioner.

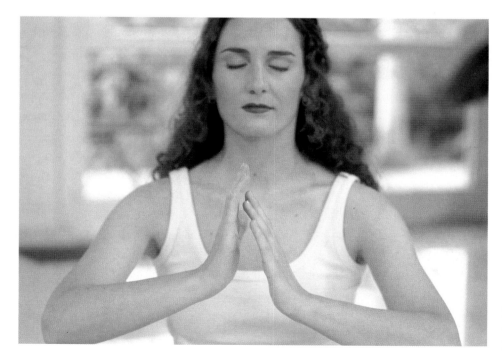

Feel the warmth emanating from your palms.

Administering Shiatsu Massages

This practical section will introduce you to the basic techniques of shiatsu. These simple massage techniques are easy to learn and have a wide range of applications. We consciously chose those techniques that allow an easy entry and corresponding success. For this reason, the techniques shown here do not belong to any particular school of shiatsu.

Preparations

Please familiarize yourself with the necessary preparations before you attempt the first massage. Also, pay attention to the specific notes and alerts for the individual treatments.

Room and Atmosphere

Shiatsu is best administered in an environment that is comfortable for your partner. You will need a space that is well ventilated, at a comfortable temperature, and free of any drafts. Such a pleasant ambience encourages relaxation. Indirect light and calm music also contribute to this atmosphere. But be sure to ask your partner about his or her wishes for

Preparations

- Work in a pleasant, warm room without distractions.
- Have a sufficiently large massage surface (such as a mat) that is not too soft, and cushions and blankets to support the positioning of body parts.
- Make sure the recipient is in a comfortable and relaxing position.
- Do the concentration exercise for the hara.
- Get in a comfortable and relaxing position, such as sitting on the legs or kneeling.
- Apply pressure perpendicular to the area that is being massaged.
- Work with both hands.
- Find your own rhythm.

this. During the massage, you should be undisturbed. Make sure that you will not be interrupted by the phone or doorbell. The space should be sufficiently large that you can move freely around your partner. Your partner can wear clothes during the massage, but the clothing should be comfortable and in no way constricting. Jewelry and other accessories should be removed before the massage.

The Proper Position

Shiatsu massages are traditionally administered on the floor. Your partner rests on a mat that is thick and not too soft. A futon is suitable, as are a number of blankets stacked together. The mat should be large enough that you can comfortably kneel on it next to your partner.

Using small cushions or rolls helps ensure a comfortable position for your partner. You can make round cushions by rolling up blankets or towels. Placing a rolled-up blanket placed under the knees will support your partner's back. The slight bend in the knees will also bend the hips and relax the abdominal muscles. At the same time, it will ensure that the lumbar spine of your partner is resting comfortably on the mat.

If you want to massage your partner's back, have him or her lie on his or her stomach. This position can be optimized using some simple additions. Place your partner's feet on a rolled-up blanket, which will relax the leg muscles. If your partner has a hollow back in this position, place a cushion under his or her stomach to straighten it.

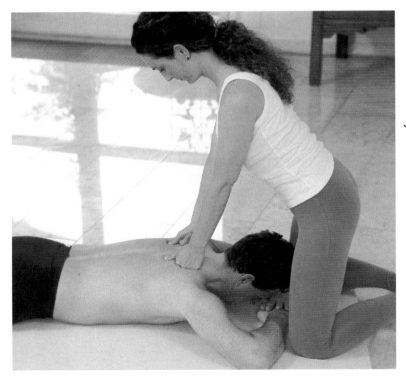

Choose a calm and pleasant environment in which to administer a shiatsu massage.

Preparing Yourself

The hara, as the seat of life energy, is important for the treatment, which explains one of the most important tenets of shiatsu: "Work from the hara." In all your movements, concentrate on your hara, which will be easier to do if you practice the hara exercise (page 144) regularly.

Pay attention to your own breathing, and be sure to inhale deeply and consciously into your abdomen. Breathing into the hara will help you find a stable balance point from which you can carry out all massage techniques.

Giving and Receiving a Massage

A shiatsu massage is a two-way process. On the one hand, you are giving a massage, but on the other, you are receiving one. As a shiatsu giver, try to feel into the body of the recipient and to see with your hands instead of your eyes. Even before the massage is over, you will receive a clear message about your effectiveness from your partner: Based on the degree of tension or relaxation of the shiatsu recipient, you will know whether your massage is having the desired effect.

Well-being and relaxation should quickly take over in your partner after a few proper techniques. You will feel his or her tension slowly dissolve under your hands.

Remaining Relaxed Yourself

To be able to give a good shiatsu massage, you will need to remain relaxed yourself and to rest within yourself. That is why it is important to prepare yourself

before the shiatsu massage. Collect yourself and imagine that you want to pass on your energy through your hands to your partner. Carry out the hara exercise, and don't begin the massage until you are feeling completely calm inside. Only in this way can you focus your attention on your hands and make them receptive to the contact with your partner's body. Be sure to remain relaxed while giving the massage, and avoid tensing your shoulders. Counter possible tension by taking the best position for each technique. Working from the hara prevents the buildup of tension inside you and helps you as a shiatsu giver to benefit from the massage as well.

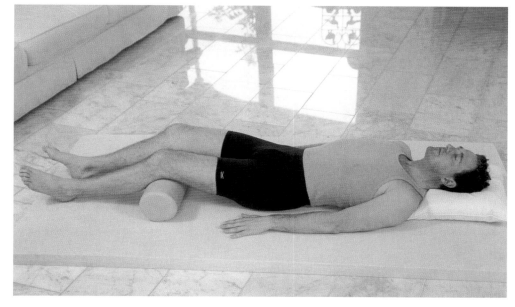

A rolled-up blanket under the knees relaxes the abdominal muscles.

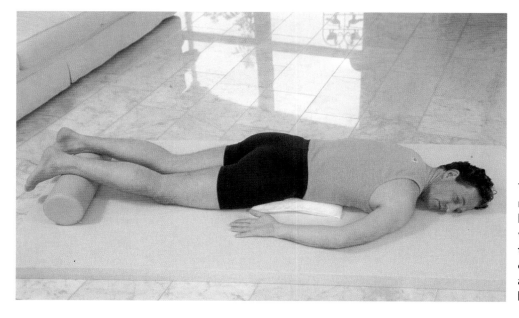

You can support a recipient lying on his or her stomach with a roll under the feet and a cushion to accommodate a hollow back.

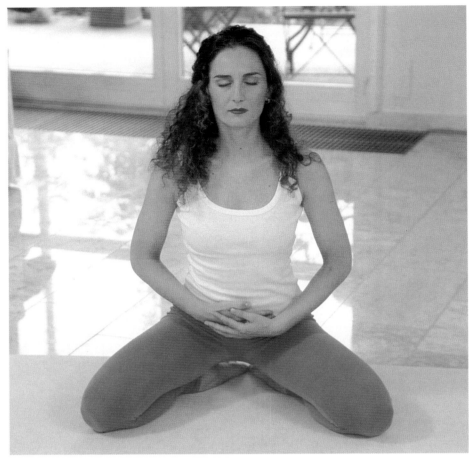

Prepare yourself for the massage by concentrating on your hara.

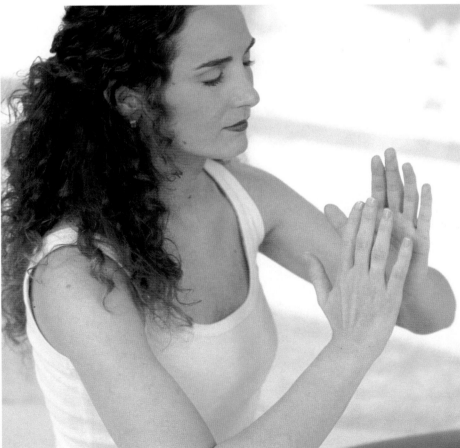

Focus all of your attention on your hands.

Using Both Hands

In shiatsu massages, you will always work with both hands. The resting hand is called the mother, or *yin* hand. It supports the active hand. The active hand is the child, or *yang* hand.

It is very important to have your resting hand in touch with your partner's body at all times. Without contact with the resting hand, the recipient will feel uncomfortable during the massage. Visualize your hands as two poles: chi can circulate only when both poles are in contact with your partner's body. If the contact is with just one pole, the cycle is interrupted.

Finding the Right Rhythm

A shiatsu massage is a constant exchange between giving and taking.

Design your massage in a harmonious rhythm. Have the individual treatment phases blend into one another, and be sure not to have interruptions between the individual treatment sequences.

Feel the calm, regular rhythm of your breathing, and massage in the same rhythm.

Together with the shiatsu recipient, you will thus soon find your own rhythm.

The Initial Position

A good starting position is important for all techniques. Most techniques are done from the heel seat. For this, you will kneel on the mat with your buttocks resting on your heels, which gently stretches your thigh muscles. The farther apart your knees are, the more stable this position will be. You can do the concentration exercise for the hara (see page 144) in this position before you begin the massage.

Another important starting position is the half-knee stand, which you develop from the heel seat. For this, rise up on your knees and bring one leg forward. The half-knee stand allows you to carry out many different exercises while staying comfortable and relaxed.

Position your body so that it is always at a right angle to the area being massaged. In this way, you will be able to use your body weight optimally without undue exertion or contortion.

Time Requirements

How much time you need for a massage depends on which body regions you will be massaging. You will need 45 to 60 minutes for a whole-body massage and less time for a partial massage. In addition, the recipient should have time after the massage to indulge a need for rest.

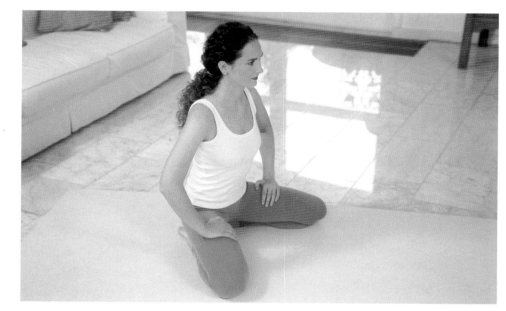

The heel seat is the basic position for many techniques.

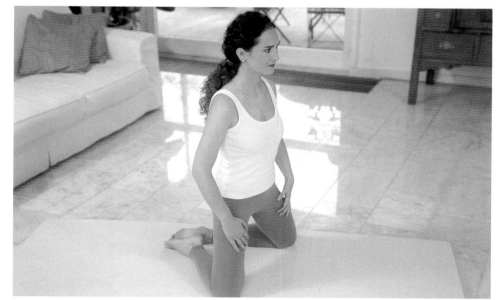

Rise up from the heel seat to your knees.

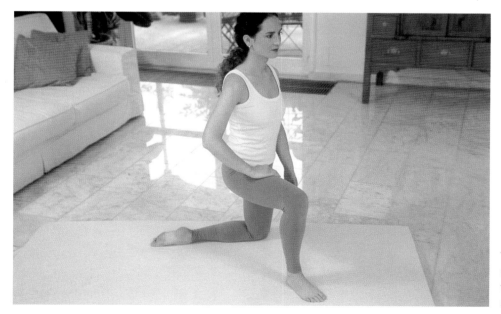

The half-knee stand evolves from the heel seat.

The Basic Techniques

Today, a dizzying array of shiatsu variations exists. And in the course of their work, therapists develop their own techniques and variations. With the basic techniques presented here you will be able to administer basic massages with ease. But don't be discouraged if everything doesn't fall into place right from the start. With patience and practice, you will master all these techniques.

Pressure Techniques

By applying pressure, you will stimulate the chi that is circulating in the body. For this reason, pressure techniques are an important shiatsu element. There are different ways of exerting pressure with the fingers, thumbs, hands, elbows, and other body parts. The following describes pressure techniques that you can use in shiatsu massage.

Pressure Points and Strength

As a novice in shiatsu massage, it is important for you to develop a feeling for where and how much pressure to apply.

Normally, pressure is exerted on certain points, which

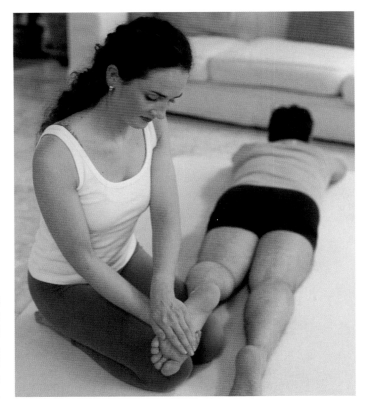

In shiatsu massage, pressure can be applied using the elbow, the individual fingers, and the flat hand.

> **Note**
> - The strength of the pressure depends on the sensitivity of your partner.
> - Apply pressure carefully while your partner is exhaling, using only gentle pressure on older people.
> - Avoid pressure techniques in areas of illness or injury.

lie along the chi paths or meridians (see page 17). For now, you don't need to know the exact location of the individual points; where necessary, we will discuss the individual points in more detail. The amount of pressure you apply depends on the sensitivity of the shiatsu recipient. Ask the recipient how he or she is experiencing the pressure. But also pay attention to his or her reactions. If your pressure is too strong, you will notice the recipient tensing or cramping up. Your partner's breathing, too, can offer clues to his or her experience. If you are pressing too hard, making it uncomfortable for the recipient, he or she is likely to hold his or her breath, interrupting the calm and relaxed breathing cycle. However, note that below the threshold at which pain occurs, there is a different kind of pain that is experienced almost as a pleasant sensation. This "welcome pain" signals that you have located the correct spot and are exerting the right amount of pressure. This pain often emanates along the paths of the meridians, which also shows that you are on the right track.

When applying a pressure technique, don't start off with maximum strength. Instead, ease into it: First make contact and then increase the pressure. Bring the exertion of pressure into harmony with the breathing rhythm of your partner; increase the pressure as he or she exhales and hold it for 3 to 7 seconds, or for a complete breathing cycle—that is, up to the next exhalation.

Pressure with the Heel of the Hand

Applying pressure with the heel of the hand creates a very pleasant and focused deep effect. A relaxed hand is important for the proper application of this technique. Place the entire hand on the body part to be massaged. Apply pressure by shifting your weight via your shoulders and outstretched arms onto the heel of the hand.

Before you use this technique, do a small exercise.

Kneel in the heel seat. Place both hands in front of you on a mat. Rise up onto all fours. You can consciously vary the amount of pressure that you are exerting with the palms of your hands by moving your pelvis and buttocks forward and back. When you move your buttocks forward, pressure increases; when you slide back, it decreases. Keep your back straight and remember your hara. Breathe into your lower abdomen, and try to make this movement out of your hara. After this exercise, practice this technique on the back of your partner's upper thigh. Apply the pressure perpendicular to the middle axis of the leg. Develop a feeling for how much weight you can put into it, keeping in mind that the pressure should be pleasant for the shiatsu recipient.

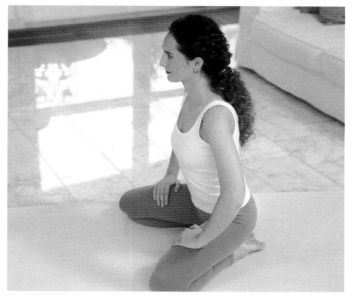

The initial position for exerting pressure is the heel seat.

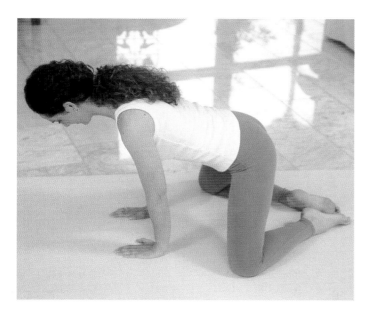

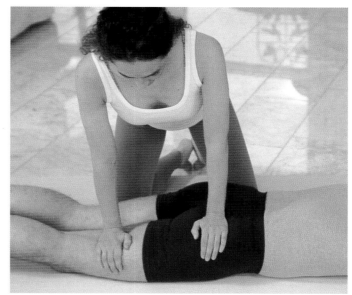

Far left: Move to all fours and apply pressure on the surface using the ball of your hand.

Practice the pressure technique on your partner.

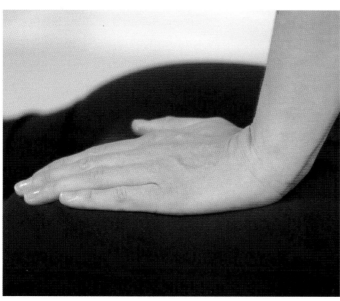

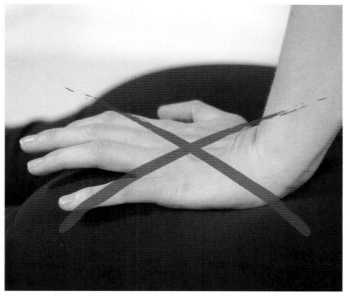
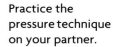

Far left: The palms adjust to the contours of the body part being massaged.

Don't open the fingers; the hand here doesn't have enough contact with the body.

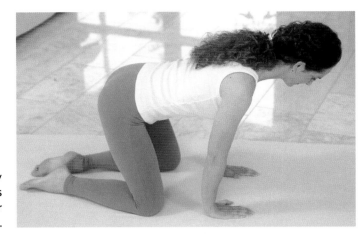

Apply pressure by moving your pelvis and shoulder girdle forward.

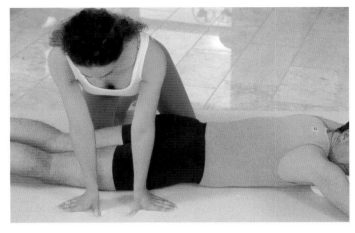

Move into position from all fours.

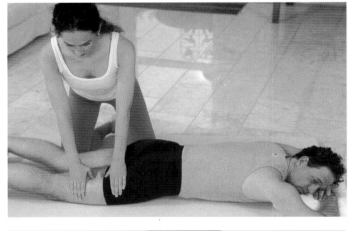

Place the thumbs on the middle axes of the legs and apply pressure when your partner exhales.

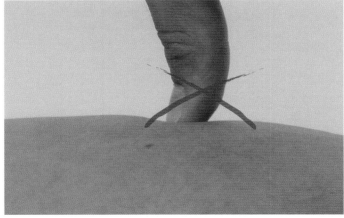

Left and right: Note the correct way to apply pressure with your thumb.

Pressure with the Thumb

With your thumb you can apply a very focused pressure on specific points. At first this technique will be exhausting and your thumb joints will need to get used to it, so don't overdo it at the beginning. Apply the pressure not with the tip of the thumb but with the whole top joint. Apply steady pressure on the designated point and avoid bouncing, circling, or vibrating movements. Increase the pressure steadily with the exhalation rhythm of your partner. By moving your pelvis and buttocks forward and back, you can regulate the strength of the pressure, just as you did with the heel of the hand. The following warm-up exercise will help you develop a feel for the thumb pressure technique.

Position yourself in the heel seat, sitting on your knees. Place both thumbs about shoulder-width apart on the mat in front of you, with the other fingers supporting each hand. From this position, move onto all fours. Shift your weight by moving the pelvis and shoulder girdle forward and back. Your arms, thumb, and other fingers should remain straight during this exercise.

After this exercise, practice the thumb pressure technique on your partner. Place your thumbs on the middle axes of the backs of the upper thighs and apply pressure as your partner exhales. Remember that the pressure should be perceived by your partner as pleasant.

Pressure with the Fingers

You can relax your partner's tense shoulder muscles by applying pressure with your finger. For this technique, your partner should lie on his or her side. Grasp the front of the upper shoulder with one hand and place the four

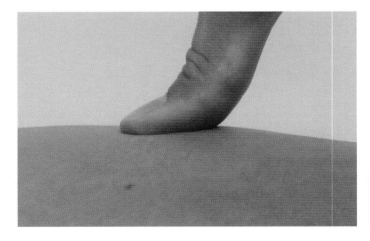

fingertips of the other hand under the middle edge of the shoulder blade. When your partner begins to exhale, move the shoulder backward while moving your fingertips underneath the shoulder blade, so that your hands are moving toward each other. Hold this position for a few of your partner's breathing cycles. This technique is very good for resolving tension in the shoulder area. Adjust the strength of the pressure to the sensitivity of your partner.

The "Tiger Mouth" Grip

You can stretch the sides of the body using the so-called tiger mouth grip. At the same time, you can exert pressure on specific places with this grip. For this technique, your partner should lie on his or her side. Open your hand in a half-moon shape, as if you were reaching for a jar. With some imagination, you can see that the hand resembles a tiger's open mouth, from which the name comes. Place the wide-open hand on the side of the upper rib cage and apply pressure on that hand by moving your pelvis forward and back. Apply pressure while your partner is exhaling and reduce it as he or she is inhaling. Move down along the ribs point by point, repeating the cycle each time: Apply pressure during exhalation and reduce pressure during inhalation.

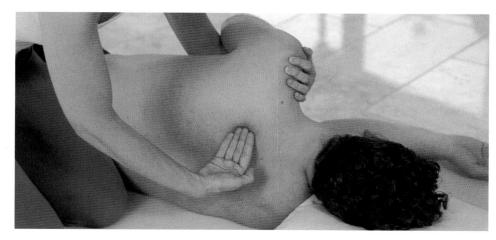

Place your fingertips below the shoulder blade with your palm facing you.

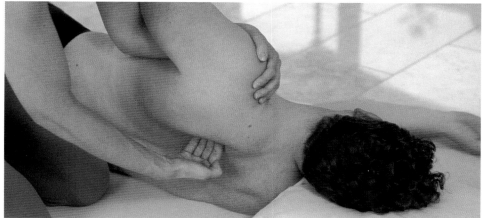

Now move the shoulder and the shoulder blade above your fingers.

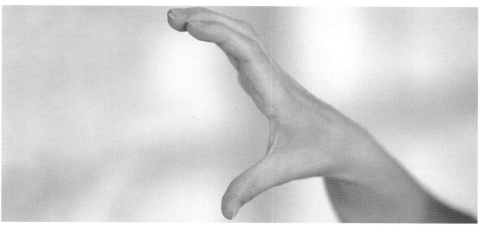

The wide-open hand resembles the mouth of a tiger.

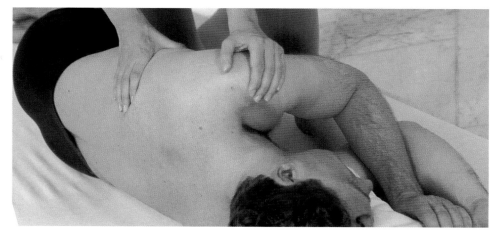

Place the wide-open hand on the ribs of the side and apply pressure when your partner exhales.

Pressure with the Elbow

Using your elbow allows you to exert stronger pressure than you can with your hands, and it relieves your hands and fingers. The elbow technique is used when large muscles are tense; it can be used on the muscles of the back,

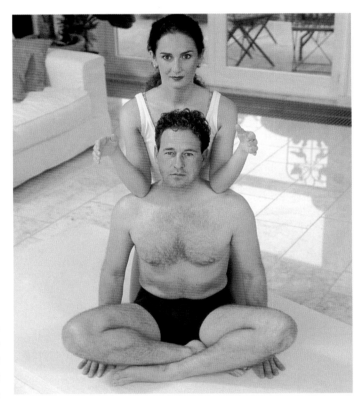

Slightly bend your elbows, relax your wrists, and place your elbows on the neck muscles.

buttocks, legs, and shoulders. To avoid causing your partner discomfort, don't bend your arm all the way, to prevent the elbow from becoming sharply pointed. When you are using your elbows on the shoulder muscles, stand or kneel behind your partner. Place the slightly bent elbows between the neck and shoulder joint on the shoulder muscles. As your partner exhales, carefully exert a vertical downward pressure. Adjust pressure depending on your partner's sensitivity. Massage all the muscles of the neck in this way. Afterward, stroke from the neck down the shoulders and arms.

Note: Do not use this technique if your partner is pregnant, as applying pressure with the elbows can cause contractions.

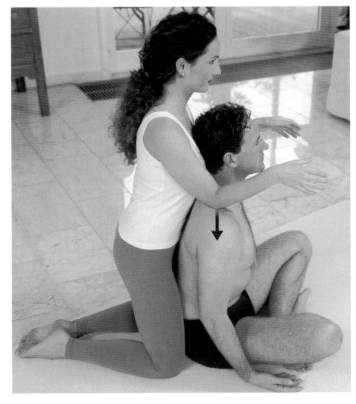

Left: As your partner exhales, carefully apply downward pressure.

Right: After you have massaged the side of the neck, stroke from the neck over the shoulders to the arms.

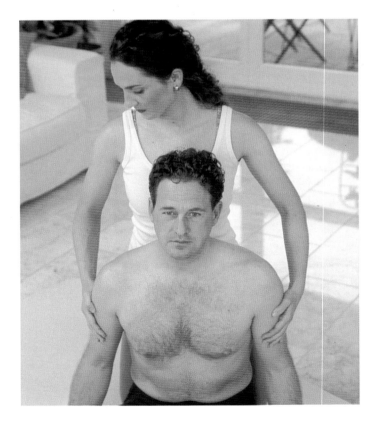

Stretching Techniques

Stretching techniques are another important component of shiatsu. They serve to relax your partner, dissolve energy blockages, and thus stimulate the unobstructed flow of chi.

This section introduces some simple and important stretching techniques.

Stretching Properly

- When stretching, pay attention to your partner's pain threshold.
- For older people or people with stiff joints, carry out stretches very carefully.
- Avoid swinging motions while stretching, as they increase muscle tension.
- Do not stretch any injured body parts.

Stretching Properly

Stretch a muscle according to the following formula: Bring the muscle to be stretched into position only until the partner starts to slightly pull. Do not exceed this point.

Remember your own posture, and keep your back straight while working from the hara. Gently increase the stretch as your partner exhales, but only to the point where no unpleasant pain occurs. Slightly release the stretch as your partner inhales. Keep this up for five breathing cycles and then return the stretched body part to its normal resting position. Avoid abrupt movements as well as bouncing, which would increase tension in the muscle—the opposite of what you are trying to accomplish.

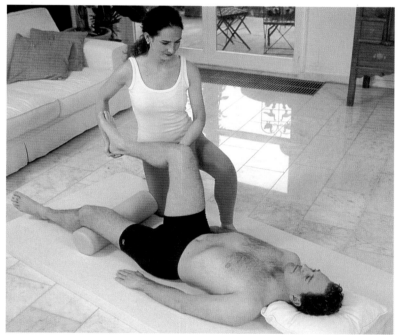

Hold the leg at the knee and heel.

Stretching the Backs of the Thighs

By stretching the backs of the thighs, you affect the energy paths that run along this area.

From the heel seat, rise into the half-knee stand, placing your outer foot next to your partner's hip. Hold your partner's knee with your outer hand and the heel with your other hand. Slowly bend your partner's leg. Shift your weight to the foot supporting your standing leg and move your partner's leg with you. Keep the leg in this stretched position for three breathing cycles. Slightly increase the stretch when your partner exhales and slightly release it when he or she inhales. If you notice that your partner is tensing against your touch, your pressure is too strong. Afterward, carefully return the leg to its resting position and repeat the stretch on the other leg.

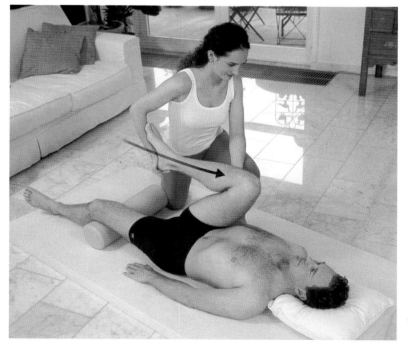

Bringing your weight forward, move the leg into the stretching position.

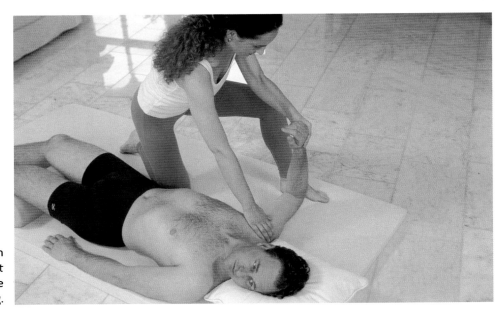

Loosen the arm in the shoulder joint through gentle swinging.

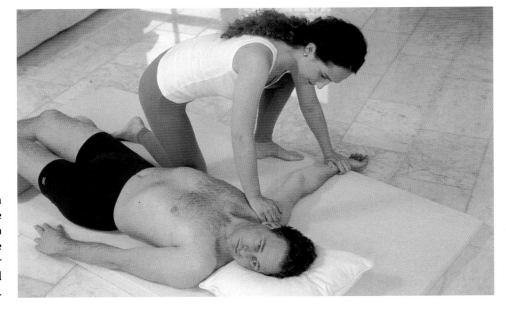

Place the arm at a right angle to the body and stretch the muscles of the upper and lower arm using the heel of your hand.

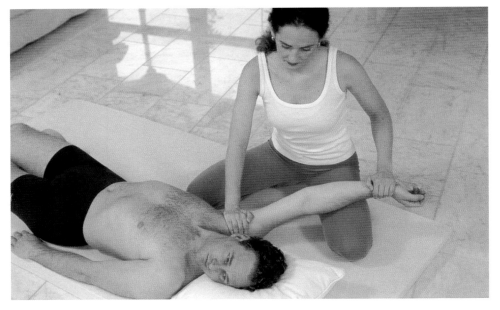

Seated next to your partner's head, place the arm over your thigh and stretch it using the heel of your hand.

Stretching the Arms

Stretch the arms in several positions to influence the flow of energy through the different meridians of this part of the body. Be sure to loosen the arm and shoulder muscles before your stretches. To do this, go into the half-knee stand and place your right hand on your partner's right shoulder. Grasp your partner's hand with your left hand. Slightly lift the right arm so that it is raised above the mat and the elbow is bent at a right angle. Move the arm back and forth with light swinging movements. Your partner should let you guide his or her arm during this exercise and should not tense against you.

Now extend your partner's arm above his or her head with the palm facing up. Your right hand remains on the right shoulder. Place the heel of your left hand on your partner's lower arm, above the wrist. Carefully move your weight forward onto your hands and in this way stretch the muscles on the inside of your partner's upper and lower arm. Then place the arm on the ground perpendicular to the rest of the body. Return your hands to their previous position and again put your weight on your hands.

Finally, sit in the heel seat next to your partner's head. Stretch your partner's arm over his or her head. Place your partner's arm on your thigh and use the heel of your hand to stretch it, as in the previous two positions.

Repeat all these stretches for the other arm.

Pressure and Stretching Shiatsu Techniques at a Glance

PRESSURE TECHNIQUES

Pressure with the Heel of the Hand

Place your hand flat on the body part to be massaged. Make sure that your palms adjust to the contours of the body. Apply pressure by shifting your weight via your shoulders and straight arms to the heel of your hand.

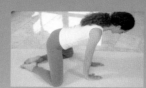
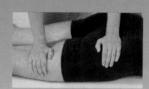

Thumb Pressure

Place the entire last joint of the thumb on the body part to be massaged and apply steady pressure on one point in rhythm with your partner's breathing. Avoid swinging, circling, or vibrating movements.

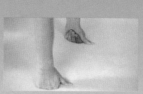
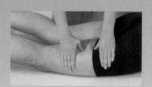

Finger Pressure

Take the front of the shoulder in one hand. Place the four finger-tips of the other hand below the middle edge of the shoulder blade. Move the shoulder back and slide your fingers under the shoulder blade, moving your hands toward each other in synchrony with your partner's breathing.

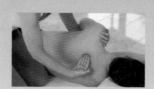
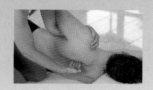

Tiger Mouth Pressure

Place your hand with fingers spread wide on the side of the upper rib cage. As your partner exhales, apply pressure with your hand by moving your pelvis back and forth. Move down along the ribs point by point.

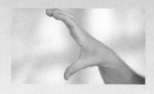
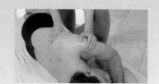

Elbow Pressure

To massage the muscles of the neck, kneel behind your partner, slightly bend your arms, and place them on your partner's shoulder muscles. Apply downward pressure as your partner exhales.

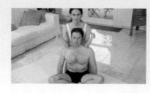
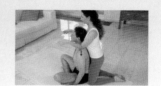

STRETCHING TECHNIQUES

Stretching the Backs of the Thighs

Take your partner's knee with one hand and his or her heel with the other. Shift your weight and bend your partner's leg. Increase the stretch as your partner exhales. Carry out the same stretch on the other leg.

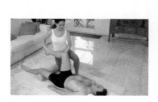
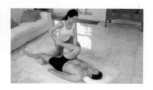

Stretching the Arms

Place your right hand on your partner's right shoulder and take his or her right hand into your left hand. Swing the raised arm. Place the arm down over the head, place your left hand on the lower arm, and stretch the muscles of the inside of the upper and lower arm. Repeat to the side of the body and then, with the arm over your thigh, above the head again. Carry out the same stretches for the other arm.

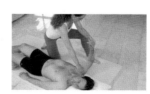
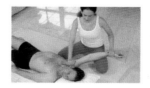

Massaging the Individual Body Parts

Using just the pressure and stretching techniques introduced so far, you are now able to administer a whole-body massage. Your massage will activate the chi that is in the lower abdomen (hara) and thus stimulate the body's ability to heal itself. However, keep in mind that this is a massage, not a medical treatment. Apply pressure as your partner exhales, and try to develop a feeling for how much pressure you can exert while having the massage remain a pleasant experience for your partner. Always work rhythmically, using smooth movements, and always keep your hands in contact with your partner. For the practitioner, shiatsu should be easy, without undue exertion; it should renew his or her energy. For the recipient, shiatsu should stimulate the body's ability to defend itself.

> **Tip**
>
> Massage from your hara (see page 144) and use your body weight for pressure techniques—do not work using your muscles alone. Relax your own body. Massage at a right angle to the surface being treated.

> **The Massage of the Back**
>
> The massage of the back happens in three steps:
> - Begin with loosening exercises.
> - Prepare your partner for the massage with stretches.
> - Apply pressure techniques with your thumb and the heel of your hand.

The Back Massage

The back is one of the body regions that most frequently experience pain. The spine, especially, as the carrying structure of the body, endures severe strain. Bad posture and exhausting activities take their toll on all related structures, such as bones, joints, and muscles, and accelerate their wear. A back massage is a perfect entry to shiatsu, since this is an area where you can apply almost all the different techniques and where you will immediately recognize whether your touch is having the desired effect. Remember to ask your partner to tell you how he or she is experiencing your touch.

Left: The bladder meridian is the longest meridian of the body and runs from the head down the back to the outside edges of the feet.

Right: Bad posture and stress on the spine often lead to back pain.

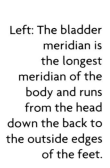

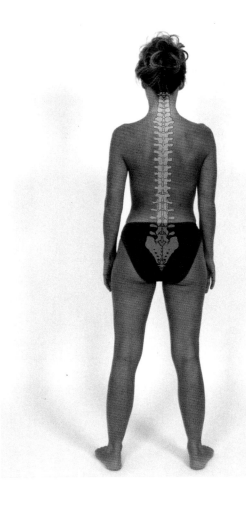

Massaging the Bladder Meridian

The bladder meridian is one of the body's twelve main pathways through which life energy, or chi, circulates. This meridian runs symmetrically on both halves of the body. It starts in the corners of the eyes and runs down the head along its sides and then down the spine, along the backs of the legs, and down into the outer sides of the feet. In the neck, the meridian divides into two branches, which run parallel to each other on the back. Many of the points you will work on during your massage lie on this meridian, and many of them play a significant role in treating back pain and the ailments of organs.

The Correct Position

Your partner should lie on his or her stomach. The mat should be large enough for your to reach your partner from all sides, with enough space for you to comfortably kneel on it. Your partner's arms should be to the sides of the body and his or her head turned to the side. In the case of neck pain, it may

be helpful to place a cushion under your partner's torso. A rolled-up towel or cushion under the feet will relax the thigh muscles.

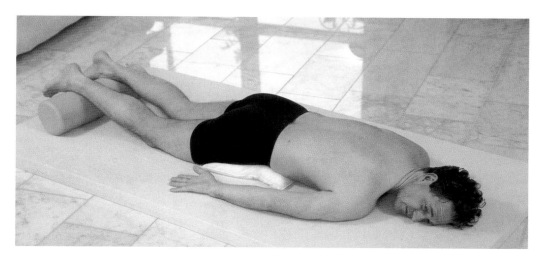

In the classic position, the arms rest next to the body and the head is on its side.

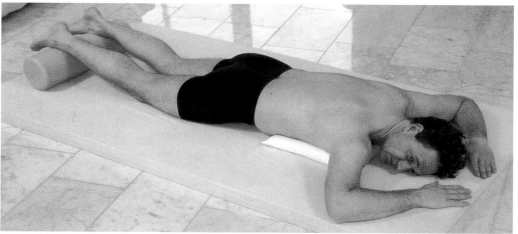

Some people prefer having their arms above their head.

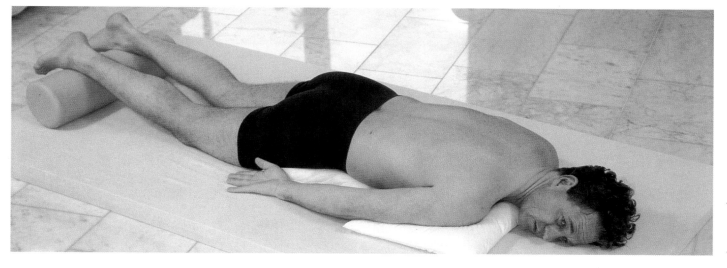

If your partner has neck pain, a cushion under the chest may make him or her more comfortable.

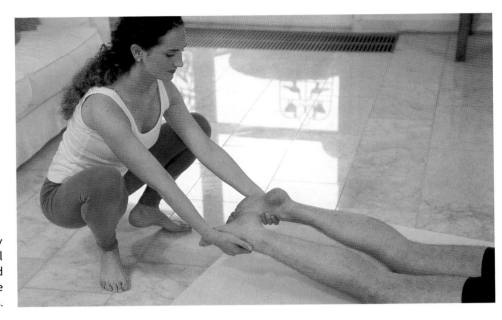

Take the feet by the ankles, pull lightly, and carefully shake the legs.

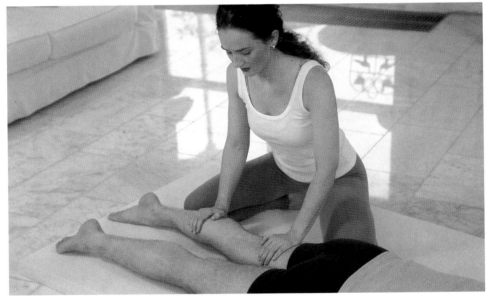

Tension in the leg can be resolved by gently rolling it back and forth.

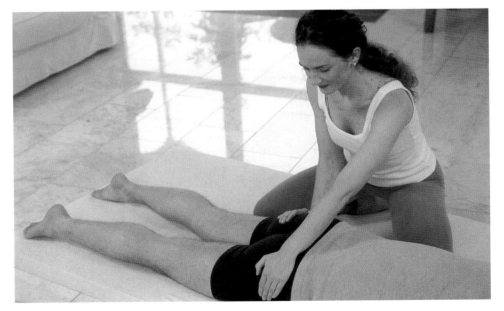

Gentle shakes or rolls in the pelvis relax the leg and back muscles.

Loosening

An overall loosening of the body is the ideal preparation for the massage.

Shaking the Legs

Take your partner's feet by the ankles and pull on both legs while shaking them with small vibrating movements. Ask your partner to relax while you do this. Carry out these shaking movements for 30 to 60 seconds, or until you can feel the tension disappearing from your partner's leg muscles.

Rolling the Legs

Kneel next to your partner's knees. Slide your hands down from the sacrum region until one rests on the calf and the other on the back of the thigh. From this position, carry out small rolling movements for 30 to 60 seconds, but without exerting pressure. Repeat this exercise for the other leg.

Rolling or Shaking the Pelvis

Sit on your knees next to your partner's pelvic region. Place your hands next to each other on the sacrum, and shake or roll the pelvic region back and forth. The movements here are small and carry over to the legs and the back.

The Stretches

Small stretches are experienced as pleasant and relaxing by many people. The following techniques help loosen and relax the different parts of the back muscles. The actual stretch occurs as a result of you shifting your body weight.

The Longitudinal Stretch

Kneel at your partner's left side. Place your right hand between your partner's shoulder blades and the left hand in the middle of the sacrum. The fingertips of the left hand should point toward the feet and the left hand should follow the contours of the sacrum. Rise up on your knees and move your buttocks toward your arms. This shifting of weight exerts pressure on your arms and you will develop a diagonal stretch. Apply weight to your partner as he or she exhales and reduce the weight by moving your buttocks back as your partner inhales.

The Diagonal Stretch

From the same initial position, place your right hand on the left shoulder blade so that your pinkie finger touches the middle and lower edge of the shoulder blade. Place your left hand on the right pelvic bone (the iliac crest). Again, apply pressure as your partner exhales by moving your body forward as you rise up on your knees and reduce pressure as he or she inhales by moving back. Perform this stretch three times. Then place your right hand on the right shoulder blade and your left hand on the left pelvic bone and stretch your partner's back three times in this direction.

The Side Stretch

To stretch the side of your partner's back, place your right hand

> **The Back Massage**
> - Have the receiver in a good position; if necessary, support the chest area with pillows.
> - Pull on the legs.
> - Gently rock the pelvis.
> - Shake the muscles of the thighs and calves.
> - Apply pressure with the ball of one thumb.
> - Apply pressure with the balls of both thumbs.

on the left shoulder blade so that the pinkie finger touches the shoulder blade and place your left hand on the side of the left pelvic bone. Rise up on your knees and stretch the left side of the back by shifting your body weight onto your arms. As always, exert pressure while your partner exhales. Carry out this stretch three times on each side of the body.

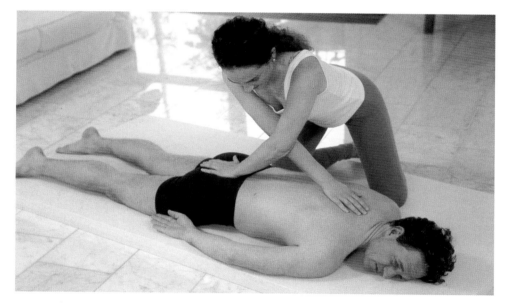

Longitudinal stretch: Stretch the back using your own body weight.

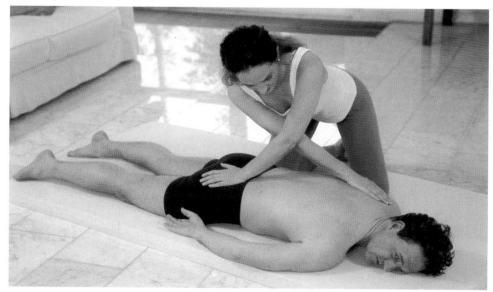

Diagonal stretch: Apply pressure by shifting your body weight.

Pressure with the Heel of the Hand

Massage the muscles on both sides of the spine from top to bottom using the heel of your hand. Start from the initial position of the heel seat, then rise up onto your knees. Place your left hand (now the resting hand) on the sacrum. Place the heel of your right hand (now the active hand) on the upper back, next to the spine. Apply pressure with your active hand by shifting your weight forward via the pelvis and buttocks. Keep your arms extended and your hands in broad contact with your partner's back. Exert pressure as your partner exhales and release and move the heel of your hand down a little bit each time your partner inhales. Massage one side of the back three times in this manner, and then do the same with the other side of the back.

Thumb Pressure with One Hand

Use the thumb pressure technique to apply pointed pressure on the muscles that run parallel to the spine. Start with pressure points at the level of the upper edge of the shoulder blade, about 2 centimeters away from the dorsal processes. Massage downward, point by point, in a line to the sacrum. Again, you exert pressure by shifting your body weight over the extended arms, and apply pressure as your partner exhales. Use only a light amount of pressure in the kidney region. The resting hand remains on the sacrum for this

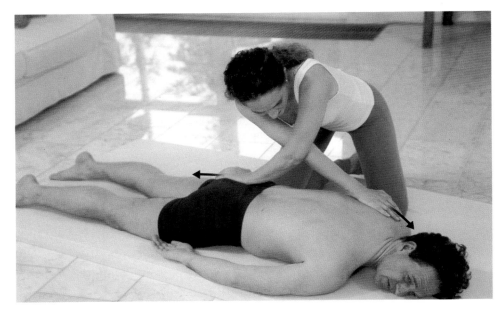

Stretching the back is the preparation for a basic massage.

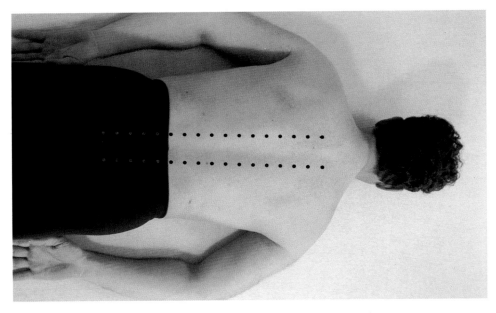

The treatment lines run from top to bottom on both sides of the spine.

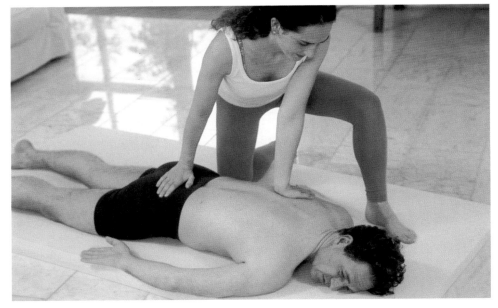

Apply pressure with the heel of your hand, and work from top to bottom point by point.

entire treatment. Massage down one side of the spine, then begin at the top again and massage the other side.

Thumb Pressure with Both Hands

You can also apply pressure using both thumbs at the same time. In this case, both thumbs are always at the same level. Sit on your knees above your partner's head. Place your thumbs on either side of the spine, at the level of the upper edge of the shoulder blades, about 2 centimeters away from the spine. Apply pressure as your partner exhales and release and move your thumbs slightly downward in the direction of the sacrum as he or she inhales. Once you have reached the highest point of the arch of the back, stop and change your position, so that you are kneeling next to the middle of your partner's back, and continue "walking" your thumbs down to the sacrum in rhythm with your partner's breathing.

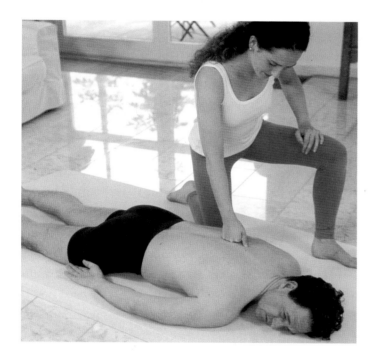

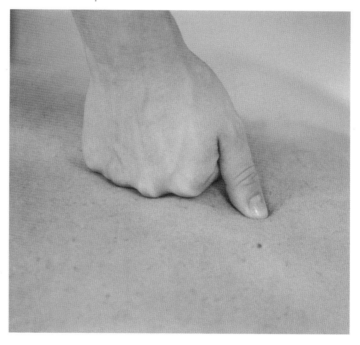

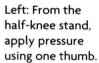

Left: From the half-knee stand, apply pressure using one thumb.

Right: Place the tip of your thumb down and support it with the other fingers.

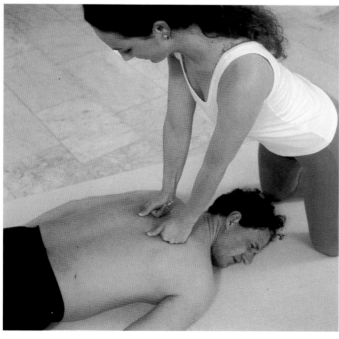

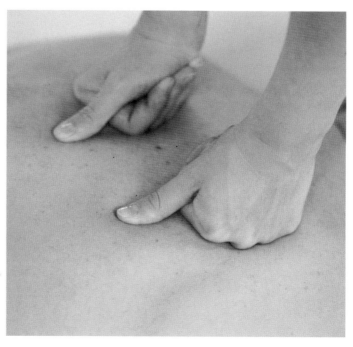

Left: If you are working with both hands, apply pressure by shifting your body weight forward and passing the pressure along via straight arms.

Right: Make sure that the thumbs are parallel to each other.

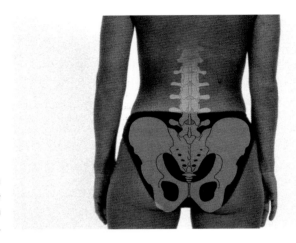

The sacrum connects the mobile spine with the pelvis.

Massaging the Area of the Sacrum

The sacrum forms the base of the spine. It consists of several vertebrae that are fused together. This is the point where the flexible spine meets the stationary, inflexible pelvis.

For this reason, the joints between the sacrum and the pelvic floor are very complicated. Often, lower back pain originates in this region. In addition, the skin above the sacrum is the reflex zone for the bladder and organs of the lower body. If one of these organs has an illness, a massage of the sacrum zone can be very pleasant.

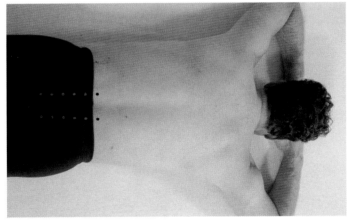

Massage the lower part of the back by . . .

> **The Sacrum Massage**
> - Apply pressure with both thumbs.
> - Apply pressure with the heel of the hand.
> - Move the sacrum "together."

Thumb Pressure with Both Thumbs

First find the holes of the sacral bone with your thumbs. They are located about 2 to 3 centimeters to either side of the middle of the sacrum. Moving your thumbs from the top down, you will feel on both the right side and the left four small indentations aligned in a row. It is possible that your partner will have an electric feeling when you apply pressure here, as these spots are the points where nerves exit from the spinal cord. These spots are also acupuncture points and lie on the bladder meridian.

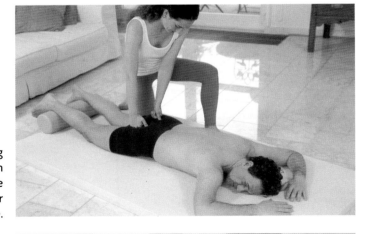

. . . applying pressure from the half-knee stand at your partner's side.

Place your thumbs on the top hole on each side. As your partner exhales, rise up onto your knees and apply pressure via your arms and shifting your body weight. Adjust the pressure based on the sensitivity of your partner. As your partner inhales, release the pressure and move your thumbs

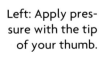

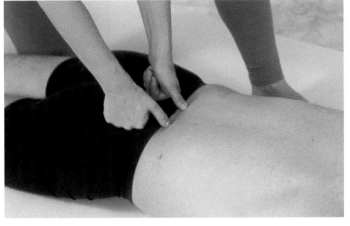

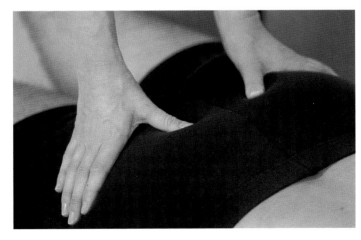

Left: Apply pressure with the tip of your thumb.

Right: In the lower sacrum region, it is easier to support your thumbs if you extend your fingers.

a little bit in direction of the coccyx. Massage the sacrum point by point in this manner.

Applying Pressure with the Heel of the Hand

After you have finished the above exercise, apply pressure on the sacrum region using the heel of your hand. To begin, sit in the heel seat next to your partner's pelvis and place the heels of your hand on either side of the spine. As your partner exhales, rise up onto your knees and apply pressure on the sacrum. As he or she inhales, release the pressure and move your hands slightly down, toward the sacrum. Continue applying and releasing the pressure in synchrony with your partner's breathing cycle until you have massaged the entire sacrum region. The pressure from the heels of your hands can be a little stronger than that from your thumbs, but it still should not be painful for your partner.

The strong pressure on the sacrum relaxes the region and often alleviates pain.

Pushing the Sacrum "Together"

Fold the fingers of your hands together. Keeping the fingers interlaced, place the palms of your hands on the sacrum. As your partner exhales, move the heels of the hands together above the sacrum. As your partner inhales, release the pressure and move your hands down. Continue this pattern until you have massaged the entire sacrum region. This technique serves to relax a tense sacrum region.

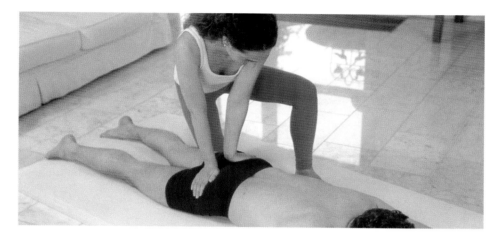

Apply pressure on the sacrum region using the heels of your hands. This alleviates pain.

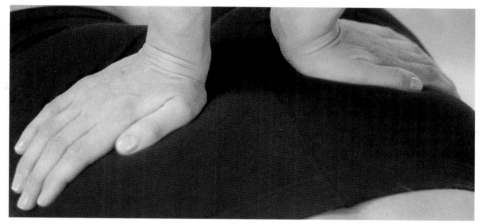

The hands make wide contact with the sacrum and the surrounding area.

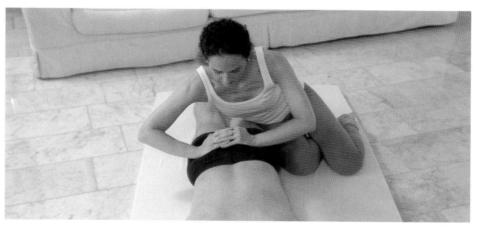

Move the heels of your hands together as your partner exhales.

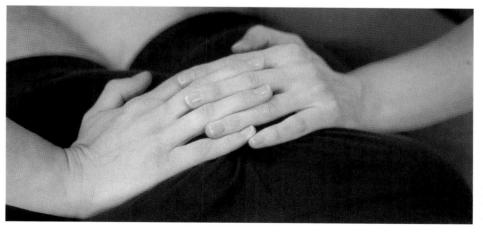

Make sure that your hands are exactly above the sacrum.

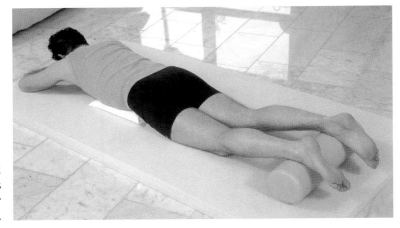

An optimal resting position is a precondition for good relaxation.

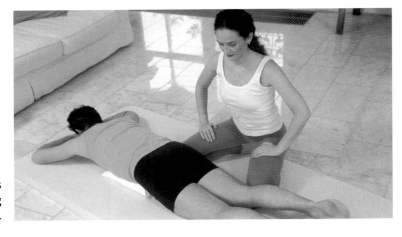

The heel seat is the basic starting position.

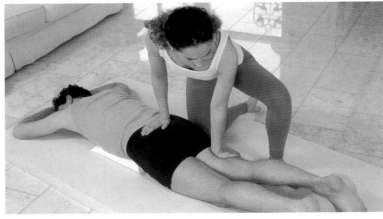

The resting hand is on the sacrum while the other transfers your weight.

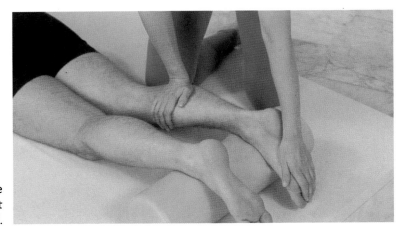

Firmly stroke the sole of the foot with a flat hand.

Massaging the Backs of the Legs

Our legs carry us through our lives. Unsurprisingly, their constant use often expresses itself in the wear and tear of our knee, hip, and foot joints. A sedentary lifestyle leads to the hardening and shortening of the muscles and tendons in the legs, which sooner or later leads to an energy imbalance in the legs.

There are six meridians on each leg that either start or end in the foot. Regular shiatsu massages loosen the muscles and tendons, improve circulation, and ultimately increase flexibility. We must not forget the feet in this context. When we walk or stand, the entire weight of our bodies rests on our feet. From an early age, feet are continuously forced into shoes that are too tight and, despite being very important, lead an uncared-for and rather poor existence. But according to the basic principles of foot reflexology, there are many reflex zones on the backs and soles of the feet that have a connection to the various parts of our bodies. For this reason, you should include the feet in a shiatsu massage.

You will massage and stretch each leg in turn and finish by stroking both feet.

> **Note**
> In the case of varicose veins or infections in the legs, do not use pressure techniques.

The Position

To massage the backs of the legs, have your partner lie on his or her stomach. Place a rolled-up towel or pillow under the ankles to support the feet and also to slightly bend the legs and knees, which helps ensure optimal relaxation. If necessary, adjust for a hollow back by placing a thin pillow under the abdomen area.

Pressure with the Heels of Your Hands

First massage the backs of the legs from top to bottom using the heels of your hands. Sit in the heel seat at about the level of your partner's knees. From this position, rise up on your knees and place the active hand below the buttocks on the middle axis of the thigh. Place the resting hand on the sacrum. As your partner exhales, apply pressure by moving your buttocks and shoulders forward. As your partner inhales, release pressure and move your hand down toward the feet a little bit. As your partner exhales, apply pressure again by shifting your body weight, and so on. Soon you will achieve a harmonious cycle in which you apply and release pressure in tandem with your partner's breathing. Skip massaging the sensitive zone on the back of the knee. You should apply stronger pressure on the thigh and reduced pressure on the calf. Massage from the buttocks to the heel in this manner. Once you have reached the heel, use your flat hand to stroke across the sole of the foot to the toes. Repeat this sequence twice.

Applying Thumb Pressure with One Hand

For applying pressure along the middle axis of the leg with one thumb, the initial position is the same as before. The resting hand is on the sacrum while the thumb of the active hand is on the middle axis of the thigh, below the buttocks. As your partner exhales, shift your weight forward onto the thumb; as he or she inhales, release the pressure. Move toward the heel point by point, again skipping the back of the knee, or at most applying very light pressure there. Since thumb pressure on the calf can be very painful at times, proceed as follows: After you have massaged from the thigh to the knee region with thumb pressure, change position so that you are in the heel seat next to your partner's feet. Place your partner's calf on your thigh and loosen it by walking both hands up and down along it.

Then hold the sole of the foot with your resting hand. With light pressure on the sole of the foot, lightly apply thumb pressure to massage and stretch the calf. The pressing and stretching should occur as your partner exhales. Massage point by point in this manner from the calf to the heel. To conclude, stroke the sole of the foot with your flat hand with some pressure.

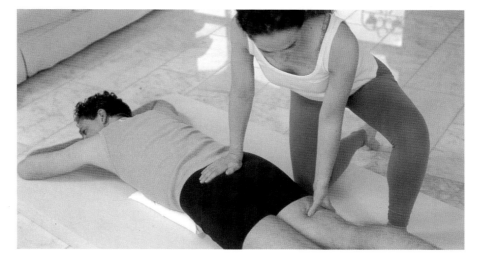

Use thumb pressure to massage from the buttocks to the back of the knee, but don't massage the knee itself.

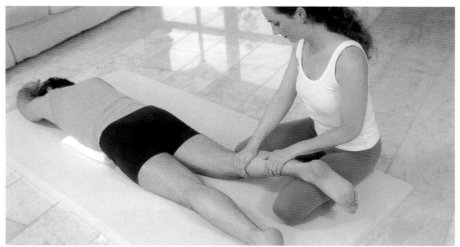

Walk the calves with both hands.

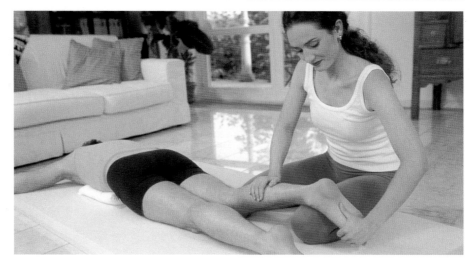

While applying pressure with your thumb, also stretch the calf muscles.

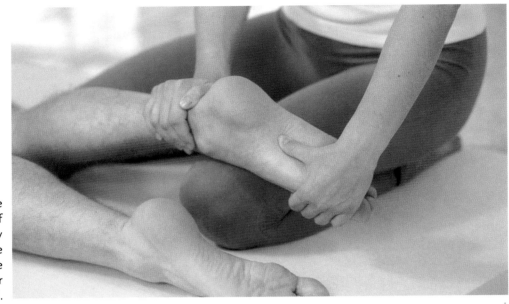

Stretching the heels and calf muscles: Apply gentle pressure on the sole of the foot with your hand.

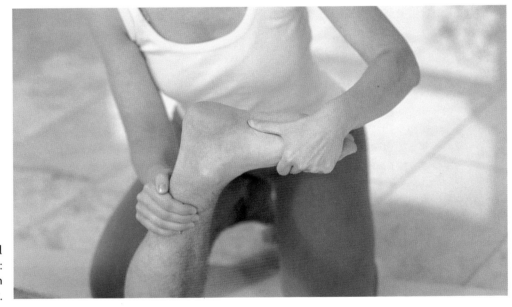

Stretching the heel and calf muscles: Repeat the stretch with the leg bent.

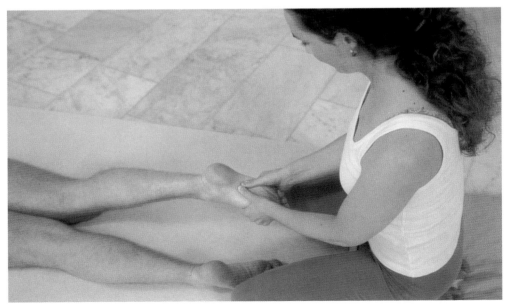

Thumb pressure: Apply pressure in points about a thumb-width apart.

Stretching the Heel and Calf Muscles

After you have applied thumb pressure on the calf muscles, you can now stretch the calf muscles. Hold the sole of the foot in one hand while holding the heel with your other hand. Apply light pressure on the sole. As your partner exhales, bend the leg so that the sole of the foot points toward the ceiling. Hold this position for several breathing cycles and then release. Repeat this stretch three times with each leg, afterward returning each leg to its resting position.

Pressure on the Foot with Both Thumbs

First use both thumbs to massage the sole of the foot. Apply pressure in several lengthwise lines over the entire sole of the foot. Take the foot into both hands and, starting in the heel region, press your thumbs point by point along your lines with the points about a thumb-width apart. Again, apply pressure as your partner exhales. Stroke the foot in conclusion.

Now go back and massage and stretch the other leg in the same way.

Pulling on the Legs

After you have massaged both legs, you should loosen them. To do this, crouch behind your partner and grasp the ankles from the outside. As your partner exhales, lightly tug on both legs by moving your pelvis backward. Keep up this tension for a few breathing cycles. Do not lift the legs during this exercise; lifting the legs could unpleasantly amplify a hollow back in the lumbar spine. The thighs should remain on the mat during this stretch. Finish by returning both legs to their resting position and stroking the feet one after the other.

The Leg Massage

- Massage the back of the leg with the heel of your hand.
- Massage the back of the thigh using thumb pressure up to the back of the knee.
- Place the calf over the thigh and massage it.
- Stretch the calf muscle.
- Apply pressure with the thumb on the sole of the foot.
- Massage the other leg in the same way.
- Pull on both legs.
- Finish with strokes.

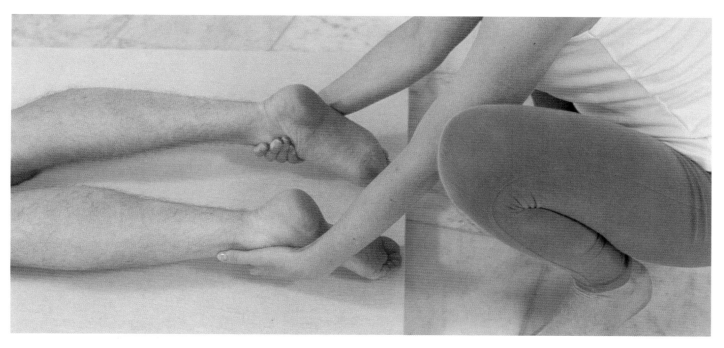

Hold the ankles from the outside so that you will have a solid grip on them while pulling.

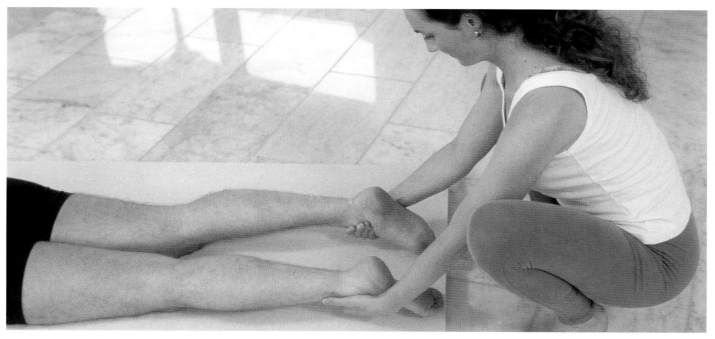

Pull by shifting the weight of your pelvis backward. Avoid lifting the legs while you pull.

Massaging the Shoulders and Neck Muscles

The shoulders are in a way the crossroads and connecting joint between the back, the arms, and the neck and throat area. Painful muscle knots often develop in this region. A simple shiatsu massage can release such tension and stimulate the flow of energy in the shoulder-arm-neck area.

The Position

For the massage described here, it is best to have your partner lie on his or her side. To allow optimal relaxation, have your partner stretch out his or her bottom leg while bending the top leg and laying it on the side of the body, supported by a rolled-up towel, a blanket, or a pillow. This support makes the position more stable. Your partner's bottom shoulder should push forward a little bit, and the bottom arm should lie in front of the body, with the elbow bent. Your partner's head should rest on a sturdy pillow so that the neck and spine are straight. You should be in the initial position, the heel seat, next to your partner's buttocks. The following pages describe techniques to treat the shoulders and the muscles on the sides of the neck.

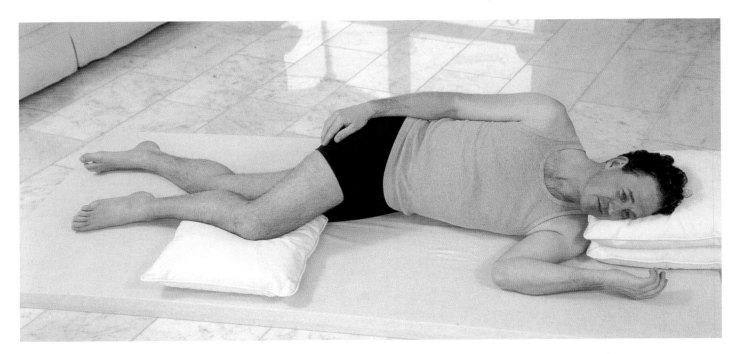

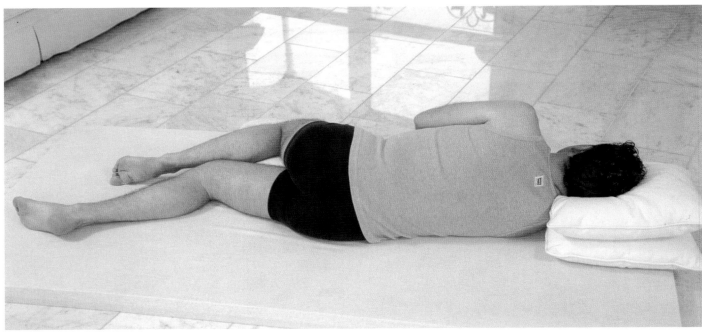

The head, top shoulder, and top leg are supported so that the entire spine forms a straight line.

Stretching the Shoulders

Cover your partner's shoulder with your hands. Move your left arm below your partner's left arm and place your left hand around the front of the shoulder. Place your other hand on the back of the shoulder and interlace your fingers. The weight of your partner's arm is now resting on your left lower arm. Once you have covered your partner's shoulder with your hands in this way, when your partner exhales, slightly pull the shoulder toward the feet by moving your upper body backward. Release as he or she inhales. Synchronize a pulling and releasing pattern to the breathing cycle of your partner.

Circling the Shoulder

Leave your hands in the same position as for the shoulder stretch. Now make large circles in a clockwise direction in such a way that the shoulder blade moves along as well. Follow this movement with your own upper body. The circling movements loosen the entire shoulder girdle.

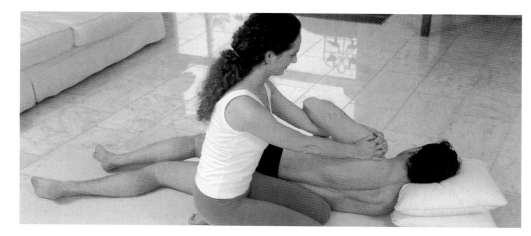

Take the front and back of the shoulder into your hands.

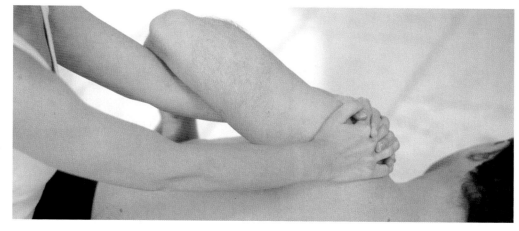

Pull the shoulder in synchrony with your partner's breathing . . .

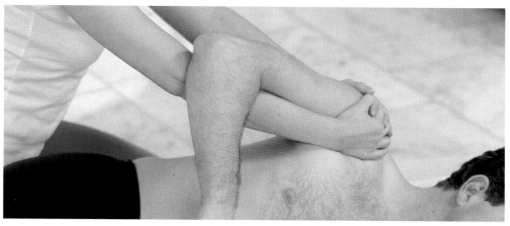

. . . by moving the weight of your upper body backward.

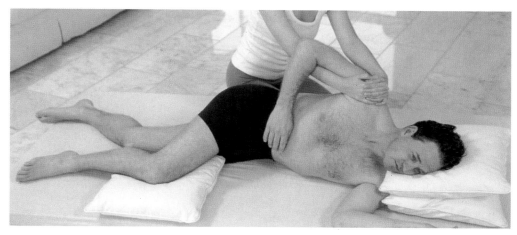

When rotating the shoulders, move your upper body with the motion.

Stroking and Stretching the Neck Muscles

Now very gently stretch the side neck muscles. Leaving your front hand on the shoulder, stroke with your other hand from the shoulder along the neck to the back of the head. At the same time, use your front hand to gently pull the shoulder down. Hold this stretch, applying slight pressure on the back of the head, for several breathing cycles. Release the pressure as your partner inhales. Perform this stretch three times in a row.

Shiatsu massage in the area of the side neck muscles can be initially painful if your partner is tense because of outside stress. But when done properly, it provides great relief. The muscles relax, and an existing headache quickly disappears.

"Cleaning the Wings"

Immediately below the shoulder blade is a broad, flat muscle that extends all the way to the shoulder joint. Massage

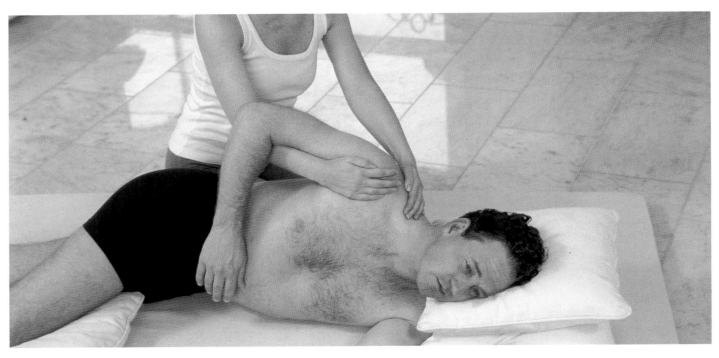

While the right hand pulls the shoulder down slightly, stroke the shoulder with your left hand.

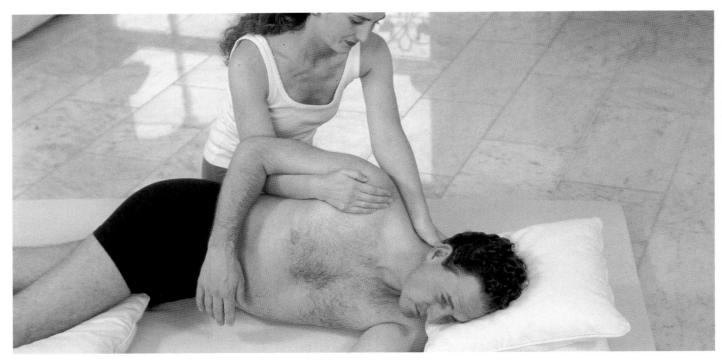

With one hand on the back of the head and the other on the shoulder, gently stretch the neck and shoulder muscles.

this muscle with your fingertips. Place the fingertips of your right hand immediately below the shoulder blade. As your partner exhales, move the shoulder to the back with your left hand. With the movement, the shoulder blade will "glide" right over the fingers of your right hand. Hold this position for several breathing cycles and then release the tension as your partner inhales.

Now have your partner turn over, and massage the shoulder and neck muscles on the other side in the same manner.

Massaging the Shoulder and Neck Muscles
- Position the recipient in a stable position with the spine straight.
- Stretch the shoulder.
- Circle the shoulder.
- Stretch the neck muscles on the side.
- Clean the wing.
- Massage the shoulder and neck muscles on the other side in the same way.

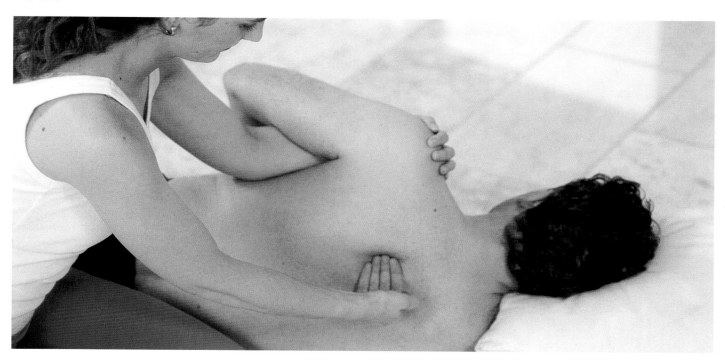

With your palm facing you, place your fingertips under the lower edge of the shoulder blade.

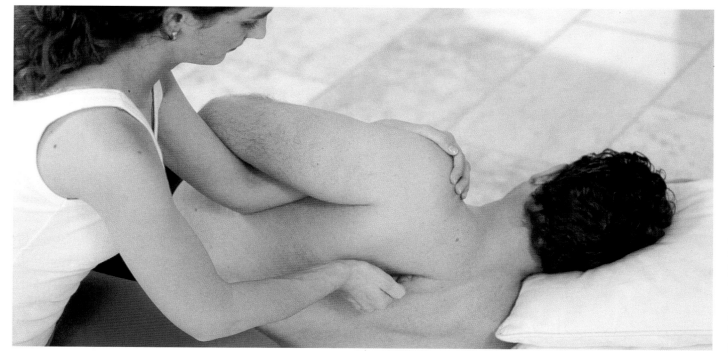

As your partner exhales, move your hands toward each other, causing the shoulder blade to slide over your fingertips.

The Hara or Abdominal Massage

Western society assigns little importance to the abdomen. It is thought of simply as the body area that houses the organs of digestion and elimination. In Eastern philosophy, however, the abdomen has a much deeper significance. The abdomen, or hara, is seen as the location of chi, our life energy. According to this thinking, a healthy hara is a prerequisite for health in the whole body. The stomach or abdominal massage shown here stimulates your chi.

> **Caution**
>
> For most people, the abdomen is very sensitive. Do not administer hara massages to pregnant women. Proceed very carefully in the case of existing pain in the lower abdomen.

The Position

The hara massage is done with your partner lying on his or her back. With some props you can relax the abdominal muscles and make the massage even more pleasurable. For this, support your partner's knees with a rolled-up blanket, which will slightly bend the knees and hip joints and relax the abdomen. Relax the abdomen further by slightly elevating the upper body, which you can do by placing one or two pillows under your partner's back. Your partner's arms should rest loose and relaxed next to his or her body.

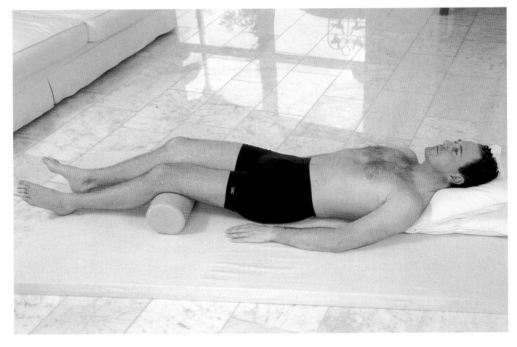

You can relax the abdominal surface by placing a rolled-up blanket under your partner's knees.

Feeling the Hara

The first step of the hara massage consists of making contact. Place one hand directly on your partner's abdomen and rest it there for a few breathing cycles. This initial contact helps prepare your partner for the coming massage.

Circular Strokes

Place both your hands on the abdomen and start making slow, clockwise circular movements. Gradually increase the size of the circles. Adjust the strength, speed, and rhythm of your strokes to the sensitivity of your partner. A good sign that you have the "right dosage" is

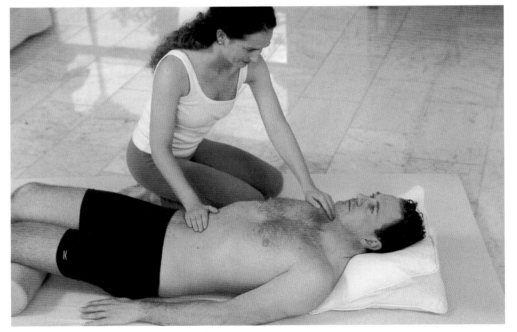

Feel the hara with your hand.

the increased relaxation of the abdomen, indicated when it becomes "softer."

"Cat's Paws"

After the circular strokes, walk your fingertips two or three times clockwise around the navel, as if your fingertips were the paws of a small cat. To do so, place your flat hand on the abdomen, bend your fingers at their base, and roll them up onto the fingertips. Then move and repeat. Pressure and touch should be very light. Do the same, after a slight delay, with your other hand, creating a fluid, rolling, harmonious movement.

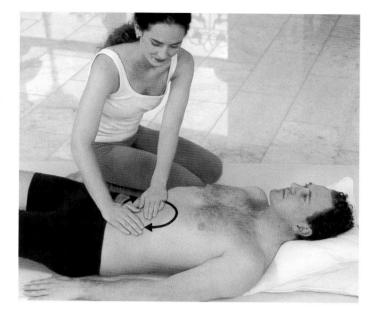

Carry out circular, clockwise movements with both hands.

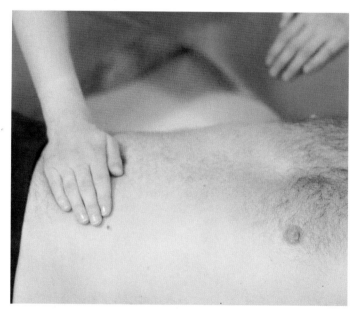

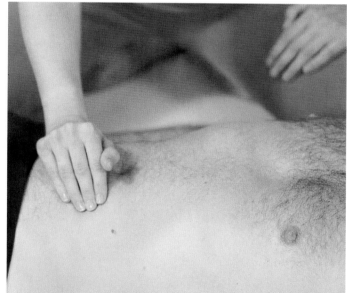

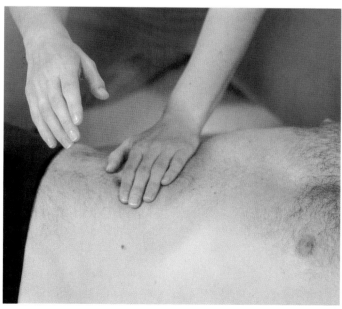

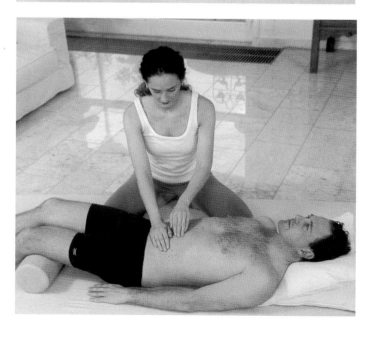

Placing the hands on the skin one after the other creates a fluid, rolling movement (cat's paws).

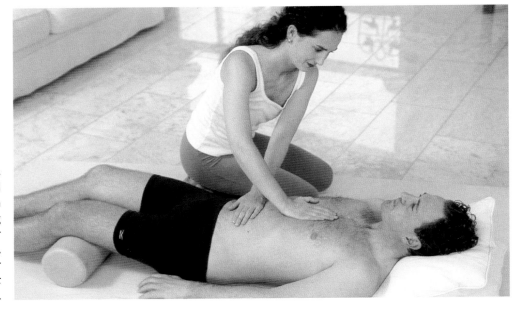

Place your hands on the upper and lower abdomen without applying pressure. As your partner inhales, move the upper hand upward bit by bit.

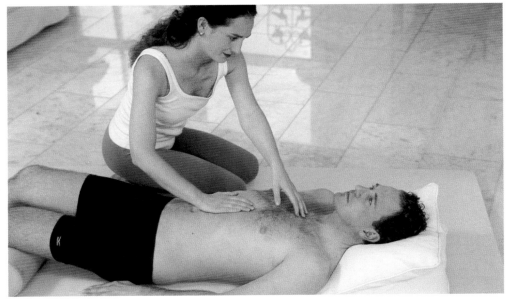

Use both hands to stroke from the rib cage to the abdomen.

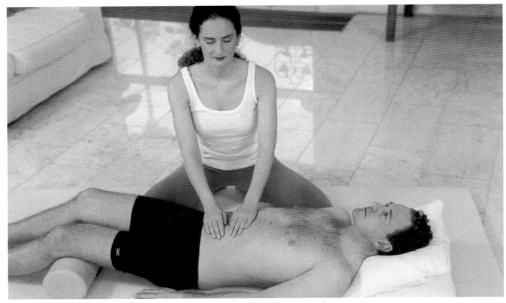

Place both hands on the abdomen and let them rest there for a few moments without applying pressure.

Deepening the Breathing

This exercise helps you direct and deepen your partner's breathing. Place one hand on the upper abdomen and the other on the lower abdomen. Slide the upper hand bit by bit from the upper abdomen past the sternum to the beginning of the neck. Move the hand upward with each intake of breath and rest the hand as your partner exhales.

Do not apply pressure with either hand.

Saying Farewell

End the hara massage by stroking your partner from the rib cage down to the abdomen, gently and slowly, with one hand after the other.

At the end, rest your hands on the abdomen for a few breathing cycles before breaking contact.

Massaging the Arms

The legs root us on the ground and are responsible for stability and movement. The arms serve to communicate. They gesticulate, hug, and receive. Their action radius is much larger than that of the legs. As on the legs, there are six energy pathways, or meridians, that run along the arms.

To massage the arms, your partner should be able to "let go" of them—that is, to let them hang loose and fully relaxed. Many people have difficulty doing this. The following loosening exercises are thus an ideal start to a massage of the arms.

As with the legs, you will massage first one arm and then the other.

The Position

The arm massage is best when the recipient is lying down. You can support his or her knees with a pillow; the upper body should rest flat on the mat. Begin by sitting on your heels at your partner's side.

Loosening

To loosen the arm, lightly and slowly shake it. For this, rise up onto your knees next to your partner. Place one hand on the shoulder joint and with the other lift your partner's arm at the wrist so that it bends at the elbow and the upper arm rises slightly above the mat. In this position, you can easily lead the arm from its base joint.

Move the arm back and forth with slight swings, and encourage your partner to consciously allow these passive movements of the arm.

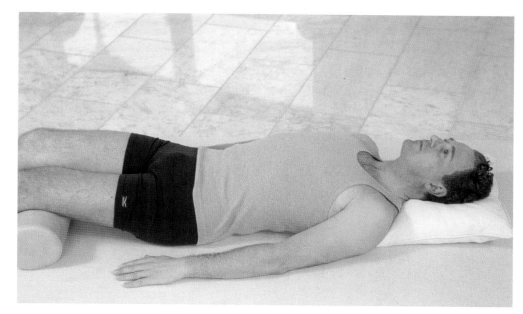

To begin the arm massage, have your partner lie down.

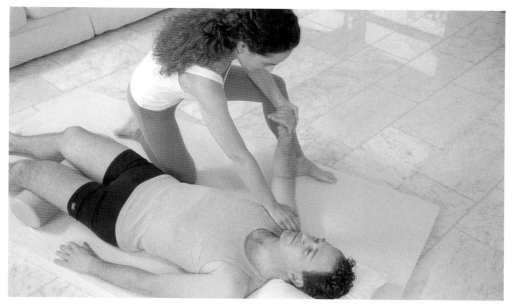

With the elbow bent, lift the arm . . .

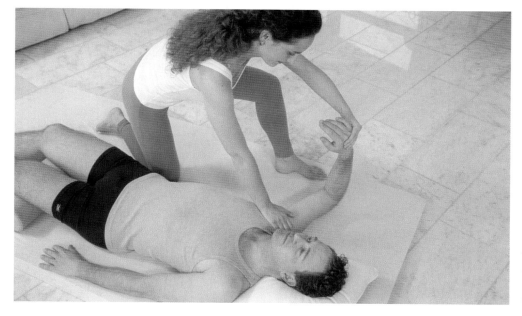

. . . and move it to the back and front with light swinging movements.

Circling the Arm

As an introduction, carry out circling movements with your partner's arm. For this, place your outside hand on the shoulder joint. With your inside hand, grasp the arm by the wrist and extend it up past your partner's head. Then bend the elbow and bring it to the side before returning the arm to its initial position by your partner's side. Repeat this movement five or six times.

Pressure with the Heel of the Hand

Extend the arm at a right angle from the body with the palm facing up. Place your resting hand on your partner's wrist and massage the inside of the arm with the heel of your active hand, moving point by point with gentle pressure from the shoulder to the hand. Do not massage the elbow region, as it is a very sensitive area. Depending on the width of your partner's arm, work in a single line or in parallel lines.

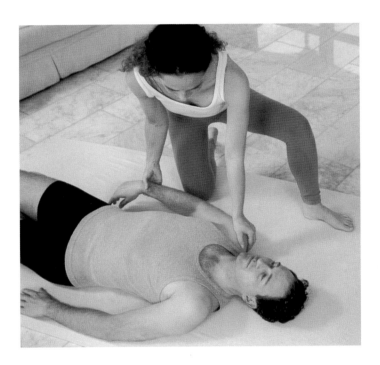

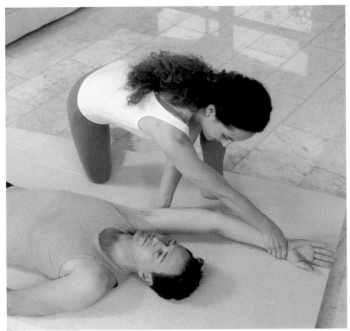

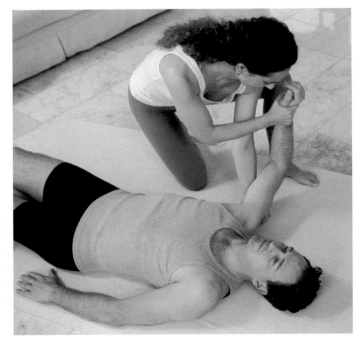

From a resting position, move the arm up, to the side, and then back down so that the elbow makes a circular movement.

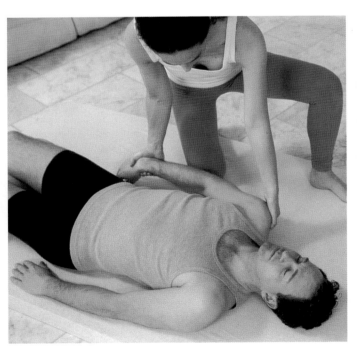

Pressure with the Thumb

You can repeat the above technique with your thumb. Your partner's arm remains extended from the body at a right angle and the palm continues to face up. Rest your right thumb on your partner's wrist. Apply point-by-point pressure from the shoulder down to the palm with your thumb in thumb-width distances. It is also possible to work with both thumbs at the same time, in which case you start from the shoulder and palm and work both thumbs in toward the elbow.

Which of the two variations you choose depends on what is more pleasant for your partner. You may also have a preference yourself.

Massage of the Arms
- Loosen the arm.
- Circle the arm.
- Apply pressure with the heel of the hand.
- Apply pressure with the thumb.
- Repeat for the other arm.

For both variations, work in several treatment lines and do not massage the sensitive elbow region.

When you have finished this technique, go back and begin loosening and massaging the other arm.

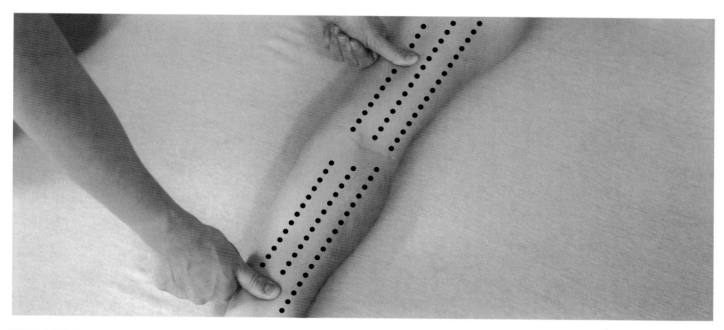

Top and bottom left: Apply pressure in several treatment lines. For each, work from the shoulder to the hand in points about one thumb-width apart.

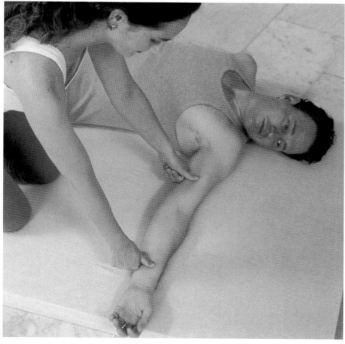

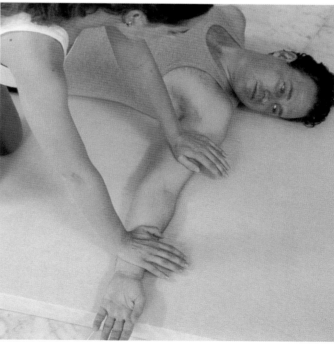

Apply gentle pressure with the heel of your hand.

Massaging the Hands

With their differentiated movements, our hands are our most important tools. The activities of the hands can be described as doing, receiving, and giving. It is hard to imagine civilization—in the sense of scientific and technological progress—being able to advance as far as it has without the differentiated range of motion offered by our hands.

As with the feet, there are many reflex zones on the hands that are connected to other parts of the body. Three meridians begin and end in the fingertips. For these reasons, shiatsu massage on the hands can be a very intense experience, much as with the foot. The introduction to this massage consists of simple loosening exercises during which your partner allows him- or herself to be led by you.

You should massage one hand completely and then go back and massage the other.

The Position

Usually the massage of the hands follows the massage of the arms. Ideally, your partner will be lying on his or her back, but if you are massaging only the hands, he or she can also be sitting upright.

Circling the Hands

This exercise serves to introduce the hands to the massage and to loosen them up. Position yourself in the heel seat next to your partner's arm. Grasp his or her lower arm below the wrist with one hand and with the other grip your partner's hand and, bending it as far into the wrist as possible while pulling gently on the hand to loosen up the wrist joint, lead it in circling movements. Circle the hand three times to the left and then three times to the right.

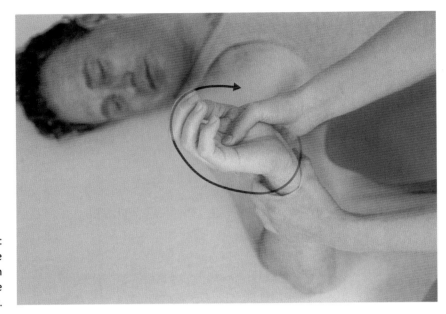

Circling the hands: Circle the hands in both directions while pulling lightly.

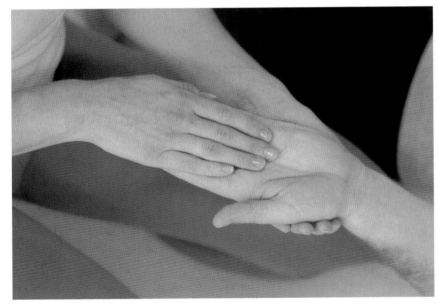

Stroking the palm: Use your fingers to stroke gently from the carpus to the fingertips.

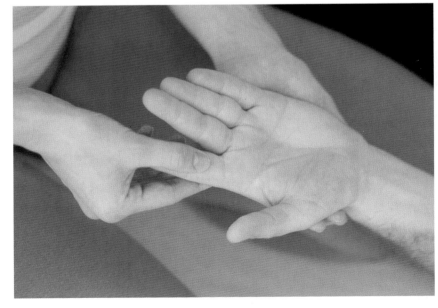

Stroking the fingers: Stroke each finger from its base up to its tip with light pressure.

Stroking the Palms and the Fingers

Hold your partner's hand with one hand and use the other hand to stroke it from the carpus across the palm to the fingertips and beyond. Then stroke each finger between your thumb and index finger from the base joint to the tip. Apply a light pressure on the base joint and use this pressure to pull along the finger. Repeat this stroke three times on each finger.

Pulling the Fingers

Grasp a finger base joint between your thumb and index finger. Use your other hand to pull that finger slightly. Exert the pull as your partner exhales and release the tension as he or she inhales. You will have optimal results by doing this stretch three times on each finger.

Thumb Pressure on the Palm

Hold the hand so that its palm faces up. In one of the spaces between the metacarpal bones, apply pressure on the palm point by point with your thumb, massaging from the carpus to the base joints. Once you have reached the base joints, start again on the carpus and repeat the massage in a new treatment line. Use this method to work the muscles between the individual metacarpal bones one after the other. Apply pressure in rhythm with your partner's breathing. Because the palm is a sensitive region, be sure to note your partner's reaction as you massage the palm and adjust the pressure accordingly.

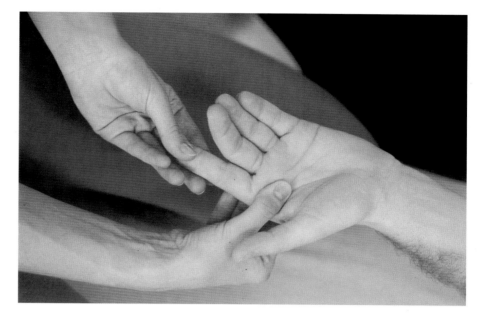

Pulling the fingers: Pull gently on each finger in synchrony with your partner's breathing.

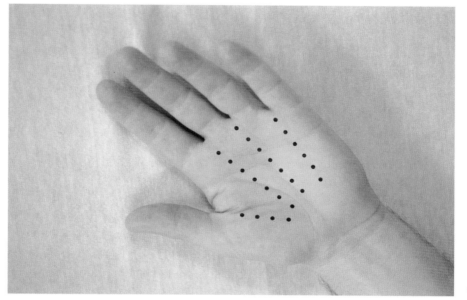

Thumb pressure: Press the muscles between the individual metacarpal bones in several treatment lines.

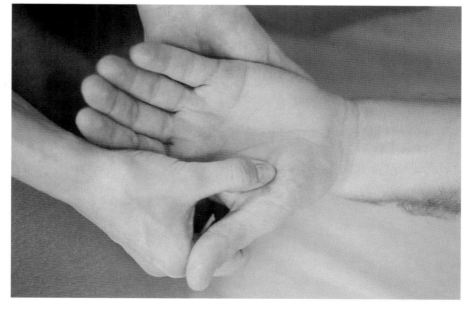

Apply pressure in rhythm with your partner's breathing.

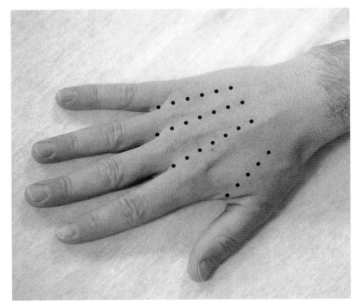

Apply thumb pressure in treatment lines running from the carpus to the base joints of the fingers.

Thumb Pressure on the Back of the Hand

Turn over your partner's hand so that its palm faces down and its back faces up.

Apply thumb pressure in the spaces between the meta-carpal bones. Massage point by point in treatment lines from the carpus up to the base joints.

The bones on the back of the hand are covered by only a very thin layer of skin, so be sure to apply only light pressure.

Stretching the Palm

Now turn your partner's hand so that the palm faces up.

Hook one pinkie into the space between your partner's pinkie and ring finger and the other pinkie into the space between your partner's thumb and index finger. Use your index, middle, and ring fingers to apply pressure on the back of your partner's hand. In this way, you are gently stretching the palm. Use your thumbs to stroke line by line from the wrist to the finger joints.

Finish the massage with strokes of the hand and fingers. Then go back and repeat the massage for the other hand.

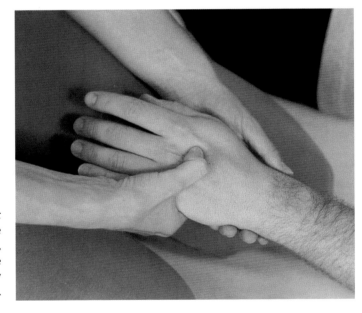

Apply only light pressure on the back of the hand, as these zones are frequently very sensitive.

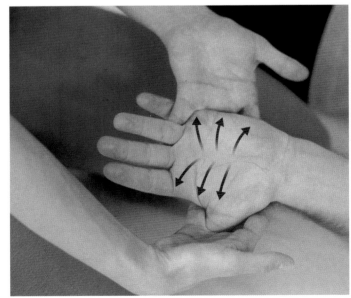

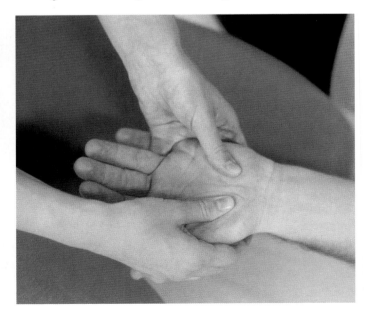

Left: Gently stretch the palm . . .

Right: . . . and stroke it from the wrist to the finger joints.

Massaging the Neck

The spine, or, to be more precise, the neck, is the connector between the head and the back. The cervical vertebrae are the most flexible parts of the spine but also the least stable. They allow the head a great range of motion. Bad posture, psychological stress, and many other problems can cause muscle tension that greatly reduces the flexibility of this zone. Neck pain is almost like a toothache, present with every small movement.

You can loosen the muscles in the neck region with a simple shiatsu massage. This massage will also stimulate the flow of energy in the neck and prevent painful tension. Your partner should lie on his or her back for this part of the massage, with his or her head lying flat on the surface, and you should position yourself in the heel seat above your partner's head.

Taking the Head into Your Hands

Take the back of your partner's head into both your hands. To do this, place your hands underneath your partner's head by rolling the head first to one side and then the other. Allow the head to rest in your hands for a few breathing cycles.

Stroking with Both Hands

Use both hands to stroke your partner from the neck to the back of the head. To do this, move your hands down in a V shape, leaving your partner's head resting on your lower arms. Now stroke across the neck to the back of the head as your partner exhales.

Stroking Hand over Hand

Place one hand on your partner's neck and stroke with it toward the back of the head. As soon as the first hand reaches the back of the head, place the second hand on the neck and move it upward. Replace the first hand on the neck and continue stroking in a fluid hand-over-hand movement, with which you are applying a slight pull.

Neck Massage
- Position the recipient on his or her back with the head flat.
- Rest the head in both of your hands.
- Stroke the neck with both hands.
- Stroke the neck hand over hand.

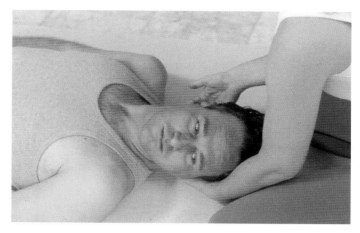

Grasp the head by first placing one hand and then the other underneath it.

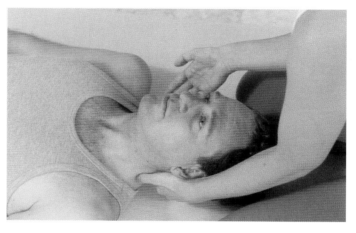

Strokes up the neck to the back of the head . . .

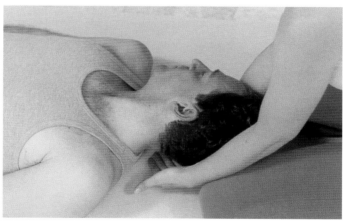

. . . are especially pleasant for neck tension.

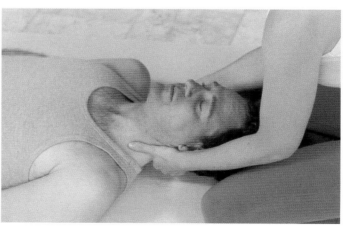

Stroke the neck hand over hand while applying light pressure.

Massaging the Head and Face

The head and facial massage is probably the most relaxing and pleasurable part of receiving a shiatsu massage. Shiatsu harmonizes and regulates the flow of energy in the meridians that run along the head and face. A pleasant side effect is that massaging the face dissolves tensions of the facial muscles and gives it a relaxed and beautiful appearance. Take a lot of time for the head and facial massage. Your partner should lie on his or her back, with the head resting directly on the mat, without a pillow. You should sit in the heel-seat position above your partner's head.

Thumb Pressure on the Middle Axis

Place one thumb on top of the other on the middle axis of the forehead, above the nose. Apply pressure point by point in rhythm with your partner's breathing, applying pressure on the exhalation and releasing on the inhalation,

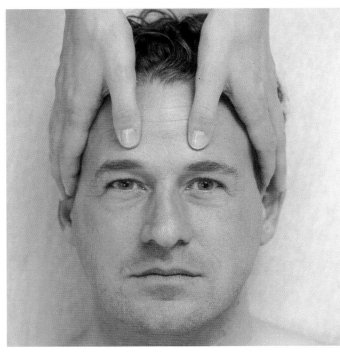
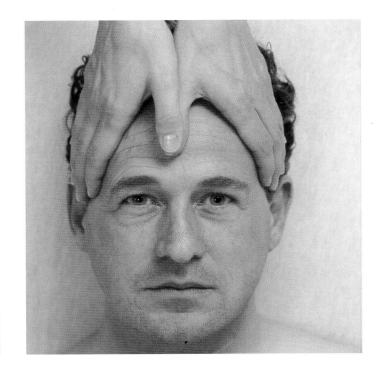
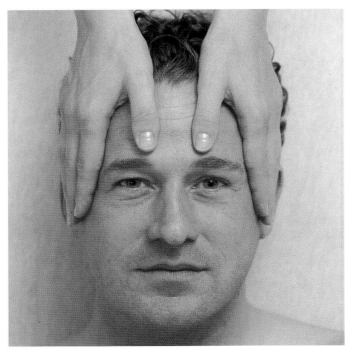
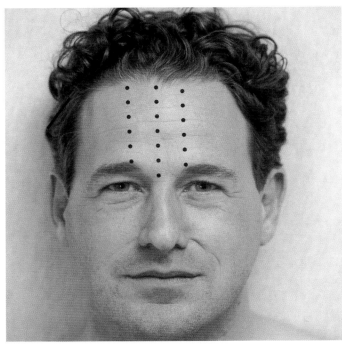

Left: Orient yourself on these treatment lines when administering thumb pressure on and to the sides of the middle axis.

Right: Apply pressure point by point on the middle axis in thumb-width steps.

Left: The pressure points parallel to the middle line often help with headaches that are located in the forehead.

Right: Begin the strokes by returning your thumbs to the forehead.

and move in thumb-width steps across the forehead to the back of the head.

Thumb Pressure to the Side of the Middle Axis

Place the thumbs about 2 centimeters on each side of the middle axis above the eyebrows. Apply pressure point by point in lines parallel to the middle axis, moving up to the back of the head. Again, apply and release pressure in rhythm with your partner's breathing.

Facial Strokes

Place your thumbs in the middle of the forehead and stroke them out to the temples while applying light pressure. Repeat this stroke under the hairline, and then again in a series of lines from the hairline to the eyebrows. Treat the whole face in this way, including the region below the eyes, the region below the cheekbone, the upper jaw region, and the chin region.

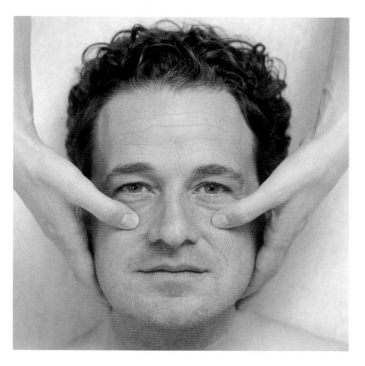

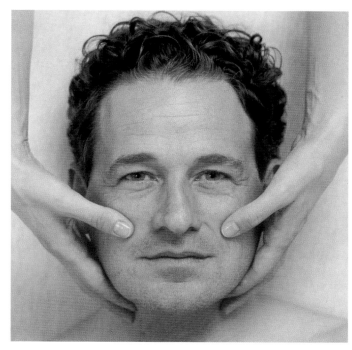

Left: Apply light strokes under the eyes, . . .

Right: . . . in the area under the cheekbone, . . .

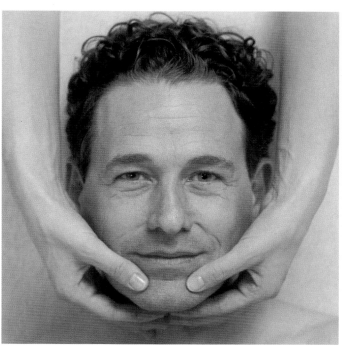

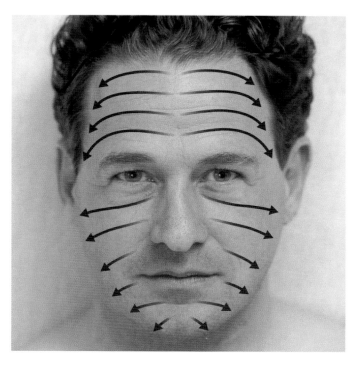

Left: . . . and finally in the chin area.

Right: The arrows outline the strokes.

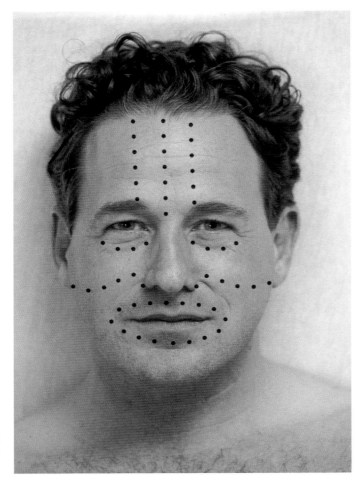

These lines map the paths of thumb pressure.

Thumb Pressure on the Face

After the strokes, administer a pressure massage using your thumbs. Walking along the same lines as for the strokes, apply pressure point by point in this order: across the forehead region, across the region above the eyes, below the cheekbones, and along the upper jaw and the chin. Below the cheekbones you can also apply pressure with your fingertips.

Concluding the Facial Massage

To conclude the facial massage, place both palms on your partner's ears. Leave your hands there for 1 to 2 minutes and then slowly remove them. This amplifies the relaxing effects of the facial massage.

Left: Apply pressure on the forehead, . . .

Right: . . . under the eyes, . . .

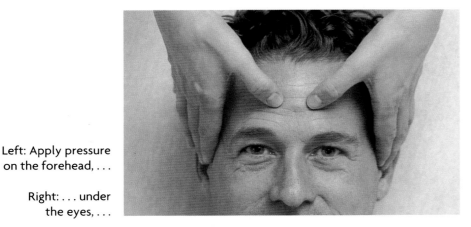

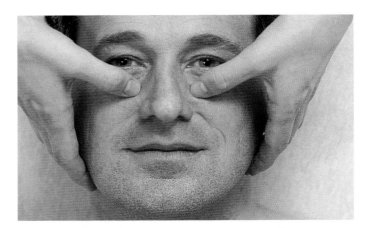

Left: . . . under the cheekbones, . . .

Right: . . . and in the chin area.

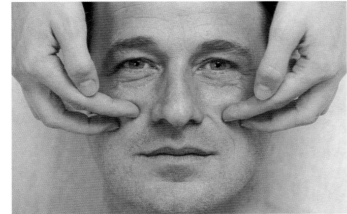

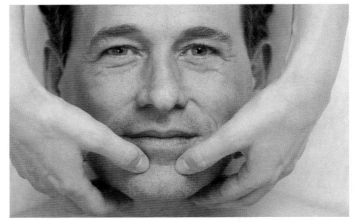

The Conclusion of the Shiatsu Massage

Sit in the heel-seat position at your partner's side. Place your hands on his or her hara. Leave them there for a few breathing cycles. Now sit at your partner's feet and place your hands on the backs of the feet, leaving them there for a few breathing cycles. Afterward, allow your partner to rest for 15 to 20 minutes. Cover him or her with a woolen blanket. The feeling of relaxation engendered by the massage can continue on long past this rest period. Advise your partner to be careful when maneuvering through traffic or the rest of everyday life. The appearance of any reactions such as anxiety and fever shows that your partner's body is responding to the massage, and they usually disappear by themselves.

Shiatsu Massage at a Glance

Massaging the Back
The back experiences pain most frequently of any body part, often because of chronic stress to it. A back massage is a good way to start a shiatsu massage. Before you begin the massage, carry out overall loosening and stretches to relax the muscles in a pleasant way.

Massaging the Sacrum
The reflex zones of the bladder and the organs of the lower body are at the base of the spine. Massaging the sacrum can thus have positive effects on these organs. Moving the sacrum "together" also relaxes this tense body area.

Massaging the Backs of the Legs
Lack of exercise can lead to an energy imbalance in the legs. Shiatsu massage improves circulation in the legs and supports the mobility of the leg joints. Massage of the backs and soles of the feet also has positive effects.

Massaging the Shoulder and Neck Muscles
Massaging the shoulders and neck muscles releases painful tensions of the muscles. The resulting relief of this area stimulates the flow of energy in the body.

Massaging the Hara (Abdomen)
In Far Eastern philosophy, the abdomen plays a much larger role than in Western society. The hara houses our life energy, or chi. A massage of the hara influences chi and leads to a feeling of healthy well-being throughout the body.

Massaging the Arms
Like the legs, the arms contain by six meridians, and thus massaging them can have a positive influence on the massage recipient. It is important that the arms of your partner be relaxed and loose. Loosening exercises are a good preparation for this massage.

Massaging the Hands
The human hands are important tools. They, like the feet, have many reflex zones through which you can influence the entire body. A massage of the hands is just as pleasant for the recipient as is a massage of the feet.

Massaging the Neck
The neck is one of the most mobile, but also one of the least stable, parts of the body. Due to bad posture and psychological stress, it can have many painful tensions. A shiatsu massage loosens the muscles and stimulates chi flow in the body.

Massaging the Head and Face
The shiatsu massage of the head and face regulates the flow of chi in the meridians. It also leads to a loosening of the facial muscles, which leaves the recipient with a relaxed, beautiful look. Take a lot of time with this part of the massage.

Saying Farewell
End the shiatsu massage by placing your hands on your partner's hara and leaving them there for a few seconds. Then place your hands on the backs of the feet and leave them there for a little while.

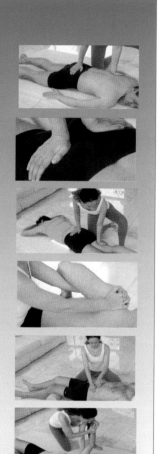
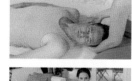
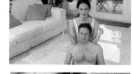
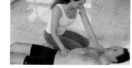

Alleviating Ailments

Aside from maintaining health and increasing overall well-being, reflex-therapeutic methods can also have a positive influence on existing illnesses. However, these methods are only complementary treatment; in no way should self-treatment or reflexology therapy replace or even delay medical treatment. This chapter describes some of the most common ailments and treatment methods for each based on the reflexology massages discussed in this book.

Allergies

The function of our immune system is to protect our body against foreign substances. Via the air we breathe, our skin, and the food we eat, pathogens and other damaging substances from our environment can enter our bodies. This is when the immune system becomes active as the body's police force: it recognizes foreign "intruders" and destroys them. For this job, it has at its disposal an array of weapons, which produce antibodies tailored specifically to the substance in question. The antibody response usually eliminates any danger. If, at one time or another, a pathogen returns to the body, the cells quickly "remember" it and immediately produce larger quantities of the needed antibody. This time around, the defense works even more quickly, sometimes without any symptoms of illness.

However, such an elaborate system is susceptible to disturbances. Often, our immune system become hypersensitive and overreacts, fending off even harmless substances in a manner that can have negative effects on the whole body. A person with such a hyperactive immune system is no less susceptible to illness than others—on the contrary, his or her body is weakened by the constant overreactions. Such overreactions of the immune system are called allergies, and the substances that cause these reactions are called allergens.

One example of an allergy is hay fever. In this case, plant particles, most often pollen, act as allergens and cause itchy, teary eyes as well as a chronic cough. Other allergens, such as certain foodstuffs, cause itchy rashes on the skin or intestinal cramps with diarrhea. Allergies can also have symptoms with life-threatening consequences, such as swelling of the mucous membranes in the mouth-throat area and effects on the circulation system up to the point of shock.

In treating allergies, there are two principal goals: One is to lessen the direct symptoms using medication and the other is to have a long-term influence on the immune system. The latter includes sensitization, a method in which the body is introduced to allergens in very small steps and thus made less sensitive to their presence. This is a promising route, especially for children and for allergies provoked by insect toxins.

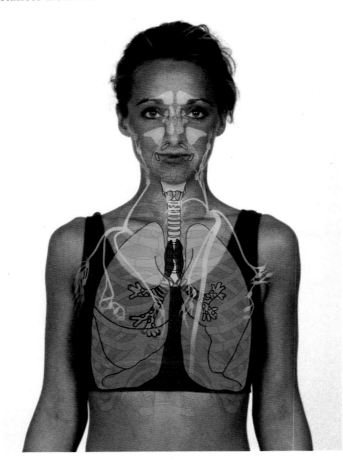

Allergic reactions often cause problems in the breathing passages.

What You Can Do

Whenever possible, avoid the allergens that cause the outbreak. Do away with exaggerated hygiene. Soap and daily showers dry out the skin, which causes it to lose its protective barrier. Use unscented laundry detergent and soaps, as perfumes tend to cause allergies. Strengthening measures—for example, regular visits to the sauna—improve the immune defenses of the mucous membranes. Maintain a balanced diet, and avoid physical and psychological stress.

How Can Reflexology Help?

Reflexology massages can alleviate acute symptoms of hay fever, such as watering, itchy eyes and a running nose. Foot, hand, and ear reflexology massages are especially well suited in the following combinations:
  * massage of the foot and ear reflex zones
  * massage of the hand and ear reflex zones

Start the treatment with a foot or hand massage and then carry out an ear massage.

Foot Reflexology Massage

The focus areas should be the zones of the eyes, the nose-throat area, the breathing passages, and the lymphatic organs.

Massage Sequence

  * Introduction: sandwich strokes.
  * Massage the head zones on the tops and bottoms of the toes with the tweezers grip, from the big toe to the fifth toe in several treatment lines.
  * Transition: sandwich strokes.
  * Massage the zones of the lymphatic system in the head and throat area using the tweezers grip, grasping the skin between the toes and gently stretching it up and down.
  * Massage the zones of the breathing passages and the lung on the top of the foot using your index finger.
  * Massaging the zones of the breathing passages and the lung on the sole of the foot using the thumb walk.
  * Conclusion: sandwich strokes.
  * Massage the other foot in the same way.
  * Stretch the heels of both feet.

Left foot

Left foot

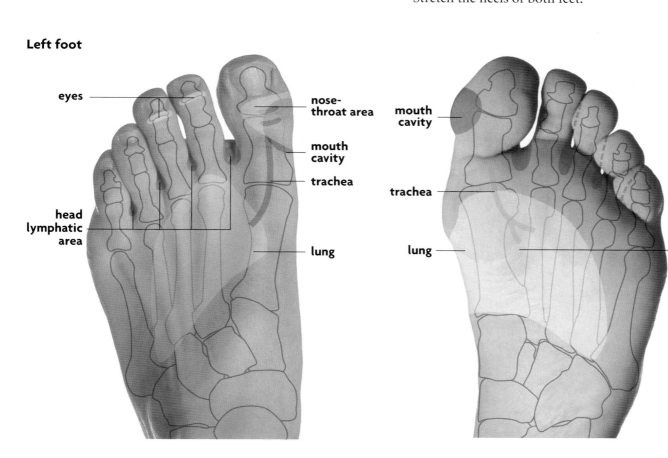

To treat allergies, locate the zones of the head and the breathing passages.

Hand Reflexology Massage

Massage of the reflex zones on the hand is analogous to the reflexology massage of the foot. The focus areas should be the zones of the eyes, the nose-throat area, the breathing passages, and the lymphatic organs.

Before you begin massaging the individual zones on the hand, you should do an overall introduction with strokes. The sandwich strokes described on page 114 are especially well suited for this. Massage first one hand and then the other. Repeat each technique three to five times on each hand. End the massage by stroking and stretching the palms.

Sequence of the Massage

- Introduction: sandwich strokes.
- Massage the head zones on the fronts and backs of the fingers with the tweezers grip, from the base of the thumb up to the pinkie in several treatment lines.
- Massage the zones of the lymphatic pathways in the head and throat area with the tweezers grip, gently stretching the skin between the fingers.
- Massage the zones of the breathing passages and the lung on the palm of the hand with the thumb walk.
- Massage the zones of the breathing passages on the back of the hand point by point using the caterpillar walk.
- Conclusion: sandwich strokes.
- Stretch the palm.
- Massage the other hand in the same way.

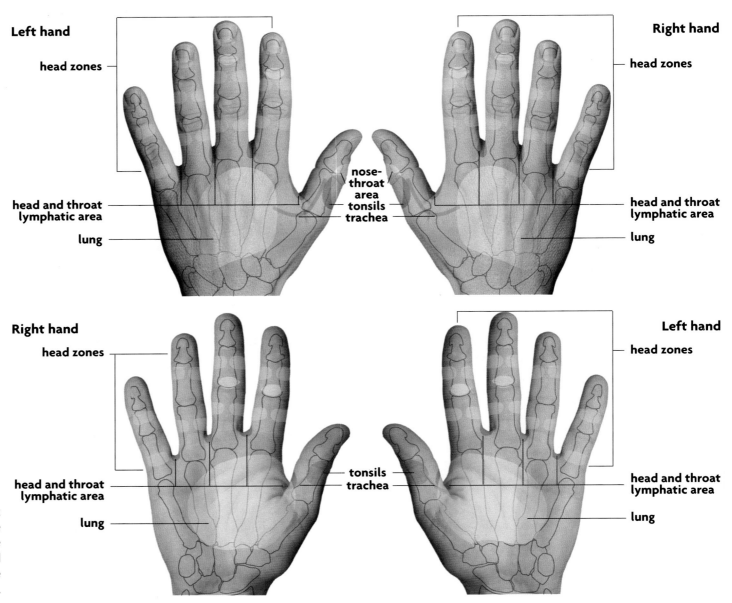

Left hand

head zones

head and throat lymphatic area

lung

nose-throat area
tonsils
trachea

Right hand

head zones

head and throat lymphatic area

lung

Right hand

head zones

head and throat lymphatic area

lung

tonsils
trachea

Left hand

head zones

head and throat lymphatic area

lung

These reflex zones on the hand can be massaged to alleviate allergic reactions.

Ear Reflexology Massage

The ear reflexology massage is well suited for use in combination with foot and hand reflexology massages. It is especially useful because of its ease of self-treatment: you can massage your own ears basically anytime and anywhere. Before you begin with a point-by-point massage, carry out some strokes that cover the whole ear to prepare it for the pointed massage. If you are massaging yourself, you can massage both ears at the same time using one hand on each ear. If you're massaging your partner's ear, finish one before turning to the other. Repeat the strokes four or five times. Press each zone or point for 5 to 10 seconds. Conclude the ear massage with strokes.

Sequence of the Massage

- Introduction: stroke with the thumb in several lines along the helix.
- Massage both lengthwise and crosswise the eye, forehead, sun, and main omega points on the earlobe.
- Massage the zones of the lung and pulmonary plexus with your index finger.
- Massage the shen men and allergy point using your thumb and the tip of your index finger.
- Conclusion: stroke with the thumb in several lines along the helix.
- Massage the other ear in the same way.

Right ear

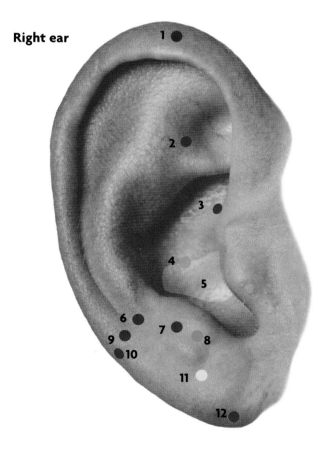

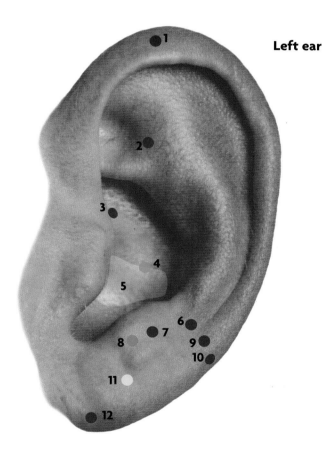

Left ear

The ear reflexology points pictured here alleviate allergy symptoms.

1 allergy point	**7 sun point**
2 shen men	**8 forehead point**
3 omega-1 point	**9 jerome point**
4 pulmonary plexus	**10 point of desire**
5 lung zone	**11 eye point**
6 polster point	**12 main omega point**

Back Pain

Today, back pain is among the most common ailments in our society. Some experts estimate that almost 80 percent of the American population will experience a back problem at some time in their lives, and one half of all working Americans report having back symptoms each year. According to statistics of health insurers, every third time an employee calls in sick and every second application for early retirement makes reference to back problems.

As discussed earlier, the spine has the shape of a double S, which enables it to support the body in a variety of sitting positions; to buffer shocks when we are walking, jumping, and running; to carry the entire weight of the body; and to allow a wide range of movements from the head to the buttocks.

The most common cause of back pain is bad posture in the spine area. Many school-aged children already suffer from a sideways bend (scoliosis), backward bend (kyphosis), or frontal bend (lordosis) of the spine. These bends are caused by the changing ways in which children spend their free time. Playing involves increasingly less movement and increasingly more sitting in front of the television or computer. The muscles that support the spine are not used enough, causing them to atrophy. At the same time, there is an excess load on the muscles of the back, neck, and shoulders, which react with tension and pain.

A sudden pain in the lumbar area after a sudden movement of bending over or getting up is called lumbago. Such a pain can be quite intense and can lead to a very restricted range of motion. The cause for this is usually degenerative damage of the disks —that is, damage caused by wear and tear—that is amplified by bad posture as well as by obesity.

If the wear and tear on the disks is very pronounced, a herniation can occur. This happens when a disk moves forward and onto the nerves that run alongside the spine, causing disruptions in sensory perceptions or paralysis in the legs. Difficulty urinating or defecating can also be a symptom of a herniated disk.

Back pain can also be a result of psychological conflicts. People with a lot of psychological stress "hang their heads" down. Their shoulders droop and they walk hunched over, carrying "the weight of the world" on their backs.

What You Can Do

Ensure that you get enough exercise in fresh air, and if necessary, reduce your body weight. Avoid prolonged periods of sitting and standing. If this is not possible—you have work obligations, for example—at least try to sit or stand with your upper body upright and to shift your weight from one foot to the other while standing. Avoid stooping over by bending your back; instead, keep your back straight and bend at the knees. If you are experiencing back pain for more than a week, see a doctor. Depending on the symptoms, he or she may be able to help you by prescribing physical therapy or medication.

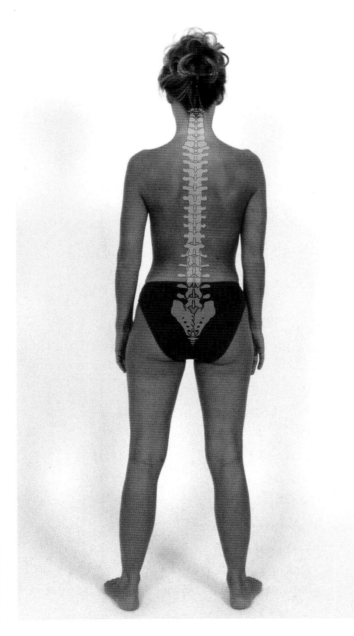

Almost 80 percent of us suffer from occasional back pain.

How Can Reflexology Help?

Shiatsu and reflexology massages are excellent measures for treating back pain. It is important to choose the method with which you are most comfortable and that at the same time is pleasant for your partner. If possible, begin with a shiatsu massage of the back, as described beginning on page 158, and of the shoulder and neck area, as described beginning on page 170. For immediate relief, you can also use ear or head reflexology, in combination with foot reflexology, to effectively alleviate pain. Head, ear, and foot reflexology massages work well in the following combinations:

- massage of the reflex zones on the head and foot
- massage of the reflex zones on the ear and foot

Foot Reflexology Massage

Foot reflexology massage is quite effective for relieving back pain. The zones of the spine are on the inside edges of the feet. The zone of the cervical spine is in the area of the base joint of the big toe, followed by the zone of the thoracic spine, followed by the zone of the lumbar spine and then the zone of the sacrum, which is in the area of the heel bone.

Sequence of the Massage

- Introduction: sandwich strokes.
- Massage the zone of the cervical spine using the thumb walk.
- Massage the zone of the thoracic spine using the thumb walk.
- Massage the zone of the lumbar spine using the thumb walk.
- Massage the zone of the sacrum using the thumb walk.
- Conclusion: sandwich strokes.
- Massage the other foot in the same way.
- Stretch both feet at the heels.

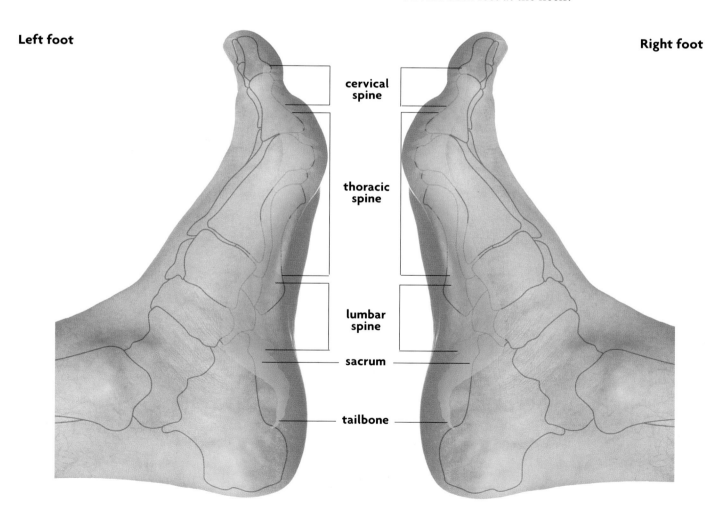

Left foot

Right foot

cervical spine

thoracic spine

lumbar spine

sacrum

tailbone

The reflex zones you will massage for back pain are located on the inside edges of the feet.

Head Reflexology Massage

Which zones to massage depends on where in the back you are experiencing pain. In the case of pain in the cervical spine, the neck, or the shoulders, massage the A or B zones. In the case of pain in the area of the thoracic spine, massage the E zone. For pain in the lumbar spine, massage the D points and D zones. Locate the painful points using the tip of your thumb and apply circling or steady pressure on the spots until the pain subsides. As the pain subsides, the back pain will do the same.

Sequence of the Massage

- Locate the pressure-sensitive zones on one side of the head:
  ▸ problems in the area of the cervical spine: A and B zones;
  ▸ problems in the area of the thoracic spine: E zone; or
  ▸ problems in the area of the lumbar spine: points D1 through D5 and the D zones.
- Massage the sensitive points with the tip of your thumb until the pain subsides.
- Massage the other side of the head in the same way.

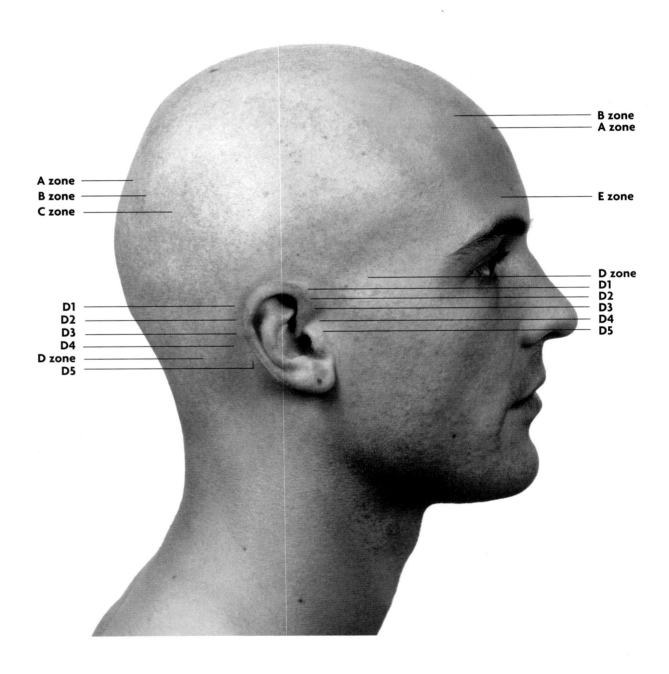

Massage the points that are sensitive to the touch in these reflex zones.

Ear Reflexology Massage

Massaging the appropriate ear zones is a quick and reliable way to alleviate back pain. The zones of the spine are located around the bend in the anthelix. The cervical spine zone is in the lower part, while the bend corresponds to the zones of the thoracic spine and the lumbar spine. The zones of the sacrum and tailbone are located in the upper area of the anthelix. The zones of the spine, with its muscles and tendons, comprise a broad band in this area.

In addition to massaging these zones, it is useful to massage the shen men, polster, and jerome points. Begin the massage by stroking the helix area in several parallel paths with your thumb. Then massage the area of the spine point by point in several parallel paths, beginning from the area of the cervical spine at the bottom and mov-

ing upward. To conclude, stroke the ear along the line of the helix in several paths. In the case of self-treatment, you can massage both ears at the same time. Carry out each stroke four or five times, and press each point for 5 to 10 seconds.

Sequence of the Massage

- Introduction: strokes with the thumb in several lines along the helix.
- Massage the spine zones point by point using the tips of the thumb and index finger in several parallel paths.
- Massage the shen men, polster, and jerome points.
- Conclusion: strokes with the thumb in several lines along the helix.

Right ear

Left ear

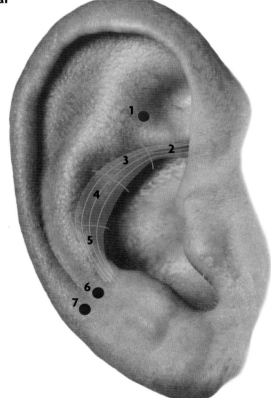

The reflex zones of the spine are located in the area of the anthelix.

1 shen men point

2 sacrum/tailbone zone

3 lumbar spine zone

4 thoracic spine zone

5 cervical spine zone

6 polster point

7 jerome point

Breathing Problems

Through the air that passes through our upper breathing passages (nose, throat, and trachea), our breathing system is in constant contact with pathogens such as viruses and bacteria. That is why many infectious diseases begin with symptoms, such as congestion, sore throat, and cough, in the area of the breathing passages. Doctors refer to a cough as bronchitis if it is provoked by an infection of the bronchi. Bronchitis is characterized by an initially dry cough that becomes productive (that is, the patient is coughing up phlegm) after a few days. Other symptoms often accompany the cough, including a light fever, headache, and pain behind the sternum. Usually the body is able to overcome bronchitis within two weeks. However, if additional bacteria attack the weakened mucous membranes, an infection of the lungs, or pneumonia, may result.

Chronic bronchitis exists if a person has a cough with phlegm almost always, and for at least three months in two consecutive years. The most common cause of chronic bronchitis is smoking. At other times, harmful substances from our environment, such as dust and exhaust fumes, can contribute to it. Chronic bronchitis has become a common illness in the United States—more than twelve million people suffer from this condition.

Treatment consists primarily of medication that causes the release of the mucus, which makes it easier to cough up and get rid of the secretions. If bacteria are found to be present, antibiotics may be called for.

Another illness that damages the mucous membranes of the bronchi is bronchial asthma. People with this illness have damage to the mucous membranes, increased phlegm production, and a sporadic contraction of the bronchi, leading sufferers to repeatedly experience severe shortness of breath. The causes for asthma are manifold and range from physical exertion, to infections of the breathing passages, to allergies. About half of all asthma patients are children under the age of ten. This condition requires medical treatment and supervision.

In treating asthma, physicians often prescribe "when-needed" medication, which is taken only to end an asthma episode, and continuing medication, which is taken on an ongoing basis to reduce the frequency of attacks. Asthma medication usually works by reducing infections and/or by temporarily expanding the breathing passages.

What You Can Do

If you are suffering from bronchitis, drink plenty of liquids to support the release of mucus. Plant-based expectorants such as menthol, eucalyptus, and thyme extracts also support the release of phlegm and work especially well for children. Applying essential oils also complements an anti-infection and expectorant treatment.

It is very important for asthma sufferers to avoid products to which they are allergic. This assumes, of course, that these products are known. They should also avoid situations that have repeatedly triggered asthma attacks. Massages and breathing techniques can help asthma sufferers regain control over their breathing.

How Can Reflexology Help?

Reflexology massages can alleviate breathing difficulties such as nasal or bronchial congestion, a persistent cough, or

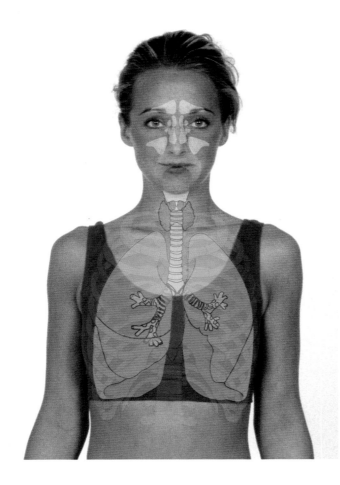

The paranasal sinuses, larynx, trachea, lungs, and bronchi make up the breathing passages.

shortness of breath. Foot, hand, and ear reflexology massages are especially well suited in the following combinations:

- massage of the foot and ear reflex zones
- massage of the hand and ear reflex zones

Start the treatment with a foot or hand massage and then carry out an ear massage. The individual directions will specify how long each zone should be massaged.

Foot Reflexology Massage

The focus areas should be the zones of the eyes, the nose-throat area, the breathing passages, and the lymphatic organs.

Massage Sequence

- Introduction: sandwich strokes.
- Massage the head zones on the fronts and backs of the toes with the tweezers grip, from the base of the big toe to the fifth toe in several treatment lines.
- Transition: sandwich strokes.
- Massage the zone of the lymphatic system in the head and throat area using the tweezers grip, grasping the skin between the toes and gently stretching it up and down.
- Massage the zones of the breathing passages and the lung on the sole of the foot using the thumb walk.
- Massage the zone of the armpit lymph nodes with the tip of the thumb.
- Massage the zones of the breathing passages, lung, and thymus on the back of the foot with the tip of your index finger.
- Conclusion: sandwich strokes.
- Massage the other foot in the same way.
- Stretch the heels of both feet.

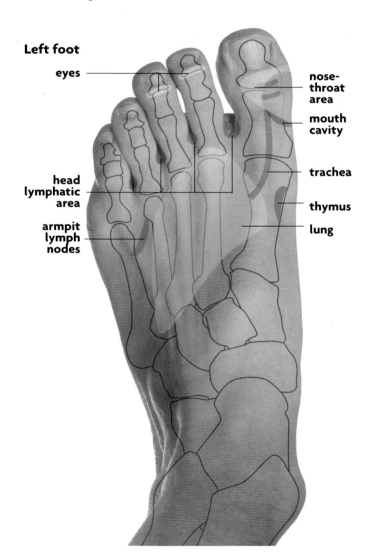

Left foot

- eyes
- nose-throat area
- mouth cavity
- trachea
- thymus
- lung
- head lymphatic area
- armpit lymph nodes

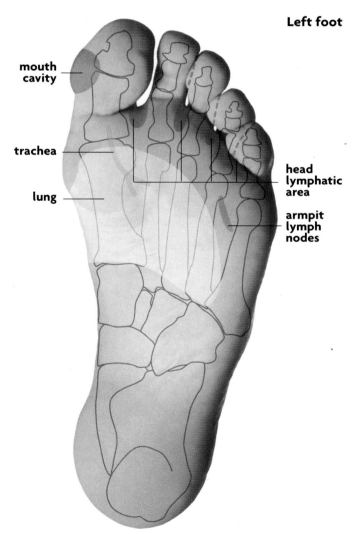

Left foot

- mouth cavity
- trachea
- lung
- head lymphatic area
- armpit lymph nodes

These reflex zones of the foot can be massaged to alleviate problems in the breathing passages.

Hand Reflexology Massage

Massage of the reflex zones on the hand is analogous to the foot reflexology massage. The focus areas should be the zones of the nose-throat area, the breathing passages, and the lymphatic organs.

Before you being massaging the individual zones on the hand, you should do an overall introduction with strokes. The sandwich strokes described on page 114 are especially well suited for this. Massage first one hand and then the other. Repeat each technique three to five times for each hand. End the massage by stroking and stretching the palms.

Sequence of the Massage

- Introduction: sandwich strokes.
- Massage the head zones on the fronts and backs of the fingers with the tweezers grip.
- Transition: sandwich strokes.
- Massage the zones of the lymphatic pathways in the head and throat area with the tweezers grip, gently stretching the skin between the fingers up and down
- Massage the zones of the breathing passages and the lung on the palm of the hand with the thumb walk.
- Massage the zone of the armpit lymph nodes between the fourth and fifth metacarpal bones with the tip of your index finger.
- Massage the zones of the breathing passages, lung, armpit lymph nodes, and thymus on the back of the hand point by point using the caterpillar walk.
- Conclusion: sandwich strokes.
- Stretch the palm.
- Massage the other hand in the same way.

Left hand

head zones

Right hand

head zones

head and throat lymphatic area

nose-throat area

tonsils

trachea

lungs

thymus

armpit lymph nodes

armpit lymph nodes

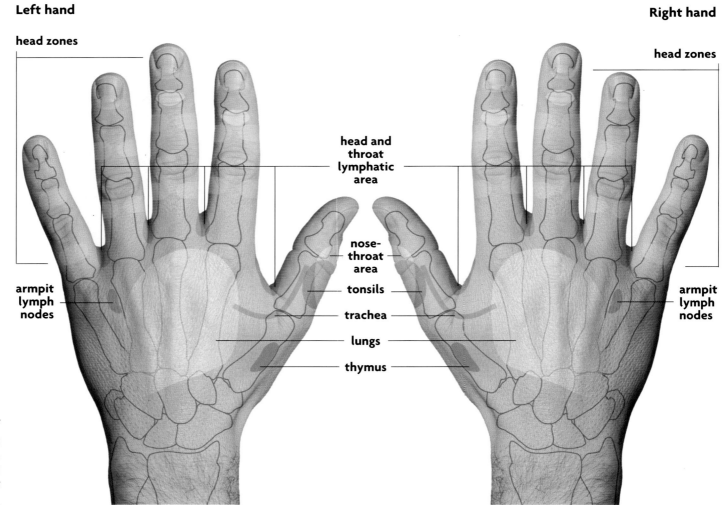

The zones of the breathing passages are easily massaged on the backs of the hands.

Ear Reflexology Massage

The ear reflexology massage is well suited for use in combination with foot and hand reflexology massages. It is especially useful because of its ease of self-treatment: You can massage your own ears basically anytime and anywhere. The focus of this ear reflexology massage is on activating the body's immune system. Before you begin with a point-by-point massage, carry out some strokes that cover the whole ear to prepare it for the pointed massage. If you are massaging yourself, you can massage both ears at the same time using one hand on each ear. If you're massaging your partner's ear, finish one before turning to the other. Repeat the strokes four or five times. Press each zone or point for 5 to 10 seconds. Conclude the ear massage with strokes.

Sequence of the Massage

- Introduction: strokes with the thumb.
- Massage both lengthwise and crosswise the antidepression point, antiaggression point, sadness-happiness point, and fear-worry point on the earlobe, and the omega-1 point.
- Massage the zones of the lung and pulmonary plexus with your index finger.
- Massage the inner-nose point between your thumb and tip of your index finger.
- Massage the shen men and sympathetic points using your thumb and the tip of your index finger.
- Conclusion: strokes with the thumb in several lines along the helix.
- Massage the other ear in the same way.

Right ear

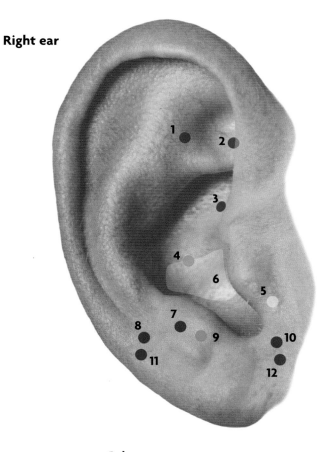

Left ear

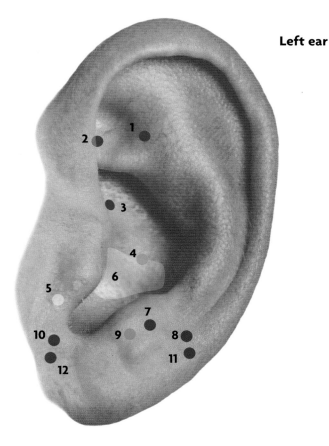

These ear reflexology points will help alleviate breathing problems.

1 shen men	**7 sun point**
2 sympathetic point	**8 antidepression point**
3 omega-1 point	**9 forehead point**
4 pulmonary plexus	**10 antiaggression point**
5 inner-nose point	**11 sadness-happiness point**
6 lung zone	**12 fear-worry point**

Digestive System Problems

The food we ingest remains for up to 4 hours in the stomach, where it is mixed with digestive juices. These juices are acidic and contain enzymes for breaking down food into its smallest components. If the sensitive stomach lining wasn't protected by a thick layer of mucus, it would be negatively affected by the aggressive acidity of the digestive juices.

Many people have had their stomach rebel in times of stress, tension, worry, or anger. We experience this reaction as pressure, and sometimes even strong, cramplike pain, in the stomach. These sensations are usually caused by a heightened production of acidic digestive juices and by increased activity in the stomach. We refer to this condition as a nervous stomach or irritated stomach. These symptoms can also be side effects of medication. If you experience these symptoms frequently, you should consult a doctor, who may prescribe medication to neutralize the stomach acid. While such medication usually helps calm the stomach, it does not treat the root cause of the problem.

Another common problem is chronic constipation. About four and a half million Americans suffer from this condition. Here, it is important to define constipation, because the frequency of bowel movements varies from person to person and depends on lifestyle and diet. Constipation can be diagnosed if stool is excreted fewer than three times per week and that stool is very hard. Lack of exercise and a fiber-poor diet are often causes of constipation. Sufferers also often don't drink enough fluid and/or frequently suppress the need to empty their intestine. Sometimes medication can depress intestinal function; this is the case with, for example, iron preparations, cough syrups containing codeine, and some sleeping pills. If constipation occurs suddenly or lasts for an extended period, you should see a doctor.

What You Can Do

It is important to complement medical treatment of the digestive system with the following measures:

- Avoid stress both at work and at home. Special relaxation exercises can be a valuable aid in this.
- Reduce your consumption of alcohol, caffeine, and spicy foods, as they increase the stomach's production of acid and can irritate the stomach lining.
- Eat primarily foods that are easy to digest, such as fresh fruits and vegetables, steamed foods, and grains. Avoid foods that are high in fats and difficult to digest.
- Eat slowly, and eat five small meals a day rather than two or three big ones.

If you suffer from stomach problems despite these measures, you can help yourself by warming your abdomen with a hot water bottle or warm towel. In addition, a cup of herbal tea (chamomile, licorice root, or melissa) can have beneficial and relaxing effects, but do not take licorice root if you have high blood pressure.

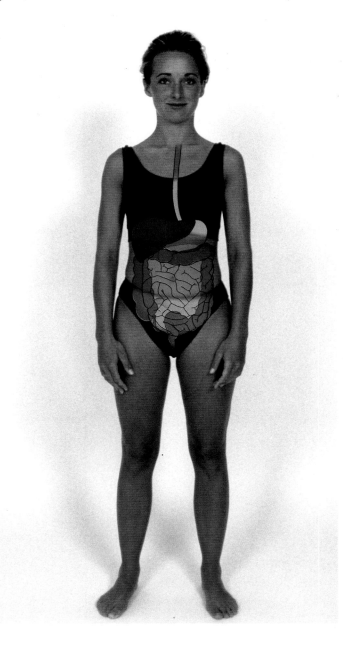

Problems in the digestive tract are often caused by functional disturbances of the stomach or intestines.

If you suffer from chronic constipation, don't use a laxative without consulting a doctor. Your intestines become used to these very quickly, exacerbating the problem. It would be better to change your diet to include more foods that are high in fiber and to drink lots of liquids (1 to 2 quarts a day).

Finally, get plenty of exercise.

How Can Reflexology Help?

Reflexology can be very effective for normalizing digestion. The shiatsu massage of the abdomen described on pages 174–175 is especially well suited for this. Carry out the abdomen massage as a basic treatment for problems in the digestive area. Foot, hand, and ear reflexology massages can also serve to harmonize the digestive system.

Foot Reflexology Massage

This foot reflexology massage has the goal of normalizing digestive function. The zones of the respective organs cover most of the feet.

Sequence of the Massage

- Introduction: sandwich strokes.
- Massage the esophagus zone using the tip of the thumb.
- Massage the zones of the digestive tract with the thumb point by point in horizontal and vertical lines.
- Conclusion: sandwich strokes.
- Massage the other foot in the same way.
- Stretch both feet at the heels.

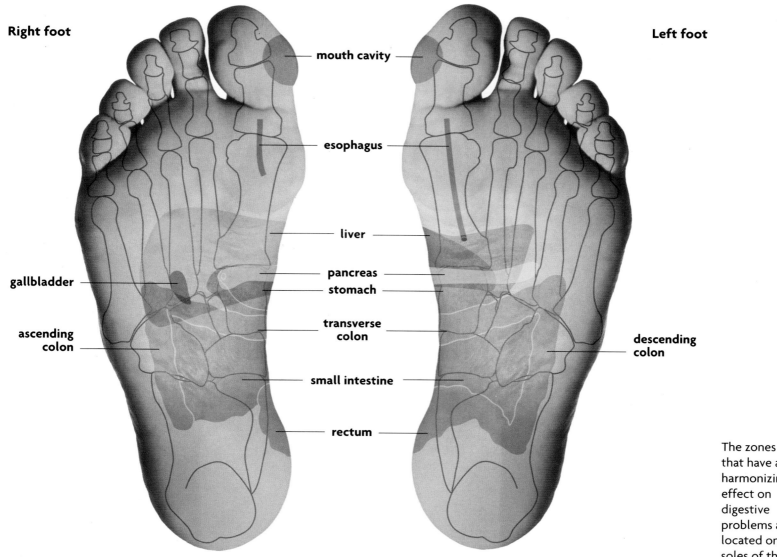

Right foot

Left foot

mouth cavity

esophagus

liver

gallbladder

pancreas

stomach

ascending colon

transverse colon

descending colon

small intestine

rectum

The zones that have a harmonizing effect on digestive problems are located on the soles of the feet.

Hand Reflexology Massage

The zones of the digestive organs extend from the area of the carpus up to the middle of the palm. Remember that the zone of the large intestine runs across both hands.

Before you begin massaging the individual zones, carry out a few sandwich strokes as an introduction to the massage. Massage first one hand and then the other. Repeat each technique three to five times.

End the massage with strokes and stretches of the palm.

Sequence of the Massage

- Introduction: sandwich strokes.
- Massage the zones of the digestive organs point by point in horizontal and vertical lines.
- Conclusion: sandwich strokes.
- Stretch the palm.
- Massage the other hand in the same way.

Right hand   **Left hand**

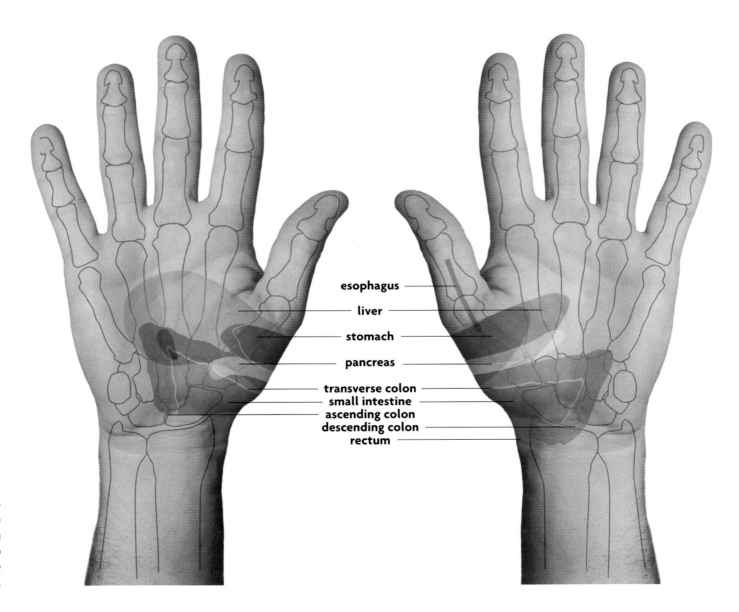

esophagus
liver
stomach
pancreas
transverse colon
small intestine
ascending colon
descending colon
rectum

Massage the zones of the digestive system on the hands to relieve digestive problems.

Ear Reflexology Massage

Massaging the zones of the digestive organs on the ear is a good complement to hand and foot reflexology massages. The zones of the stomach and the small and large intestines run around the helix root. The zones of the spleen and liver are located at the back edge of the inner auricle near the inside edge of the anthelix. Before you begin massaging these zones, carry out four or five strokes along the helix. Press the individual zones or points for 5 to 10 seconds each.

Sequence of the Massage

- Introduction: strokes of the thumb in several lines along the helix.
- Massage the zones of the digestive organs with the index finger point by point around the helix root.
- Conclusion: strokes with the thumb in several lines along the helix brim.

Right ear

Left ear

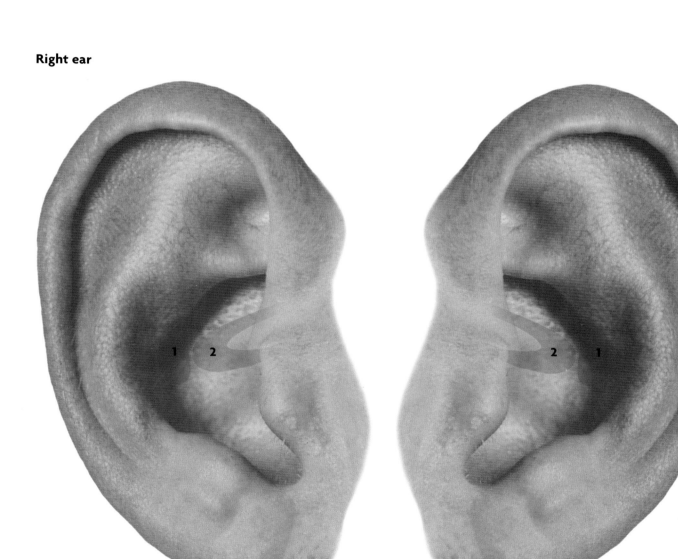

For digestive problems, massage the zones of the digestive tract and the gallbladder.

1 liver-gallbladder zone $\qquad$ **2 digestive tract zone**

Endocrine System Disturbances

The endocrine system comprises all the organs of the body that produce hormones and release them into the body's circulatory system. They include the thyroid, the adrenal cortex, and the pancreas, which produces insulin (see below). If these organs work too little or too much, our hormone levels will be too low or too high, causing disruptions in the body.

For example, an overactive thyroid leads to the increased production and secretion of thyroid gland hormones into the blood. This causes all metabolic processes to run at a high speed, leaving the sufferer with a rapid heartbeat, sweating, shaking, internal anxiety, and weight loss. Conversely, a thyroid that works too little leads to a slowing down of the body's processes and is characterized by a loss of appetite, increased body weight, and fatigue.

The term *metabolism* refers to all chemical processes inside the body in which food is turned into the body's own substances. Metabolism serves the growth of the organism and the provision of energy to all life processes. On a simplified level, these processes can be divided into protein, fat, and carbohydrate metabolisms. If these processes don't work as they are supposed to, metabolic disorders may result. For example, the disruption of the fat metabolism can cause adiposis or anorexia, a disrupted carbohydrate metabolism can cause diabetes, and a disrupted protein metabolism can cause gout.

Type-1 diabetes is caused by insufficient production of the hormone insulin in the pancreas. This type of diabetes usually surfaces in childhood or puberty. Early warning signs of the illness are increased appetite and thirst while losing weight and urinating frequently. In children, a sudden loss of concentration and noticeable fatigue are common symptoms.

Since insulin is a life-necessary hormone, type-1 diabetics receive external doses of insulin that are injected under the skin several times a day. At the same time, these diabetics have to pay close attention to their diets so that they have adequate levels of insulin in their bodies compared to the amount of carbohydrates they ingest. Diabetics measure their blood sugar levels several times a day to control this factor.

Another cause of diabetes is the inability of the body to react to the insulin the pancreas produces. This is called type-2 diabetes, and it is more common among adults, especially obese ones.

What You Can Do

Type-2 diabetics have to learn to reduce their body weight to a normal level through a better diet. A better diet in this sense refers to less processed sugar, more fiber, and less fat. This dietary change alone can normalize blood sugar levels in many cases. If this does not suffice, a physician may prescribe medication that will lower blood sugar levels. Sometimes type-2 diabetics, like type-1 diabetics, need to inject insulin.

Over- and underfunctioning of the thyroid are common illnesses.

How Can Reflexology Help?

Reflexology massages can be used to complement the medical treatment of hormonal problems. Reflexology massages aim to harmonize the excretion of hormones. Ear, foot, and hand reflexology massages can be used in the following combinations:

- massaging the foot and ear reflex zones
- massaging the hand and ear reflex zones

Begin with the foot or hand massage and then carry out an ear massage.

Foot Reflexology Massage

The focus here is on the zones of the thyroid, pancreas, and adrenal glands.

Sequence of the Massage

- Introduction: sandwich strokes.
- Massage the thyroid zone, in the area of the base joint of the big toe, using your thumb.
- Transition: sandwich strokes.
- Massage the pancreas zone in horizontal lines using your thumb.
- Transition: sandwich strokes.
- Massage the zone of the adrenal glands, at the base of the second metatarsal bone, using your thumb.
- Conclusion: sandwich strokes.
- Massage the other foot in the same way.
- Stretch both feet at the heels.

Right foot   **Left foot**

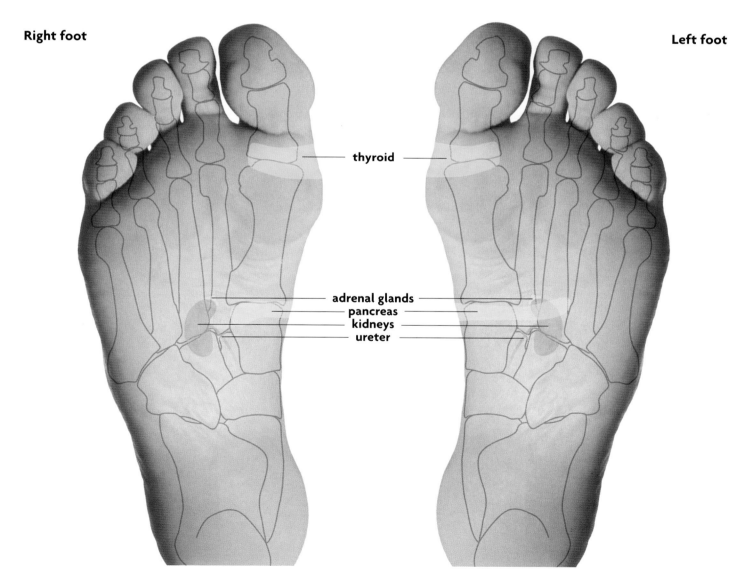

thyroid

adrenal glands
pancreas
kidneys
ureter

To address functional disturbances of the endocrine system, locate the appropriate zones on the soles of the feet.

Hand Reflexology Massage

The massage of the reflex zones on the hand has the same focus as the foot reflexology massage. After you have carried out a few strokes that encompass the whole hand, massage the zones of the thyroid, adrenal glands, and pancreas. Massage first one hand and then the other. Repeat each technique three to five times. End the massage with strokes and stretches of the palms.

Sequence of the Massage

- Introduction: sandwich strokes.
- Massage the thyroid zone with the tips of your thumbs.
- Massage the pancreas zone with the tips of your thumbs.
- Massage the zone of the adrenal glands with the tips of your thumbs.
- Conclusion: sandwich strokes.
- Stretch the palm.
- Massage the other hand in the same way.

Right hand

Left hand

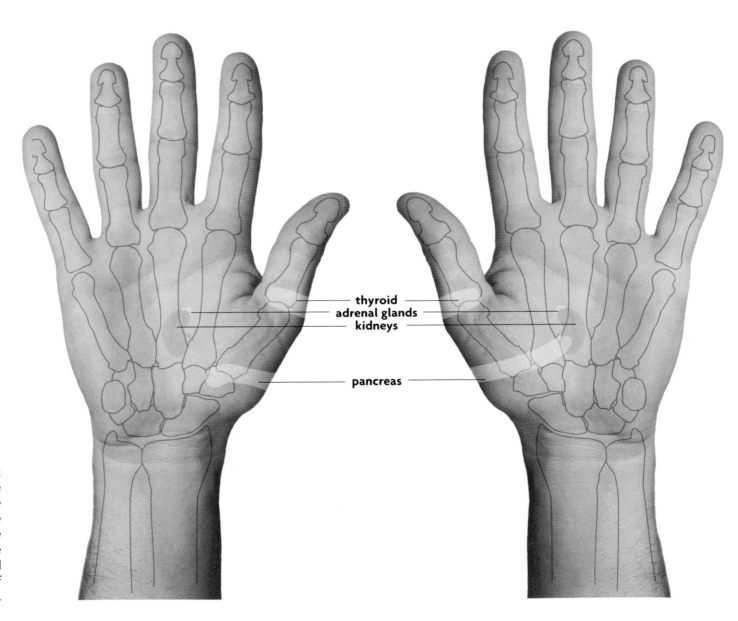

thyroid
adrenal glands
kidneys

pancreas

The reflex zones of the endocrine glands are located in the heel of the thumb and the middle of the hand.

Ear Reflexology Massage

The ear reflexology massage complements the foot or hand reflexology massage. It is especially well suited for self-treatment.

Begin with a few strokes that encompass the whole ear to prepare it for the massage of the individual points. To stimulate the function of the glands, massage the points of the adrenal glands and thyroid. Using the tip of the index finger, massage the liver and gallbladder zones inside the auricle. End the ear massage with strokes.

Carry out each stroke four or five times. Press the individual zones or points for 5 to 10 seconds each. In the case of self-treatment, you can massage both ears at the same time using one hand on each.

Sequence of the Massage

- Introduction: strokes with the thumb in several lines along the helix.
- Massage the points of the adrenal glands and thyroid between the tips of the thumb and index finger.
- Massage the liver-gallbladder zone inside the auricle with the index finger.
- Conclusion: strokes with the thumb in several lines along the helix.
- Massage the other ear in the same way.

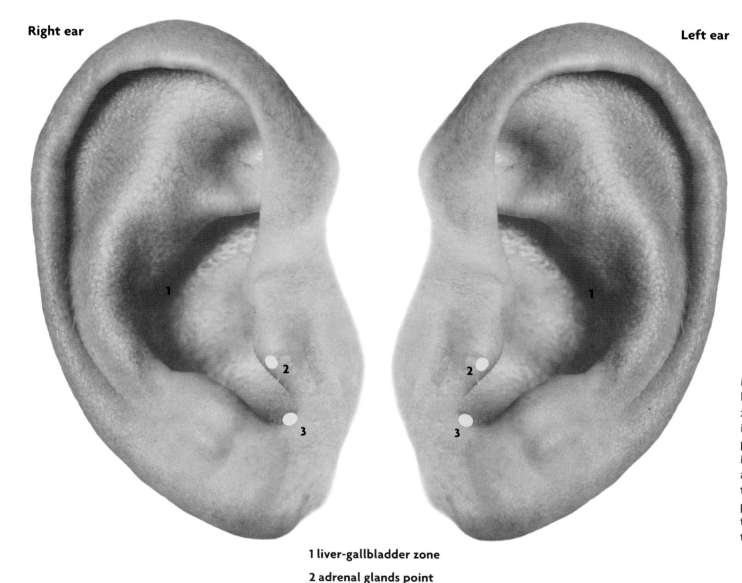

Right ear

Left ear

Massaging the liver-gallbladder zone also influences the pancreas. Massaging the adrenal and thyroid gland points stimulates the functions of these glands.

1 liver-gallbladder zone

2 adrenal glands point

3 thyroid gland point

Headache

Almost every person in the world suffers from occasional headaches. As long as they are of short duration and bearable intensity, they do not require medical treatment. However, one third of the population experiences these symptoms frequently, strongly, and sometimes for prolonged periods of time, significantly reducing their quality of life.

Headaches can be a symptom of a health problem, such as tense muscles, infection, an infectious disease, or a tumor. They are also known to be side effects of a number of medications—for example, those that treat heart problems and blood thinners. Taking painkillers for prolonged periods of time can—paradoxical as this may sound—cause headaches. Among sensitive people, seemingly insignificant changes in air pressure, weather, or diet can cause a headache. Continuing stress, lack of sleep, or bad posture can also be a factor.

On the other hand, headaches can also occur as an illness in their own right. These types of headaches are called tension headaches, cluster headaches, and migraines.

The tension headache is the most common of the three types. In the United States nearly 75 percent of all people suffer from this usually less severe headache, which extends to both sides of the head. It was formerly speculated that the cause of this headache was heightened tension in the neck muscles. Today, however, we know that this explanation holds true for at most only half of all cases. Other factors could be psychological stress and disturbances in the hormone activities of the brain.

A cluster headache is a severe headache that is usually confined to one side of the head and tends to recur in a series of attacks. This is a rather rare type of headache; between one and four Americans per thousand exerience cluster headaches. They predominantly affect men. The cause of cluster headaches is not clear.

A migraine is a headache that can last up to four days. Migraines most often occur on one side of the head and are usually accompanied by nausea and vomiting, balance problems, sensitivity to light, and disturbances to vision and the sense of smell. The cause is blood circulation problems in the brain that lead to tension and then weakening of the vessel muscles in the head. Migraines are more common for women than for men.

What You Can Do

Depending on the intensity of the pain, the frequency of the attacks, and the duration of an individual attack, you may require medication prescribed by a doctor to treat these headaches. However, you can contribute to the success of the treatment significantly by

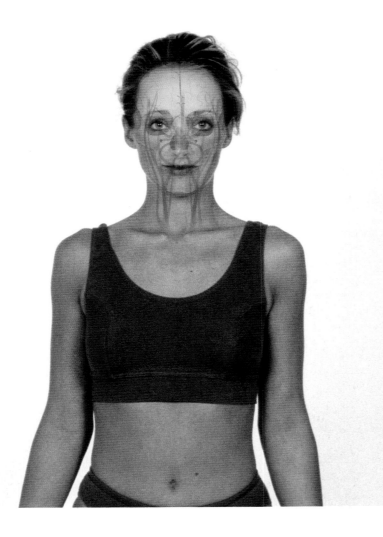

Sudden headaches are caused by cramping and subsequently flaccid blood vessels in the head.

adjusting your lifestyle to make attacks less frequent and shorter in duration. Make sure that you get enough sleep and exercise and that you are eating regular meals. Note whether you tend to experience headaches after eating certain foods.

Keep a diary in which you note all external circumstances that occurred around the time of a headache attack. In the future, try to avoid similar situations. You might also try learning a few relaxation techniques, for example autogenic training or progressive muscle relaxation according to Edmund Jacobson. Consume alcohol and nicotine, if at all, only in low levels, as they may cause headaches. Finally, it is important to pay attention to your posture to avoid having tense muscles.

How Can Reflexology Massage Help?

Reflexology massage is well suited to reducing or ending headache attacks. The uses of reflexology massage are as manifold as the causes of headaches. All the types of massage described in this book can help alleviate headaches. In the end, you should choose the method that works best for the sufferer. The different types of massage can be combined without any problems. Your massage will be most successful if you are very comfortable with the method you choose and your partner has an open mind about it.

If possible, base your treatment on a shiatsu head massage as described beginning on page 184. Acute headaches can be influenced effectively with head reflexology massage, but ear and foot reflexology massages are also effective measures.

Sequence of the Massage

- Locate pressure-sensitive points in the A zone.
- Massage the A zone of one side of the head with pointed or circular pressure.
- Apply pressure until the pain in the zone subsides.
- Massage the other A zone in the same way.

Head Reflexology Massage

Head reflexology massage is effective for relieving strong, acute pain. Usually points in the A zone will become sensitive in this case. Touch the sensitive spots with the tip of your thumb and massage the points using either steady pressure or circular movements. This treatment can be slightly unpleasant, but it is highly effective. Massage first one and then the other A zone.

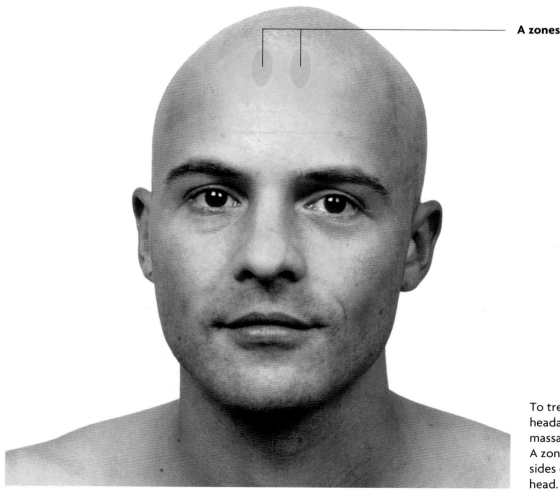

A zones

To treat headaches, massage the A zone on both sides of the head.

Ear Reflexology Massage

In the case of a headache, a number of points on the ear may be sensitive. That makes a good base treatment—that is, the thorough stroking of the ear in several paths along the helix—especially important.

There are a number of points in the area of the earlobe. Massage this area point by point in lines that run vertically and horizontally, applying pressure with the tips of your index finger and thumb. Then massage the polster, jerome, shen men, and sympathetic points.

Sequence of the Massage

- Introduction: strokes with the thumb in several lines along the helix.
- Massage the earlobe with the tips of the thumb and index finger in vertical and horizontal lines.
- Massage the polster, jerome, shen men, and sympathetic points with the tips of the index finger and thumb.
- Conclusion: strokes with the thumb in several lines along the helix.
- Massage the other ear in the same way.

Right ear

Left ear

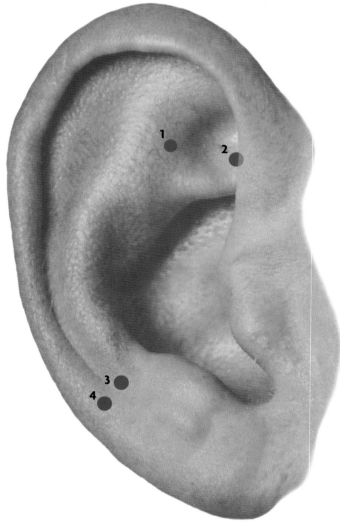
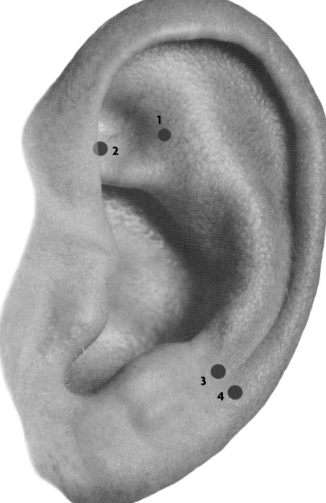

These reflex points on the ear can alleviate a headache.

1 shen men point

2 sympathetic point

3 polster point

4 jerome point

Foot Reflexology Massage

The focus is on the zones of the head, neck, and shoulders. Begin with some introductory sandwich strokes. Then take the front of the foot between both hands and shake it to loosen the zone of the shoulder girdle. Then massage the head zones on the tops and bottomss of the toes using the tweezers grip, beginning at the base of the big toe and moving point by point toward the tips of the toes. Finish your massage with some strokes.

Sequence of the Massage

- Introduction: sandwich strokes.
- Shake the front of the foot to loosen the shoulder girdle.
- Massage the head zones on the fronts and backs of the toes, beginning at the base of the big toe, with the tweezers grip.
- Conclusion: sandwich strokes.
- Massage the other foot in the same way.
- Stretch both feet at the heels.

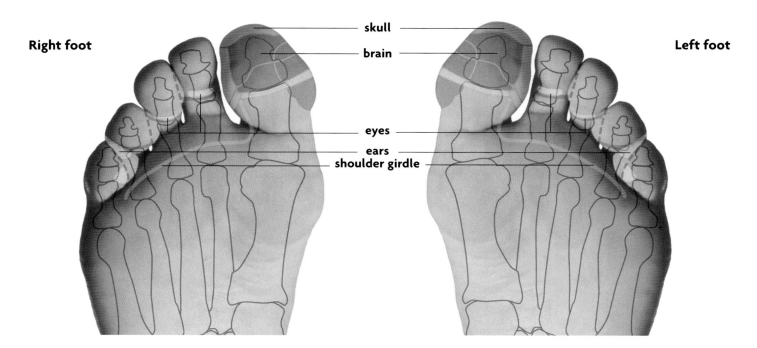

Right foot
Left foot

skull
brain
eyes
ears
shoulder girdle

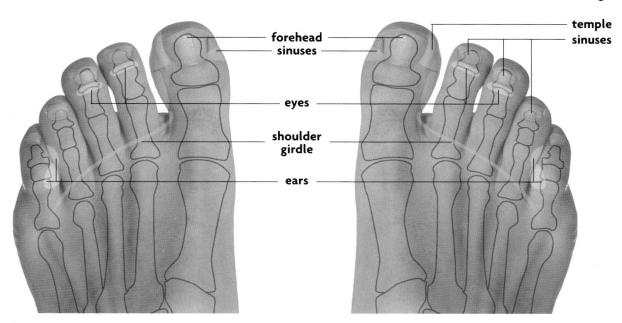

Left foot
Right foot

forehead
sinuses
eyes
shoulder girdle
ears
temple
sinuses

Massage the head zones on the tops and bottoms of the toes.

Heart and Circulatory Problems

The body of an adult contains between 5 and 6 liters of blood. The blood circulates through a large system of arteries and veins. Blood in the arteries is rich in oxygen and supplies organs and tissues. To supply all destinations equally it has to be pumped from the heart into the circulation system at a certain pressure. This pressure is usually measured in units of millimeters of mercury (mm Hg). A blood pressure of 120/80 mm Hg has been shown to be optimal. An adult who at rest has a blood pressure above 140/90 mm is said to have high blood pressure or hypertension. This can have a number of causes.

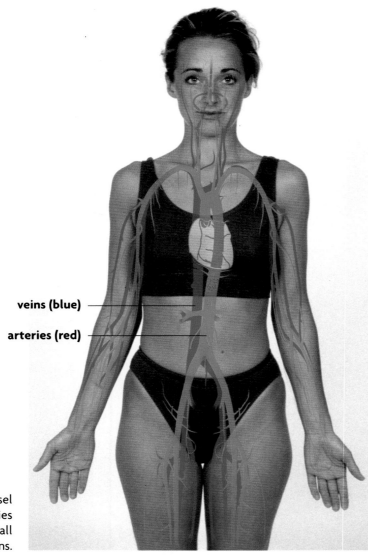

veins (blue)

arteries (red)

A complex vessel system supplies blood to all tissues and organs.

High blood pressure can be a symptom of an illness. However, the more common situation is that high blood pressure is an independent illness for which no specific cause can be found. A number of risk factors can lead to high blood pressure, including too much salt in the diet, not enough potassium in the diet, obesity, stress, and genetic predisposition. Prolonged high blood pressure that is not treated can cause irreparable damage to many organs essential to life, including the heart and kidneys, and permanent damage to blood vessels in the brain and eyes, as well as to the coronary arteries. Consequences can include heart attack and stroke. A number of medications exist to treat high blood pressure. However, they can lower high blood pressure effectively only over time and if the patient also works on it him- or herself through lifestyle changes.

Another important illness of the heart and circulatory system is the constriction of the coronary arteries. This means that the blood vessels that surround the heart in a ring, whose function is to supply the heart with oxygen, tighten or, in extreme cases, close up altogether. The result is a lower circulation of blood through the heart, which in turn can lead to disruptions in the heart rhythm or even cause a heart attack. In developed countries, such consequences of tightening of the coronary arteries cause 30 percent of deaths and are in fact the most common cause of death. What causes the coronary arteries to tighten? When fatty streaks of excess cholesterol are deposited on the blood vessel walls, the vessels become harder, narrower, and less flexible. In the worst cases, the fatty deposits enlarge and thicken to form rough-edged plaques that irritate the smooth lining of the arteries, causing cells to die and scar tissue to form, which contributes to the progressive constriction of the arteries over time. The consequences are noticeable for patients only when over 70 percent of the vessels are constricted. The length of the asymptomatic period means that prevention is very important.

What You Can Do

If necessary, normalize your body weight. You will see that this can lower blood pressure without any medication. Avoid foods high in fat and reduce your daily salt intake—5 grams of salt a day is sufficient. Eat plenty of fruits and vegetables because these foods are good sources of potassium. If you smoke, quit. Get enough exercise, and try to learn how to cope with stressful situations. This can be done by learning relaxation techniques, such as autogenic training.

How Can Reflexology Help?

Reflexology massages can supplement medical treatment. You can use foot, hand, and ear reflexology massages to this end. Foot or hand reflexology massages form the basis of this complementary therapy, and massage of the ear reflex zones can be done as a follow-up or in between as self-massage.

The goal of these massages is to bring about general relaxation as well as to dissolve psychological tension.

Foot Reflexology Massage

After a general introduction of strokes, the foot reflexology massage should focus on the head zones, the heart zone, and any sensitive zones. The zone of the solar plexus should be massaged using steady pressure.

Sequence of the Massage

- Introduction: sandwich strokes.
- Massage the head zones on the toes.
- Massage the heart zone with the thumb tip.
- Massage the solar plexus zone using steady pressure.
- Conclusion: sandwich strokes.
- Massage the other foot in the same way.
- Stretch both feet at the heels.

Right foot   **Left foot**

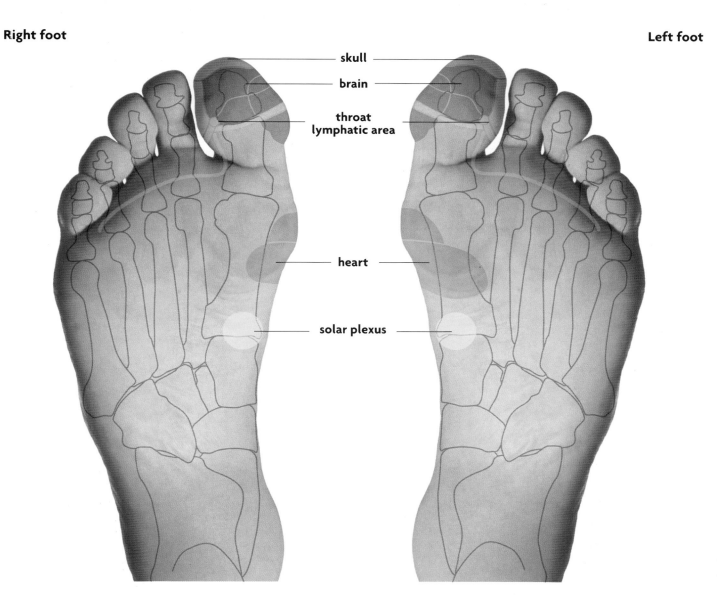

skull
brain
throat
lymphatic area
heart
solar plexus

To alleviate heart and circulatory problems, massage the head, heart, and solar plexus zones on the soles of the feet.

Hand Reflexology Massage

As with the foot massage, the hand massage should focus on the zones of the head, heart, and solar plexus. Pay attention to sensitive zones on other parts of the hand as well, and massage with steady pressure any you may find. Scars on the hand require special attention. Carefully touch the tissue surrounding the scar. If you encounter sensitive zones in this area, massage them with steady pressure.

Sequence of the Massage

- Introduction: sandwich strokes.
- Massage the head zones on the fronts and backs of the fingers.
- Massage the heart zone with the thumb tip.
- Massage the zone of the solar plexus using steady pressure.
- Conclusion: sandwich strokes.
- Stretch the palm.
- Massage the other hand in the same way.

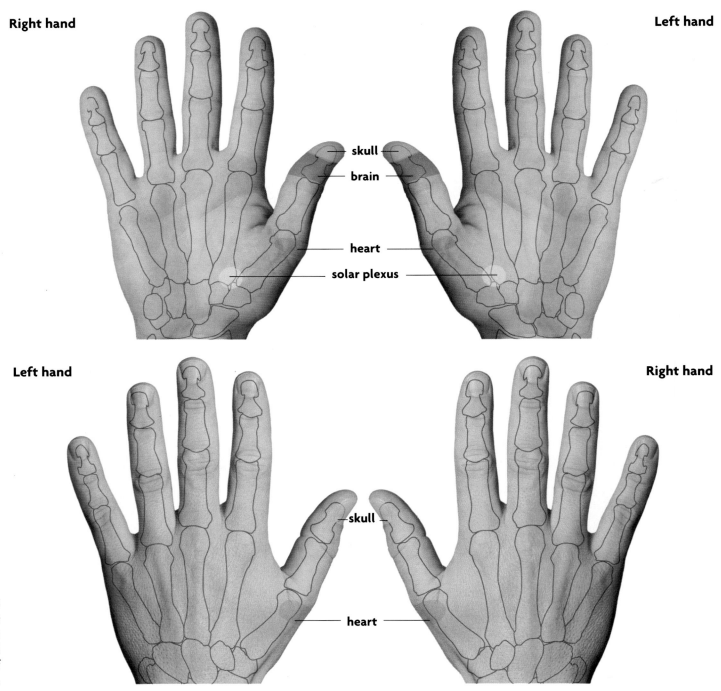

Right hand

Left hand

skull
brain
heart
solar plexus

Left hand

Right hand

skull

heart

The head zones should be massaged on the backs as well as the palms of the hands.

Ear Reflexology Massage

The ear reflexology massage can be combined with foot or hand reflexology massage. Its effect is a harmonizing of the body functions. If the goal is to influence high blood pressure, the heart and polster points should be the focus. Begin with strokes that cover the whole ear to prepare for the point massage. If you are massaging yourself, you can massage both ears at the same time using one hand for each ear. If you're massaging your partner's ears, finish one before turning to the other. Repeat each stroke four or five times. Apply pressure on the individual zones or points for 5 to 10 seconds at a time. Conclude the ear massage with strokes.

Sequence of the Massage

- Introduction: strokes with the thumb in several lines along the helix.
- Massage the heart point in the auricle with the tip of the index finger.
- Apply pressure on the polster point with the tweezers grip.
- Conclusion: strokes with the thumb in several lines along the helix.
- Massage the other ear in the same way.

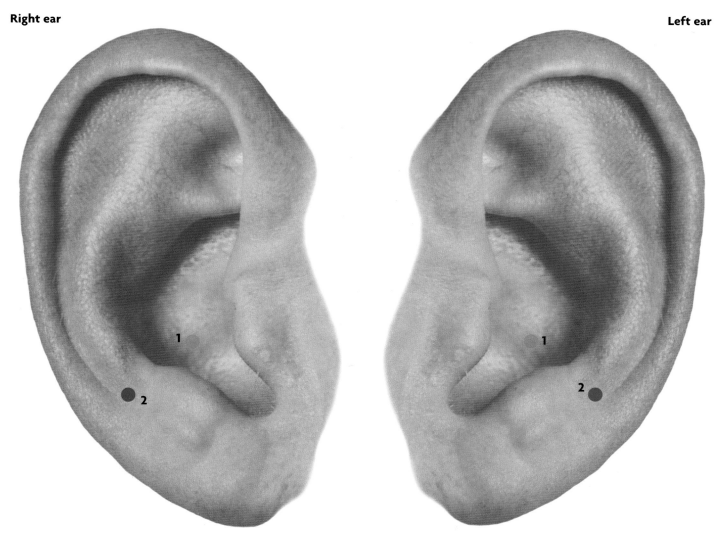

Right ear

Left ear

To remediate high blood pressure, massage the heart and polster points.

1 heart point

2 polster point

Hip Joint Ailments

Wear and tear is a frequent cause of joint pain. In the hip, the head of the thighbone rests in the socket of the pelvic bone. The joint they form is surrounded by a membrane called a synovial or joint capsule. The capsule produces synovial fluid, which cushions the joint. Muscles and tendons stabilize the joint, on which a large part of our body weight rests. On the joint surface, a protective cartilage layer covers the bone. If this cartilage is worn down, the bones rub directly against each other, causing pain and reducing the range of motion. Doctors refer to this condition as hip arthrosis (*arthros* means "joint" in Greek). With increasing age, more people (men and women equally) suffer from this condition. Treatment depends on the severity of the case. If there are signs of inflammation such as reddening and warming, or if the joint is swollen, doctors diagnose the condition as active arthrosis. In this case, the joint should be rested whenever possible. However, it must not be continually immobilized, as this may make the joint inflexible. Beyond this, cold treatments such as cold towels can help. Pain and anti-inflammatory medication may also be necessary.

If hip arthrosis exists without the inflammatory signs described above, it is considered a resting arthrosis. In this case, warmth treatments such as hot packs, UV lights, and warm baths are pleasant. In addition, under qualified instruction, exercises should be carried out with the goal of strengthening the muscles in the joint area.

If the changes caused by wear and tear have progressed too far, surgery is usually required to restore mobility.

What You Can Do

Get plenty of exercise. This keeps your muscles strong, the cartilage tissue filled with blood, and the joint flexible.

Avoid overexerting yourself or placing improper stress on the joint. Stress to the joint can result from obesity or from engaging in extreme sports. Improper stress can occur when the joints are overused in one particular way, whether through sedentary or active causes. Low-impact sports such as swimming and cycling can counteract negative stress.

Maintain a balanced diet, which has a positive influence on your joints.

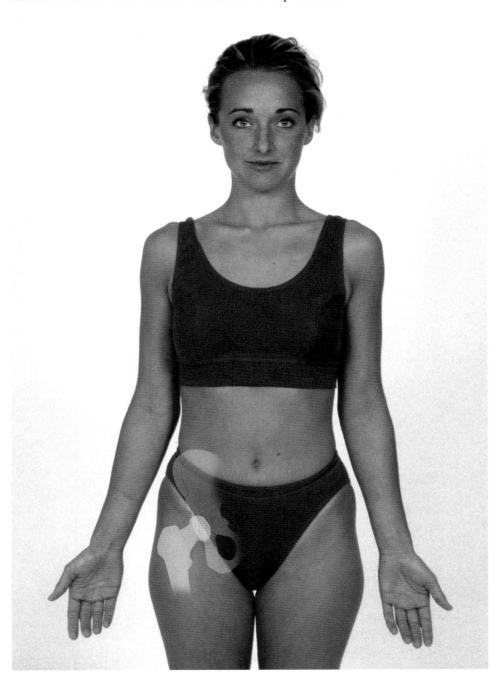

Problems in the hip area are often a result of too much or inappropriate physical stress.

How Can Reflexology Help?

For ailments of the hips, the main symptoms are pain and a reduced range of motion. Pain can be especially well influenced through reflexology massages, especially with head, ear, and foot reflexology massages. The following combinations are especially beneficial:

- massage of the head and foot reflex zones
- massage of the ear and foot reflex zones

Head Reflexology Massage

In the case of acute pain in the hip joint, the D zone or one of the D points often becomes sensitive to pressure. Iden-tify any sensitive points and massage them with the tip of your thumb. For this, you have two possibilities: rubbing/circling and pressing (see page 139). Continue massaging the sensitive points until the pain disappears. At the same time, you will notice a significant alleviation of symptoms in the hips. Head massage can be done on a partner or as self-treatment.

Sequence of the Massage

- Locate painful points.
- Massage the points with pressure or with rubbing or circling movements.

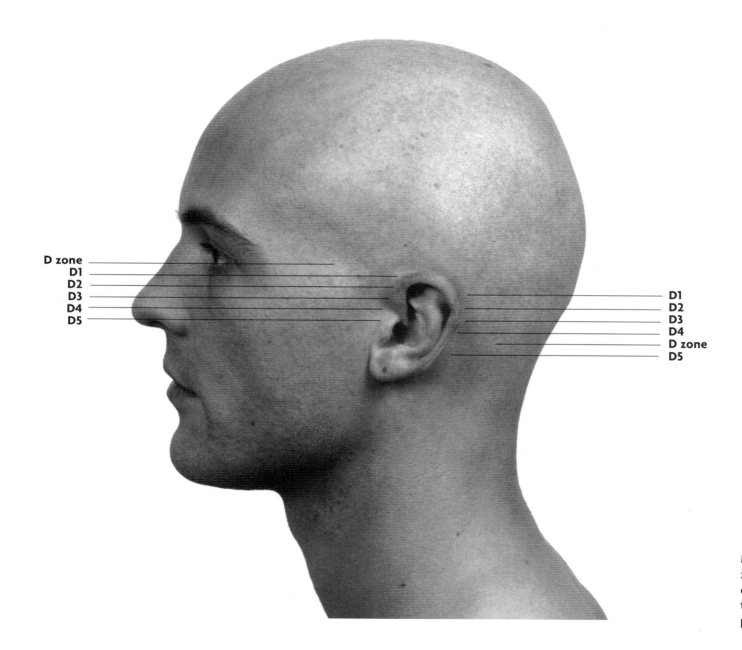

D zone
D1
D2
D3
D4
D5

D1
D2
D3
D4
D zone
D5

Massage the D zone and points on the head to treat hip problems.

Ear Reflexology Massage

Massaging relevant points on the ear is also a very effective way to treat ailments in the hip area. Ear reflexology massage is slightly more gentle than the head reflexology massage just described. The massage begins with an overall introduction using strokes that encompass the whole ear. Afterward, massage the appropriate points of the hips. If you are massaging yourself, you can massage both ears at the same time using one hand for each ear. Repeat the individual strokes four or five times and press the individual zones or points for 5 to 10 seconds. Conclude the ear massage with strokes.

Sequence of the Massage

- Introduction: strokes with the thumb in several lines along the helix.
- Massage the shen men, hip, jerome, and analgesia points between the tips of your thumb and index finger.
- Conclusion: strokes with the thumb in several lines along the helix brim.
- Massage the other ear in the same way.

Right ear

Left ear

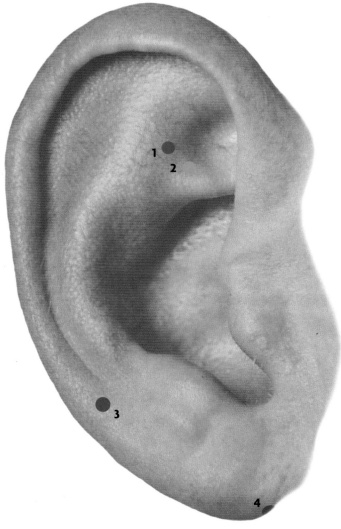
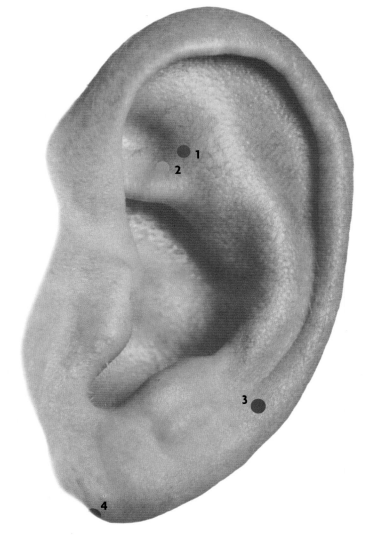
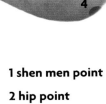

These reflex points of the ear can be massaged to relieve hip pain.

1 shen men point

2 hip point

3 jerome point

4 analgesia point

Foot Reflexology Massage

Especially for chronic ailments in the hip area, it is helpful to massage the respective foot reflexology zones. This massage can be done on a partner or as self-massage. First set the stage for the massage using sandwich strokes and then apply steady pressure with the tip of your thumb to massage the zone of the hip joint. This zone is located on the outside edge of the ankle and extends in a band around the zone of the top of the thigh.

Conclude the massage with strokes and then massage the other foot in the same way. Repeat each grip three to five times. Conclude the foot reflexology massage by stretching the feet at the heels.

Sequence of the Massage

- Introduction: sandwich strokes.
- Apply steady pressure to the zone of the top of the hip using the thumb tip.
- Conclusion: strokes hand over hand.
- Massage the other foot in the same way.
- Stretch both feet at the heels.

Right foot

Left foot

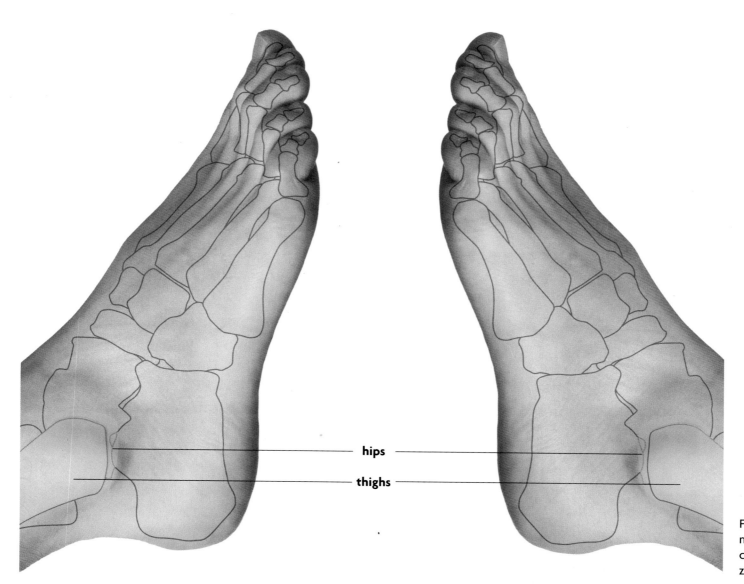

hips

thighs

For hip problems, massage the corresponding zone on the foot.

Hormonal Changes

For most of their lives, humans undergo hormonal changes. These changes are more frequent and more significant for women than they are for men. They begin for both sexes at puberty. Later, through pregnancy and childbirth, many women experience strong hormonal changes in rapid succession that have strong effects, both positive and negative, on quality of life. From about forty-five years of age onward, hormone levels start to decline. The onset of this decline is sometimes earlier in men. The decline is continuous and very gradual, which means that for several years, sufficient levels of hormones are produced so that the effects are only rarely noticeable. Possible effects for men include erectile dysfunction and an enlarged prostate. The prostate, which is normally about the size of a chestnut, can increase in advanced age up to the size of a tennis ball due to hormonal changes. The enlargement causes difficulty in urinating as well as the need to urinate more frequently. Should you have such symptoms, see a doctor to rule out other illnesses with similar symptoms, such as a prostate infection and even prostate cancer. In its early stages, the treatment of a benign enlargement of the prostate can be effected with medication. If the enlargement has advanced very far, the prostate may be removed either partially or as a whole through surgery. Preparations of stinging nettles and rye pollen can help as complementary therapeutic supplements. Pumpkin-seed preparations are also sometimes recommended, though their effectiveness remains contested.

Among women, the lower hormone levels are usually noticed over several years. During this period of menopause, menstruation becomes increasingly irregular until it finally stops altogether, marking the end of fertility. Far more unpleasant for women are the accompanying symptoms, such as hot flashes, insomnia, nervousness, and mood swings. For many women, menopause coincides with the time when their children are leaving home; they lose their roles as mothers and have to reorient themselves. For some this is a positive; however, for many it is not. These difficulties affect the mood of many women, leading to what is sometimes called menopause depression. How is it treated? There are a number of plant-based medications that have noticeable effects for "female problems." For example, preparations of chaste tree and snake herb have hormonelike effects and thus reduce symptoms that are caused by the reduction in female hormones.

What You Can Do

If you are suffering from an enlarged prostate, you can support medical treatment by eliminating spicy foods and excessive caffeine and alcohol consumption from your diet. Be sure to drink enough liquids (water, noncaffeinated tea, mineral water) in order to maintain soft stool.

For menopause problems, you can contribute to the success of treatment by indulging yourself: treat yourself to plenty of exercise in fresh air, keep a balanced diet, and ensure sufficient liquid intake. Valerian, melissa, and hops tea preparations are effective against sleeping problems, and sage helps mitigate hot flashes and sweats by reducing sweat production, as well as by its disinfectant properties. If your symptoms are so severe that these treatments don't help, a doctor may be able to offer help, after a thorough examination, through hormone treatment.

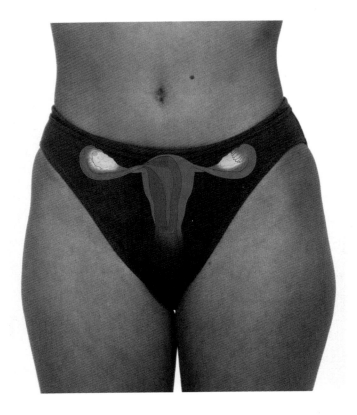

During menopause, the ovaries reduce the production of hormones.

How Can Reflexology Help?

Negative symptoms of menopause such as hot flashes, excessive sweating, and insomnia can be positively influenced through foot, hand, and ear reflexology massages. Good effects can be had by combining foot and ear or hand and ear reflexology massages.

Foot Reflexology Massage

To influence the symptoms effectively, massage the zones of the genital organs. Before you massage the individual zones, begin with some strokes. Massage first one foot and then the other. Repeat each technique four or five times.

Sequence of the Massage

- Introduction: sandwich strokes.
- Massage the zones of the ovary and the fallopian tube on the outside edge of the foot.
- Massage the zones of the uterus and the fallopian tube on the inside edge of the foot, below the ankle.
- Massage the zone of the ovary on the outside edge of the foot, below the ankle.

- Massage the zones for the male genital organs on the inside edge of the foot.
- Conclusion: sandwich strokes.
- Massage the other foot in the same way.
- Stretch both feet at the heels.

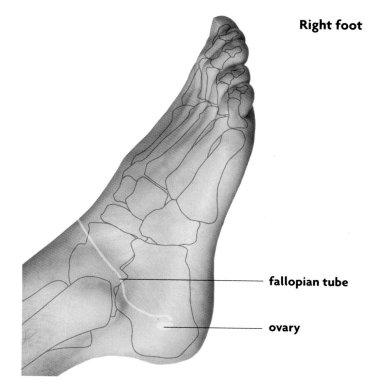

Right foot

fallopian tube

ovary

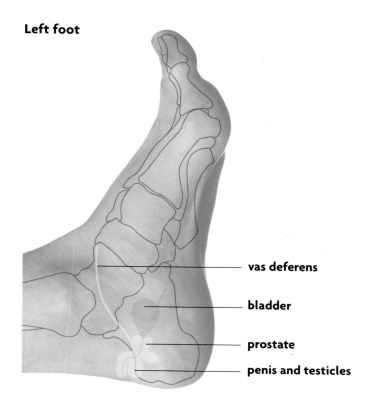

Left foot

vas deferens

bladder

prostate

penis and testicles

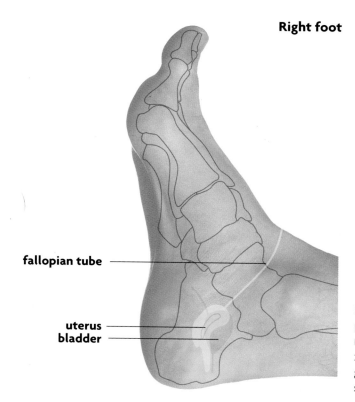

Right foot

fallopian tube

uterus
bladder

For hormonal problems, massage the zones of the genitals on the sides of the feet.

Hand Reflexology Massage

The symptoms of menopause can be alleviated by massaging the genitals zones on the hand. These zones are located on either side of the lower carpus. To begin, stroke your partner's hand. Then massage one hand, followed by the other.

Repeat each technique three to five times. End the massage with strokes and stretches of the palms of the hands.

Sequence of the Massage

- Introduction: sandwich strokes.
- Massage the zone of the genital organs below the carpus on the thumb side of the hand.
- Conclusion: sandwich strokes.
- Stretch the palm.
- Massage the other hand in the same way.

Note: The reflex zones of the genital organs for both men and women are located in a very small area on the hands.

Right hand

Left hand

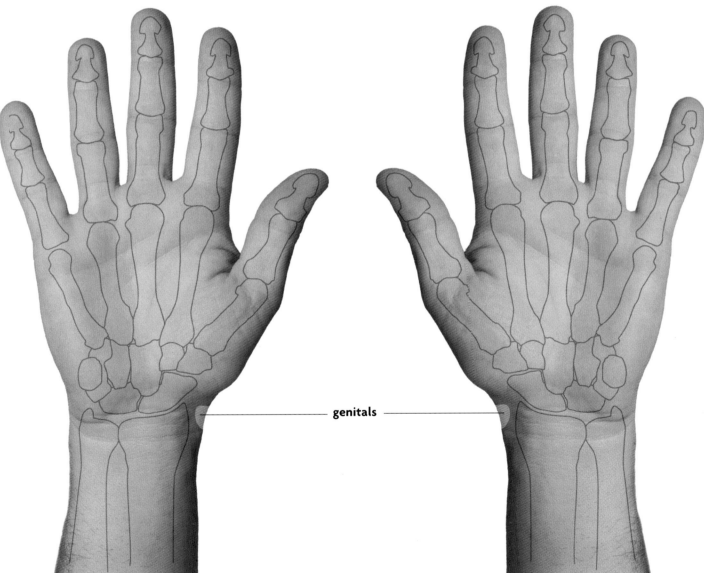

genitals

These reflex zones of the hand can be massaged to remediate hormonal problems.

Ear Reflexology Massage

The ear reflexology massage supplements a hand or foot massage. An advantage of ear reflexology massage is that it is very well suited for self-treatment: you can massage your ears at any time and in any place. Before you massage the individual zones point by point, carry out a few strokes that encompass the whole ear to prepare it for the coming massage. Conclude the massage with strokes. If you are massaging your own ears, you can massage both at the same time, using one hand for each ear. Carry out each technique four or five times.

Sequence of the Massage

- Introduction: strokes with the thumb in several lines along the helix.
- Massage the earlobe in both lengthwise and crosswise paths.
- Massage the head zone on the anthelix upward, point by point, between the tips of your index finger and thumb.
- Massage the plexus urogenitalis point between your thumb and the tip of your index finger.
- Conclusion: strokes with the thumb in several lines along the helix.

Right ear

Left ear

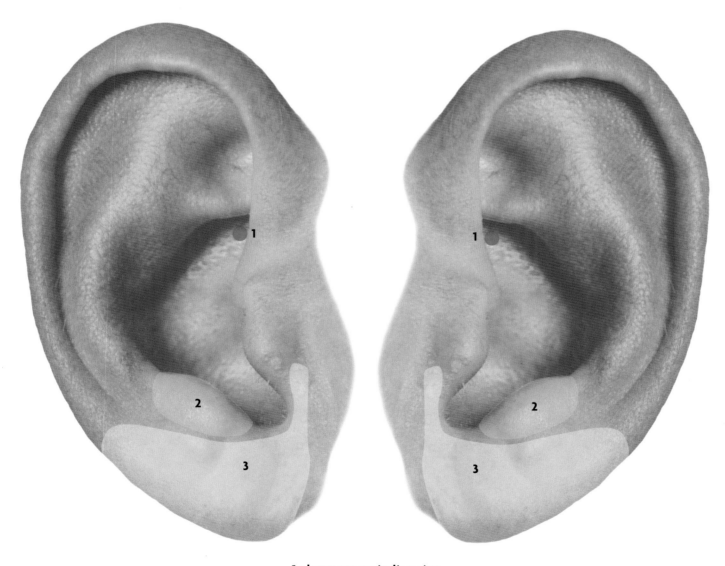

To relieve hormonal problems, massage the zones of the head and sensory organs and the plexus urogenitalis point on the ears.

1 plexus urogenitalis point
2 head zone
3 sensory organs zone

Knee Pain

In the human body, the knee has to withstand extreme stress: like the hip, it carries a large part of our body weight. In addition, it buffers shocks, such as when we are running or jumping, by absorbing a multiple of our body weight. To fulfill this role of shock absorber, the knee joint has buffers called menisci (singular: meniscus). These are half-moon-shaped cartilage disks that lie in each knee between the thigh and the calf bones. The menisci can be worn down or damaged, and when we make severe turns with the knee they can also be torn, or even torn off entirely. Depending on the severity of such an injury, a meniscus may have to be surgically removed.

The posterior (back) and especially the anterior (front) cruciate ligaments ensure the stability of this important joint. The posterior cruciate ligament is well protected and is only rarely injured; tears in the anterior cruciate ligament are relatively common, however, occurring in contact sports such as judo and soccer as well as in skiing.

Here, too, the truth is that the more stress this structure has withstood, the more easily it will tear. In old age, small external forces or twists often suffice to cause injury to the meniscus or cruciate ligament. Such an injury requires medical attention. Do not attempt to manipulate an injured knee—you may end up causing more damage than you heal.

What You Can Do

An injured knee will often swell. Swelling can have a variety of causes, including wear and tear, excessive stress, infection, and sprains. Usually in these cases the knee is painful and can hardly be moved. It is best to rest the joint: elevate your leg and apply cold towels to the knee area. If the swelling does not subside within one day, see a doctor.

How Can Reflexology Help?

Pain in the knee can be influenced through reflexology massage. Head, ear, and foot reflexology massages are especially effective.

The head reflexology massage is the most effective, but it is also slightly less pleasant to undergo.

Head Reflexology Massage

During head reflexology massage, you will focus on the knee points. These are on the side of the neck, diagonally behind the earlobe, near the prominence of the bone. Touch this area and locate points that are sensitive to pressure. Place your thumb tip on these points and apply pressure

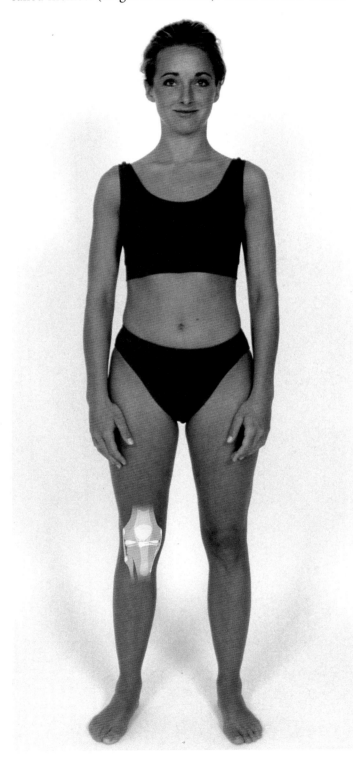

Problems in the knee are often caused by too much or inappropriate stress on the knee joint.

in small, circular movements. If these are too unpleasant, you can also work with steady pressure. Apply the pressure perpendicularly until the pain in this zone subsides. With the subsiding pain, your partner will note a reduction of the pain in the knee.

Sequence of the Massage

- Locate pressure-sensitive points behind the ear near the prominence of the bone.
- Massage the knee points with circular movements or using steady pressure until the painful zones disappear.
- Massage the other side of the head in the same way.

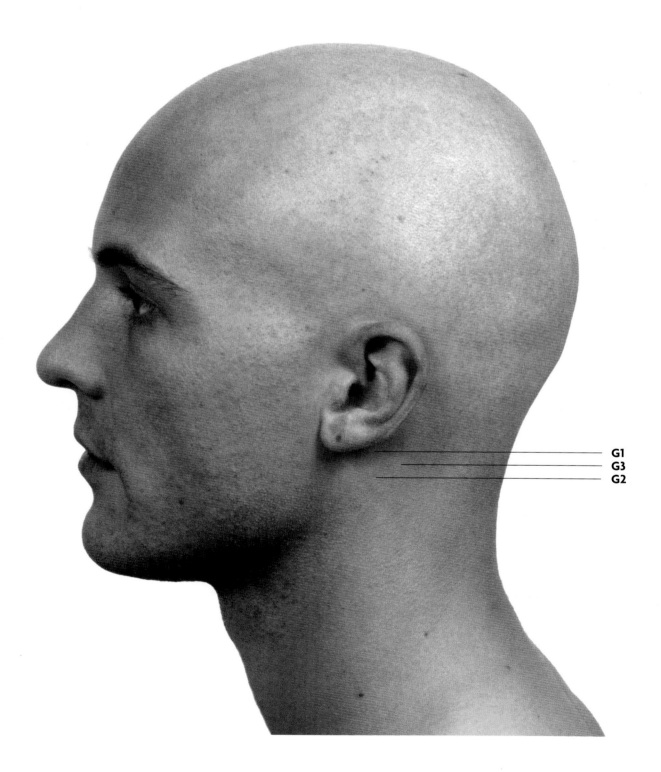

G1
G3
G2

Massage these points on both sides of the head to alleviate knee pain.

Ear Reflexology Massage

Ear reflexology massage, too, is well suited for alleviating knee pain. First administer a basic treatment by stroking the ear with the thumb tip along the helix in several paths. Then press the knee, shen men, jerome, and analgesia points in the upper anthelix, helix tail, and earlobe for 10 seconds each.

Sequence of the Massage

- Introduction: stroke with the thumb tip in several paths along the helix.
- Massage the knee, shen men, jerome, and analgesia points between the tips of your thumb and index finger.
- Conclusion: stroke with the thumb tip in several paths along the helix.
- Massage the other ear in the same way.

Right ear

Left ear

French and Chinese teachings offer two different points to massage on the ear to target the knee.

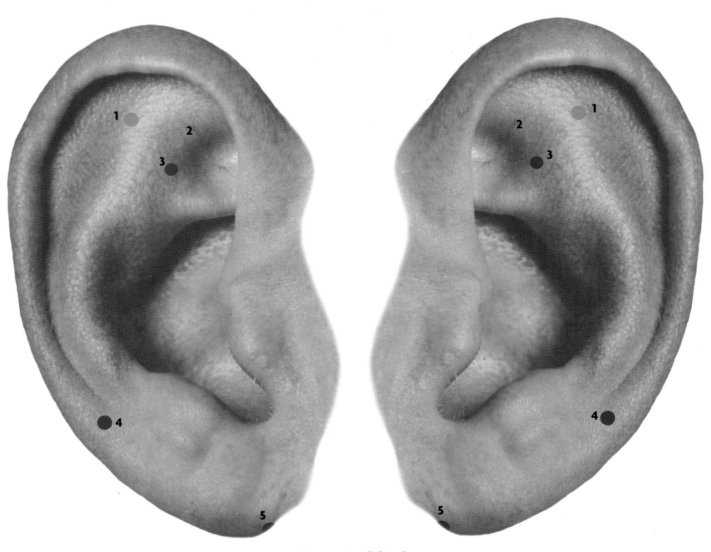

1 knee point (China)

2 knee point (France)

3 shen men point

4 jerome point

5 analgesia point

Foot Reflexology Massage

Foot reflexology massage can be combined with either of the two types of massage described above. Begin with the head or ear massage, then proceed to the foot massage. The zone of the knee is located slightly above the ankle joint on the front of the shin. After a few introductory strokes, search this area for sensitive zones and massage them with the tip of your index finger. Conclude with a few strokes.

Sequence of the Massage

- Introduction: hand-over-hand strokes.
- Locate sensitive spots in the knee zone.
- Massage the zones of the thighs and knees using the tip of your index finger.
- Conclusion: hand-over-hand strokes.
- Massage the other foot in the same way.
- Stretch both feet at the heels.

Left foot

Right foot

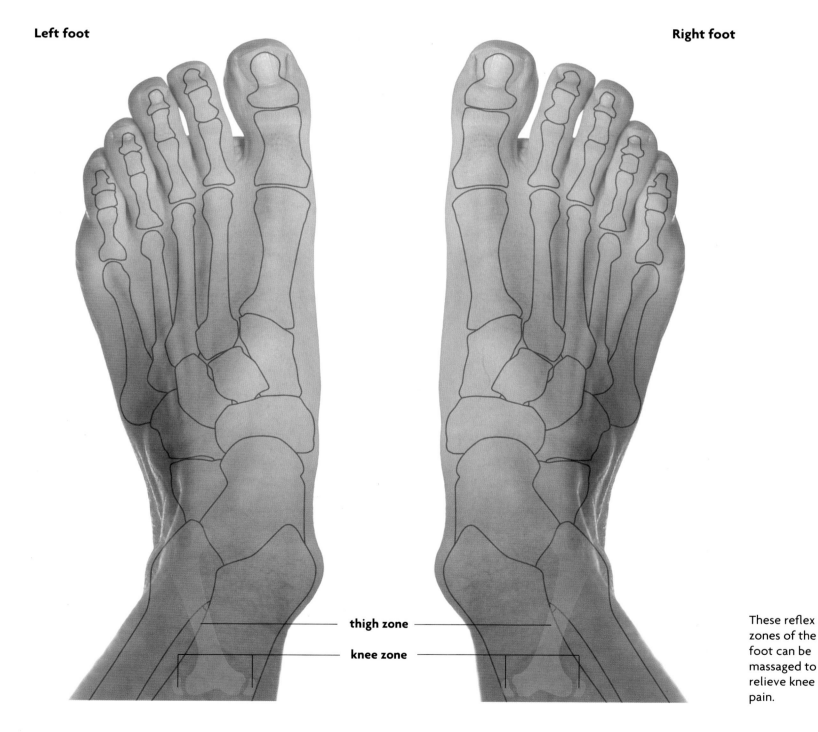

thigh zone

knee zone

These reflex zones of the foot can be massaged to relieve knee pain.

Menstrual Problems

Menstrual problems are relatively common and usually can be treated with natural healing methods. But what exactly do we mean when we talk about menstrual problems? To begin, there is painful menstruation, in which menstruation is accompanied by strong pulling pains and cramps, which can sometimes extend to the back or the legs. Women suffering from these symptoms feel ill and experience dizziness and fatigue. These symptoms can be caused by infections or malignant growths (myomas) in the uterus. Especially among young girls, menstruation can be painful. This pain often has psychological causes: they are leaving the simple world of childhood and entering the unknown terrain of adulthood.

Changes in the bleeding itself are also referred to as menstrual problems. They include both excessively strong and excessively weak bleeding. The cause here is usually changes in the structure of the mucous membranes of the uterus, which are affected by hormones as well as by psychological factors.

If menstruation stops altogether, we speak of amenorrhea. This phenomenon is very normal in times of change, such as during puberty and menopause, as well as after childbirth or after a woman has stopped taking birth control pills. Obviously, the most common cause for the absence of menstruation is pregnancy. But amenorrhea can also be a sign of a metabolic problem (for example, diabetes or a thyroid gland illness) or a functional disturbance in the reproductive organs.

A common condition that is also included in the category of menstrual problems is premenstrual syndrome, or PMS. This term refers to a variety of symptoms that affect many women two to three days before their period. Sufferers describe headaches and difficulty sleeping, food cravings, constipation, depression, nervousness, and water retention in the breasts, which often causes them to become painfully heavy. Usually these symptoms disappear when menstruation begins. Many years passed before these symptoms were defined as a medical syndrome and efforts got under way to help those women affected.

What You Can Do

As a general rule, you should consult a doctor for any menstrual problems that last over at least two cycles. Keep a calendar in which you record the time, duration, and flow of your period.

Among plant-based therapeutic supplements, borage, lady's mantle, chaste tree, valerian, and silverweed are well known for their balancing and relaxing effects for women. And of course it is important to maintain a healthy and balanced diet that is not too high in salt. Also, try to take some time for yourself and not to be always there only for others. In the interest of pursuing this last point, a massage can increase well-being and relaxation.

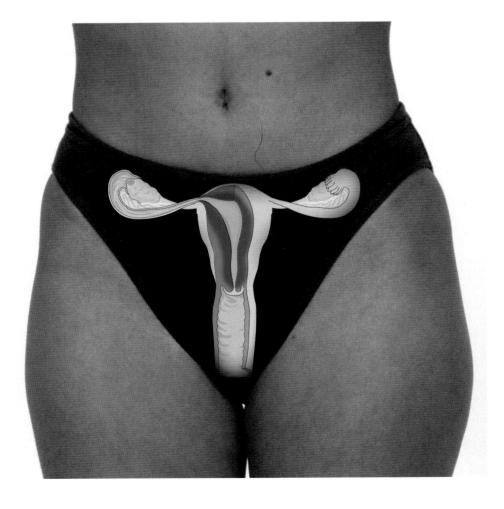

The cause of very heavy or very weak bleeding is changes in the structure of the mucous membranes of the uterus.

How Can Reflexology Help?

Ailments such as pain, difficulty sleeping, depression, and anxiety as part of menstrual problems can be positively influenced by reflexology massages. If possible, carry out a shiatsu massage of the back and sacrum, as described beginning on page 158, as a basic treatment. Massage of the sacrum region has been shown to have especially positive effects on the female abdomen. Other options include foot, hand, and ear reflexology massages.

Foot Reflexology Massage

Before beginning the massage, make sure the recipient's feet are warm; if necessary, use a warm footbath or hot water bottle to warm them. The focus of the massage is on the zones of the head, reproductive organs, and genitals.

Sequence of the Massage

- Warm up the feet.
- Introduction: sandwich strokes.
- Massage the head zones.
- Transition: sandwich strokes.
- Massage the zones of the reproductive organs and genitals with the tip of the index finger.
- Massage the zone of the ovary.
- Conclusion: sandwich strokes.
- Massage the other foot in the same way.
- Stretch both feet at the heels.

Left foot

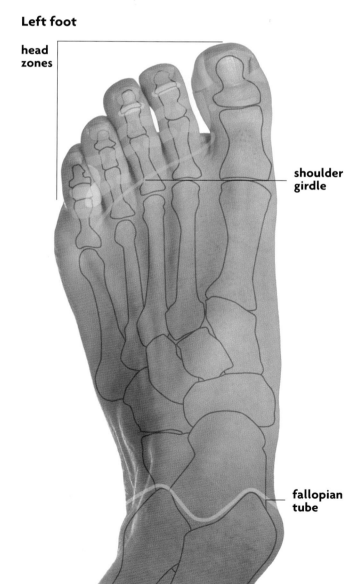

head zones

shoulder girdle

fallopian tube

Right foot

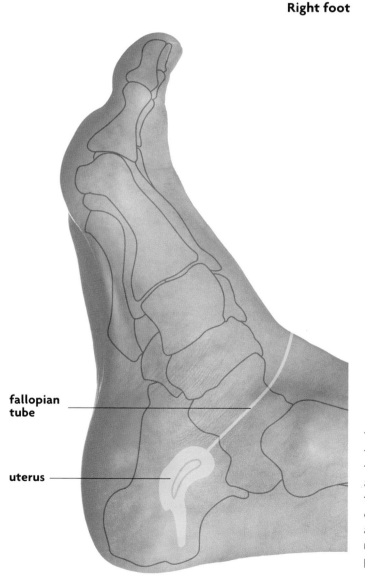

fallopian tube

uterus

The zones of the genitals and the head zones are important for massages designed to alleviate menstrual problems.

Hand Reflexology Massage

The hand reflexology massage follows the pattern of the foot massage. Massaging the reflex zones on the hand is especially good for self-treatment. The hands should be warmed up before the massage. Begin the massage by stroking both hands and then massage the head zones and the zones for the reproductive organs. The zones for the reproductive organs are located below the thumb in the area of the carpus. Repeat each technique three to five times. Massage the other hand in the same way.

Sequence of the Massage

- Warm up the hands.
- Introduction: sandwich strokes.
- Massage the head zones on all fingers using the tweezers grip.
- Transition: sandwich strokes.
- Massage the zones of the reproductive organs, above the carpus on the outer edge of the hand.
- Conclusion: sandwich strokes.
- Stretch the palm of the hand.
- Massage the other hand in the same way.

Right hand

Left hand

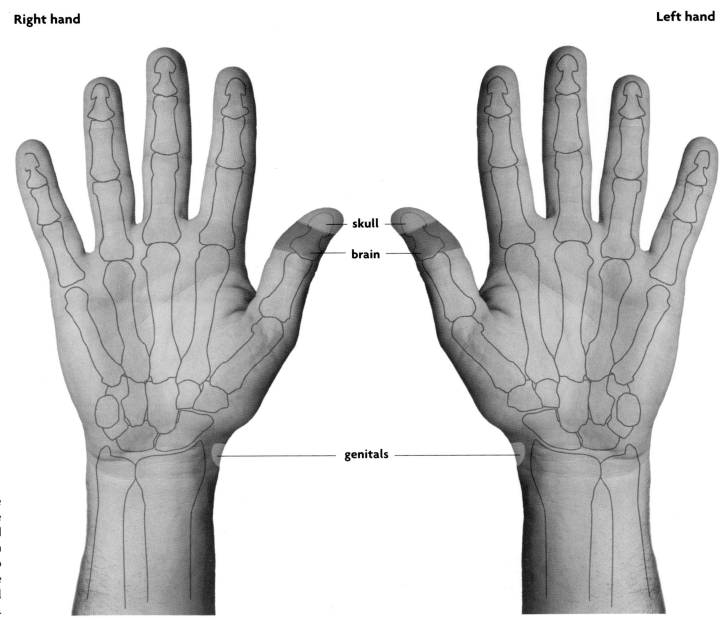

skull

brain

genitals

Massage the zones of the head and genitals on the hands to alleviate menstrual problems.

Ear Reflexology Massage

Ear reflexology massage is well-suited for self-treatment as well as for treatment of a partner. Stroke the ear along the helix in several paths with your thumb. Massage the ovary, uterus, plexus urogenitalis, and sympathetic points using the tips of your thumb and index finger. Then massage the earlobe in horizontal and vertical lines. Apply pressure on each point for 5 to 10 seconds.

Sequence of the Massage

- Introduction: strokes with the thumb in several lines along the helix.
- Press the uterus, plexus urogenitalis, ovary, and sympathetic points between the tips of the thumb and index finger.
- Massage the earlobe point by point in horizontal and vertical lines.
- Conclusion: stroke the helix in several lines with your thumb.
- Massage the other ear in the same way.

Right ear　　　　　　　　　　　　　　　　　　　　　　　　**Left ear**

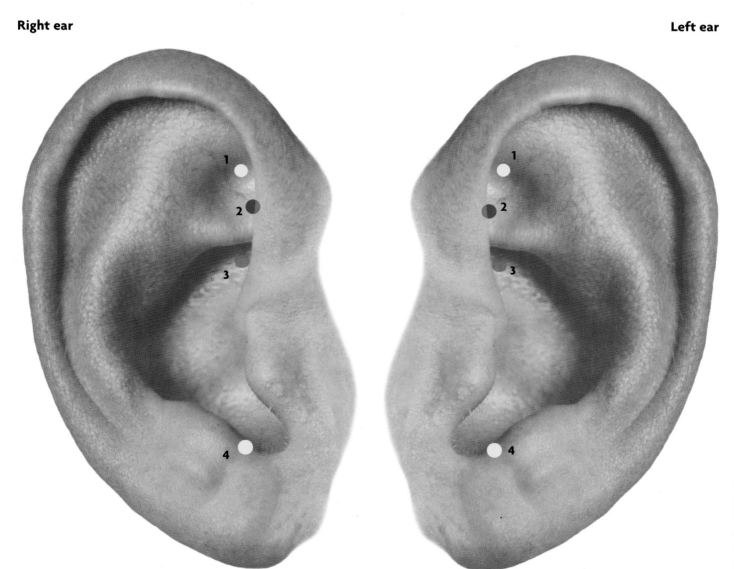

Massage the points indicated here to alleviate menstrual problems.

1 uterus point

2 sympathetic point

3 plexus urogenitalis point

4 ovary point

Shoulder Pain

Pain in the shoulder joint or in the areas close to the joint is usually an indication of wear and tear of the related structures. The shoulder is made up of several small joints. The main joint is the humeroscapular joint—that is, the joint in which the head of the upper arm bone (humerus) rests in the socket of the shoulder blade (scapula). The socket of this joint is very shallow, which allows the arm a large range of motion. This range of motion, however, comes at a price: no joint is as easily dislocated as is the shoulder. The reduced stability of this joint is also related to the fact that the connections between the joint are made up largely of muscles and not, as is the case for the hip joint, of tendons.

Doctors refer to pain in the shoulder joint as omalgia. It can have a number of causes, from infections, to degenerative changes (those caused by wear and tear), to torn tissues in the muscles.

Inflammation in the shoulder can affect the joint itself (arthritis) or the bursas (bursitis). These responses can occur especially if the joint was under extreme stress for a short period, as may be the case during athletic activity or other physical labor (hanging curtains is one such activity).

The top of the upper arm is surrounded by a band of muscles that rotate the arm inward and out. Some of these muscles run through a small canal of bone created by the shoulder blade. This tight area is very sensitive to wear and tear. Picture a rope that is always pulled over a sharp edge—over time, it will wear down. Excessive stress on these muscles has a similar effect. The body reacts to this stress by swelling, which causes pain when the arm is lifted or turned or even lain on at night. This condition is called impingement syndrome. If the stress on the muscles continues for an extended period of time, more and more muscle fibers will become damaged, until finally the entire band tears. Experts refer to this as a rotator-cuff rupture. This rupture can occur suddenly and is accompanied by a loud sound and severe pain. More frequently, however, small parts of these muscles will tear over a period of months or years.

Another cause for pain and reduced mobility in the shoulders can be the so-called frozen shoulder, which is common especially among older people. This occurs when an inflammation of the capsule surrounding the ball joint is followed by a weakening of the muscles of the rotator cuff. This leads to a severely reduced range of motion accompanied by moderate to severe pain.

What You Can Do

In the case of persistent or recurring shoulder pain, you should consult a doctor. In these cases, timely medical attention can save you from a long duration of suffering. You can support medi-

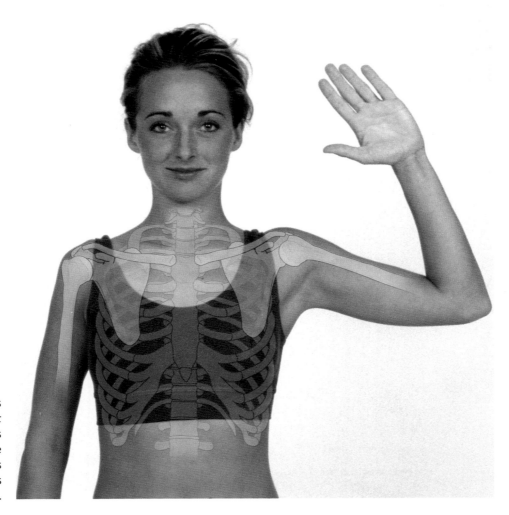

The shoulder is among the most flexible joints but is also the least stable. It is prone to injuries and ailments.

cal treatment by paying attention to your posture and by avoiding, where possible, extreme strain on the shoulder girdle. Heat treatments in the form of hot towels can help, but discuss such treatments with a doctor first, since not every type of shoulder injury reacts positively to warmth. Herbal teas are a proven complementary remedy. They are especially good for preventing joint pain. Teas made of willow bark, birch leaf, and dandelion root are well known for their ability to alleviate muscle and joint pain.

How Can Reflexology Help?

For acute shoulder pain, head, ear, and foot reflexology massages all help. You can begin with a head reflexology massage.

Head Reflexology Massage

Shoulder pain can be treated effectively using head reflexology massage. Locate the sensitive points in the B and C zones and massage these points with the tip of your thumb using steady pressure or circling movements. Apply pressure until the pain disappears. This will also noticeably alleviate shoulder pain.

Sequence of the Massage

- Locate sensitive points in the B and/or C zones.
- Massage the zones with steady pressure or circling movements using the tip of your thumb.
- Carry out the same massage on the other side of the head.

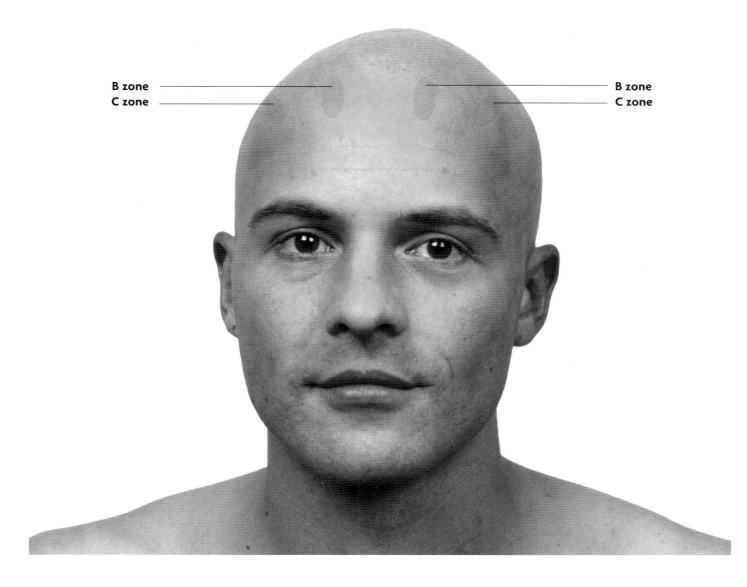

B zone

C zone

B zone

C zone

Shoulder pain often causes the corresponding reflex zones on the head to become more sensitive.

Ear Reflexology Massage

On the ear you will massage the point for the shoulder joint; it has a direct effect on the shoulder. Furthermore, you will massage all the points that have general pain-relieving and harmonizing properties: shen men, polster, and jerome. Also massage the zone of the thoracic spine. For the introduction and conclusion, carry out strokes along the helix that encompass the whole ear. Press the individual zones or points for 5 to 10 seconds each. In the case of self-massage, you can massage both ears at the same time.

Sequence of the Massage

- Introduction: strokes with the thumb in several lines along the helix.
- Massage the shoulder point between the thumb and index finger.
- Massage the zone of the thoracic spine point by point.
- Massage the shen men, jerome, and polster points between the tips of your thumb and index finger.
- Conclusion: strokes with the thumb in several lines along the helix.
- Massage the other ear in the same way.

Right ear

Left ear

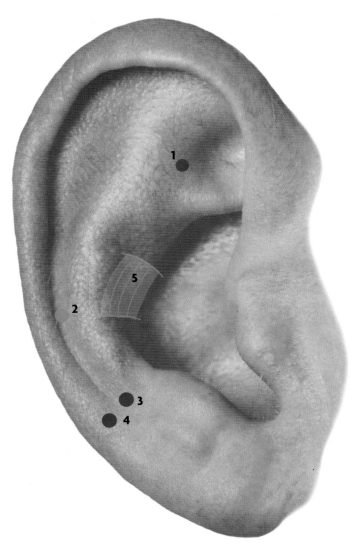
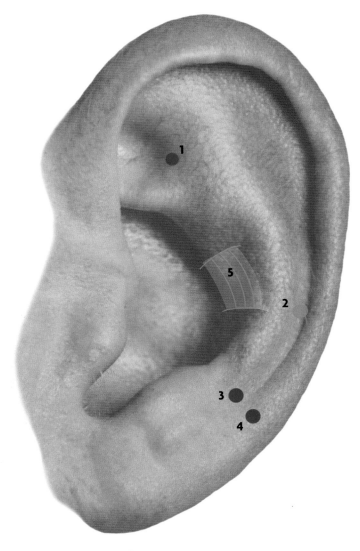

Massage these points on the ear to treat shoulder pain.

1 shen men point
2 shoulder joint point
3 polster point

4 jerome point
5 zone of the thoracic spine

Foot Reflexology Massage

For shoulder problems, massage the zones of the neck, cervical spine, shoulder, and shoulder girdle. Before you begin a point-by-point massage of the individual zones, carry out a few sandwich strokes that encompass the whole foot. Then loosen the foot by gently shaking it (see page 55). For this, take the front of the foot between your hands and gently shake it back and forth, creating a small vibrating movement that travels along the whole body. Finish the massage with strokes. Massage first one foot and then the other, and then stretch the heels. Repeat each technique three to five times.

Sequence of the Massage

- Introduction: sandwich strokes.
- Shake the front of the foot.
- Massage the neck zone and the cervical spine zone with the tip of the thumb.
- Massage the zones of the shoulder and shoulder girdle in horizontal and vertical lines.
- Conclusion: sandwich strokes.
- Massage the other foot in the same way.
- Stretch both feet at the heels.

Right foot

Right foot

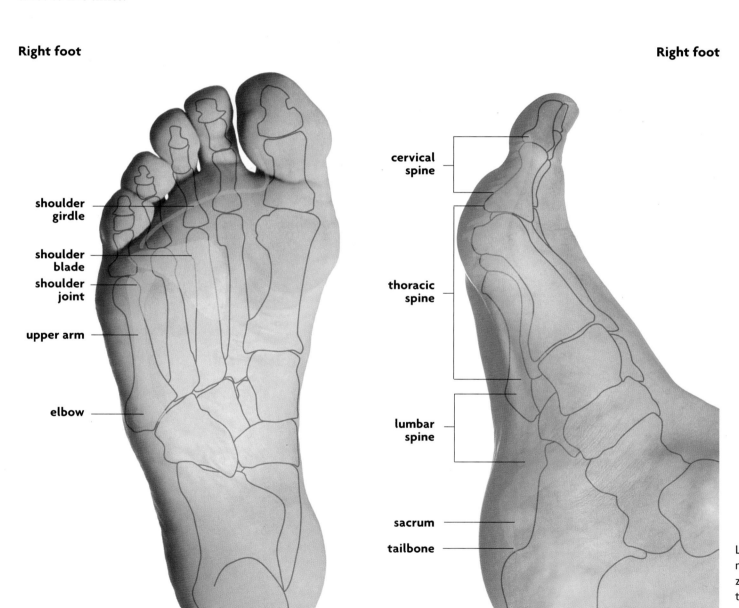

shoulder girdle
shoulder blade
shoulder joint
upper arm
elbow

cervical spine
thoracic spine
lumbar spine
sacrum
tailbone

Locate and massage sensitive zones on both the soles and the sides of the feet to relieve shoulder pain.

Sleep Problems

About forty million Americans, close to 15 percent of the population, suffer from sleep disorders. Sleep is a life necessity to regenerate body and soul, and sleep problems quickly lead to irritation or nervousness, as well as loss of concentration and a reduction in performance ability. We assume that young adults need seven to eight hours of sleep a day, while for older people five to six hours a day will suffice. This is important especially in the context of older people frequently complaining of suffering from sleep problems.

Doctors differentiate between the problem of falling asleep and the problem of staying asleep. In the case of the problem of falling asleep, sufferers remain awake for a long time after going to bed. In the case of the problem of staying asleep, sufferers fall asleep normally, but they wake up frequently during the night and again early in the mornings. Both problems are referred to as insomnia. Parasomnia is another sleep disorder. It encompasses symptoms such as sleepwalking, nightmares, and bedwetting. It frequently affects children and can significantly reduce the quality of sleep, with or without waking.

The causes of sleep problems are manifold. Frequently they are illnesses, such as when people are unable to sleep because of pain or because of psychological symptoms such as depression. It is a sign of our times that flexible working hours, working in shifts, and constantly increasing performance pressure make it more and more difficult for people to find and maintain a steady wake-sleep cycle. The increased consumption of stimulants such as caffeine drinks, medication, and drugs also has negative effects on our sleep patterns.

Frequently, no cause is found for sleep disorders. Nonetheless, sleep disorders cause a significant amount of suffering, as problems often continue for extended periods and begin to dominate the life of the sufferers. A vicious cycle can result: The sufferer goes to bed certain that he or she won't be able to fall asleep, which means that he or she has a disturbed relationship with sleep itself. In treating sleep disorders, doctors often prescribe sleeping pills. Specialists insist, however, that such medication should always be combined with behavioral therapy, for only this combination will lead to long-term improvement. First, it helps to find out how much sleep the sufferer actually requires. Behavioral therapy that allows the sufferer to practice a conscious relaxation—for example, autogenic training—can be helpful.

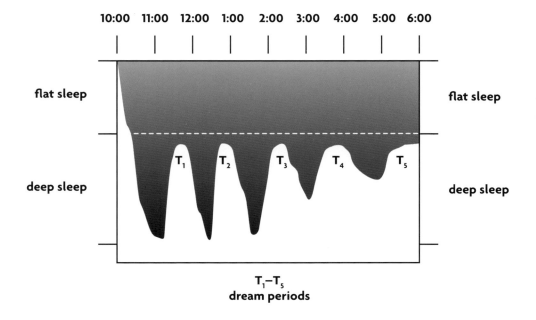

Sleep is characterized by phases of varying depths.

What You Can Do

Make sure that you get enough exercise during the day, since adequate exercise is likely to generate a healthy sleepiness for the night. Do not drink stimulating drinks from the early afternoon onward. Create a comfortable sleeping environment. The bedroom should be quiet and dark, and the optimal temperature is between 57 and 64 degrees Fahrenheit (14 to 18 degrees Celsius). Before going to bed, take a warm footbath and drink warm milk or herbal tea, especially melissa, hops, or lavender. If you still have difficulty falling asleep, do not stay awake in bed for more than 30 minutes. Instead, get up and read until you find yourself feeling sleepy. It is very important not to take psychological problems to bed with you. If you have a problem on your mind, carry out relaxation exercises—for example, autogenic training—before going to bed.

How Can Reflexology Help?

The cause of sleep problems in many cases is stress. Reflexology massages reduce stress and help the body regenerate. As such, reflexology massages, when carried out regularly, can help you fall asleep and stay asleep. Often, reflexology massages are as effective as sleeping pills, and can even replace them entirely. The following combinations are especially well suited for treating sleep disorders:

- massage of the foot and ear reflex zones
- massage of the hand and ear reflex zones

Shiatsu therapy has also had great success in treating sleep disorders. Here, you should focus on the back massage (page 158) as well as the head and facial massages (page 184).

Foot Reflexology

The emphasis of the massage is on soft, stroking techniques that encompass the entire foot. Massage of the head zone and solar plexus zone is good for reducing tension and nervousness.

Sequence of the Massage

- Warm the feet (with a hot water bottle or footbath).
- Introduction: sandwich strokes and hand-over-hand strokes.
- Massage the head zones using the tweezers grip.
- Massage the solar plexus zone using steady pressure.
- Conclusion: sandwich strokes and hand-over-hand strokes.
- Place your hands on the soles of the feet.

Right foot

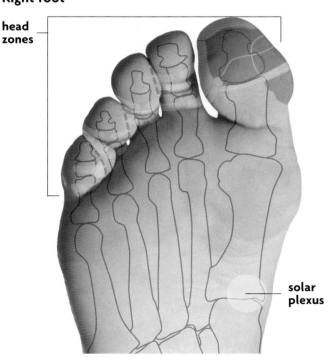

head zones

solar plexus

Right foot

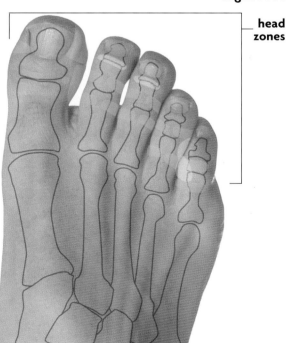

head zones

To relieve sleep problems, massage the zones of the head and solar plexus on the feet.

Ear Reflexology

For the ear massage, the focus is on strokes and on massaging the points that balance the autonomic nervous sytem. As an introduction, carry out lengthwise strokes and then massage the jerome, polster, and sympathetic points. Press each of these points between your thumb and index finger for 5 to 10 seconds. Then massage the earlobe in horizontal and vertical lines. Conclude with strokes encompassing the whole ear.

Sequence of the Massage

- Introduction: strokes with the thumb in several lines along the helix.
- Massage the polster, jerome, and sympathetic points.
- Massage the earlobe point by point in horizontal and vertical lines.
- Conclusion: strokes with the thumb.
- Massage the other ear in the same way.

Right ear　　　　　　　　　　　　　　　　　　　　　　　**Left ear**

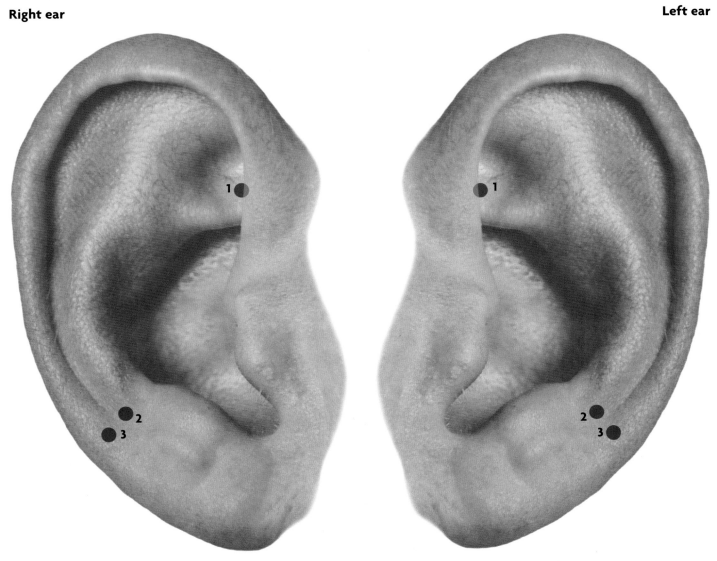

Massaging the jerome, polster, and sympathetic points has overall effects that can help with sleeping problems.

1 sympathetic point

2 polster point

3 jerome point

Hand Reflexology

For the hand massage, the same principles apply as for the foot massage. Warm up the hands before the massage. Stroke the hands of your partner with both hands, then massage the head zones in the upper part of the hand. Treat the zone of the solar plexus using steady pressure, and conclude with some sandwich strokes.

Sequence of the Massage

- Warm up the hands.
- Introduction: sandwich strokes.
- Massage the head zones on the palm and back of the hand using the tweezers grip.
- Massage the solar plexus using steady pressure.
- Conclusion: sandwich strokes.
- Stretch the palm.
- Massage the other hand in the same way.

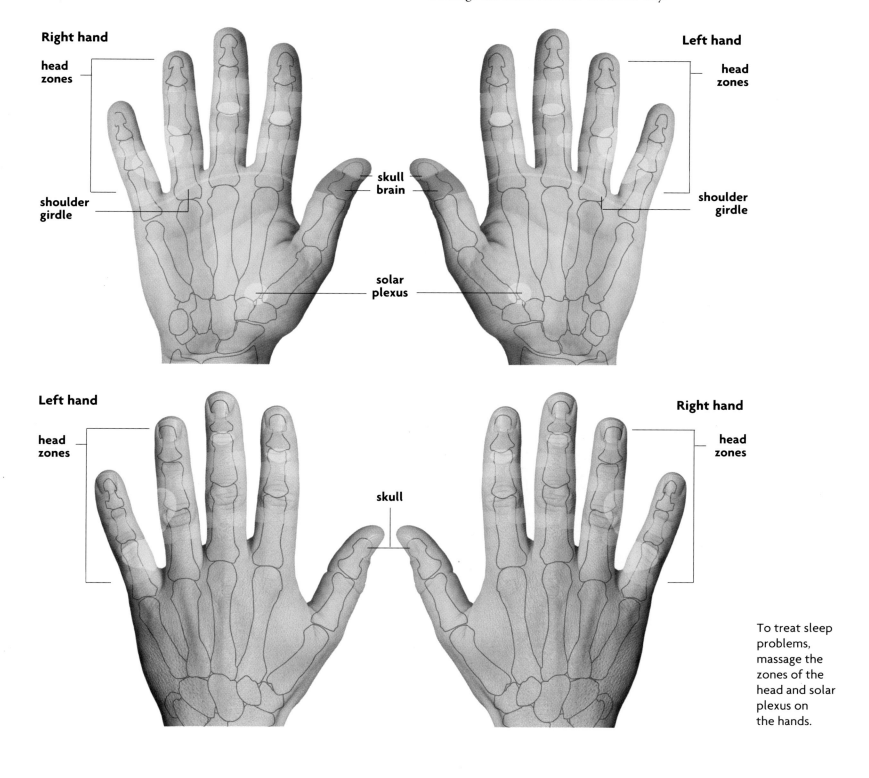

Right hand
head zones
shoulder girdle
skull brain

Left hand
head zones
shoulder girdle

solar plexus

Left hand
head zones

Right hand
head zones

skull

To treat sleep problems, massage the zones of the head and solar plexus on the hands.

Urinary Tract Ailments

Reflexology is a worthwhile complementary treatment for a number of ailments of the urinary tract. One of the most common illnesses of the bladder is an infection called cystitis. It is characterized by a frequent need to urinate despite low levels of urine and is often accompanied by strong pains during urination. This infection is usually caused by bacteria that enter the bladder from the intestines, and it occurs more easily if the affected person does not drink enough fluids, causing the bladder to be not very well rinsed. Since the urethra is very short in women, they suffer from bladder infections much more frequently than men. If you are experiencing any of the symptoms described here, you should consult a doctor immediately. He or she will test your urine for bacteria and, if necessary, prescribe antibiotics to treat the infection.

The so-called irritated bladder can have the same indications as a bladder infection, but they are less severe.

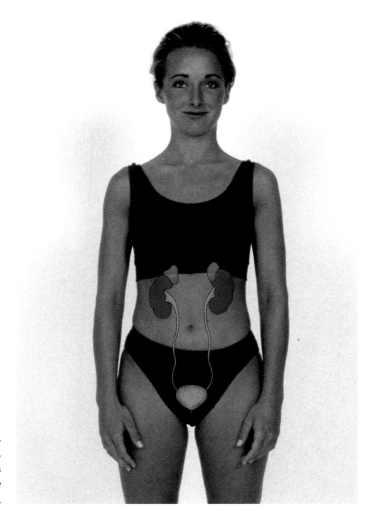

The kidneys, ureter, bladder, and urethra make up the urinary tract.

However, in the case of irritated bladder, no pathogen of an infection is present. The cause of irritated bladder is a mistake in the steering system of the body that notifies the brain when the bladder is full. This leads to the frequent need to urinate, even if the bladder is hardly filled. In this case, too, it is important to consult a doctor to rule out the possibility of an infection. Treatment of irritated bladder can usually be done with herbal or homeopathic methods that relax the bladder muscles. Pumpkin seeds, for example, are especially effective.

However, ailments of the urinary tract are not confined to the lower urinary tract. Different chemical substances in urine can lead to the formation of stones that are deposited in the kidneys. They can remain here for long periods without causing problems. However, if a stone travels in the direction of the bladder, it must pass through the narrow ureter. It stretches the walls of the ureter, causing strong, coliclike pains. These are sometimes accompanied by nausea, vomiting, or blood in the urine. In this case, a doctor should be consulted as soon as possible. Treatment differs and depends on how the stone is made up. Some kidney stones can be broken up with sound waves, while others can be dissolved with medication. Muscle relaxants can support the quick excretion of small parts.

What You Can Do

In the case of a bladder infection, you can support the treatment by drinking at least 2 to 3 liters of liquids per day. Preparations of stinging nettle herb, juniper, bearberry leaf, and horsetail grass have proved successful as complementary therapeutic supplements. Avoid spicy foods, alcohol, and caffeine during a bladder infection, as they can further irritate the bladder.

In the case of irritated bladder, too, you can help by drinking plenty of liquids. Empty your bladder only at certain times as a sort of training. Gymnastic exercises for the pelvic floor, warm sitz baths, and relaxation exercises are also useful.

If you've been diagnosed with kidney stones, it is especially important to drink enough liquids. If you experience kidney stones repeatedly, you may need to adhere to a special diet. Definitely consult an expert in this case.

How Can Reflexology Help?

In the case of acute and recurring ailments in the urinary tract, reflexology can help by positively influencing pain in the area of the bladder and the connecting urinary tract. Foot and ear reflexology massages as well as shiatsu can be used here, and all three treatments can be combined with one another.

Foot Reflexology Massage

The focal points should be the zones of kidney, ureter, and bladder. The kidney zone is about the size of a bean and is located at the base of the third metatarsal bone. The ureter zone runs diagonally from the kidney zone to the inside of the heel. The bladder zone is about two finger-widths below the lower edge of the ankle, slightly toward the heel.

It is very important that the feet of your partner be warm for the massage. A warm footbath can also be an ideal introduction.

Sequence of the Massage

- Warm footbath.
- Introduction: sandwich strokes.
- Massage the kidney zone on the sole of the foot with the thumb tip.
- Massage the ureter zone on the sole of the foot with the thumb walk.
- Massage the bladder zone on the inside edge of the foot with the thumb tip.
- Conclusion: sandwich strokes.
- Massage the other foot in the same way.
- Stretch both feet at the heels.

Left foot

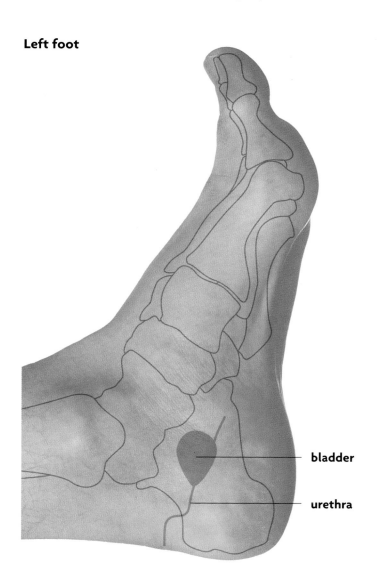

bladder

urethra

Left foot

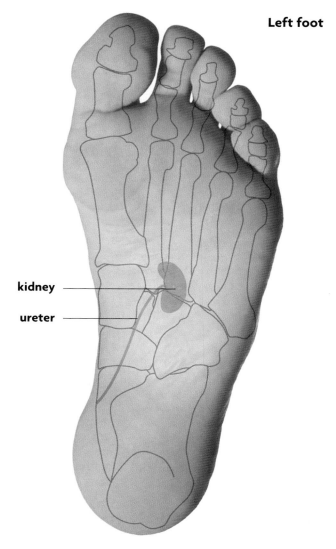

kidney

ureter

The reflex zones of the urinary tract run from the middle of the sole to the inside ankle.

Ear Reflexology Massage

Ear reflexology massage is very well suited for the treatment of urinary tract ailments, especially when combined with foot reflexology massage.

The points and zones of the pelvic organs are located in the upper part of the deep auricle. The kidney-bladder area is an elongated zone, in contrast to the kidney point, which covers a much smaller area and is located inside the kidney-bladder area.

Introduction and preparation consists of strokes that encompass the whole ear. If you are massaging yourself, you can massage both ears at the same time. If you're massaging your partner's ear, finish one before turning to the other. Repeat each stroke four or five times, and press the individual zones or points for 5 to 10 seconds each. Conclude the massage with strokes.

Sequence of the Massage

- Introduction: strokes with the thumb in several lines along the helix.
- Massage the kidney-bladder area, the kidney point, and the zones of the urethra and the plexus urogenitalis in the upper part of the auricle with the tweezers grip.
- Conclusion: strokes with the thumb in several lines along the helix.

Right ear

Left ear

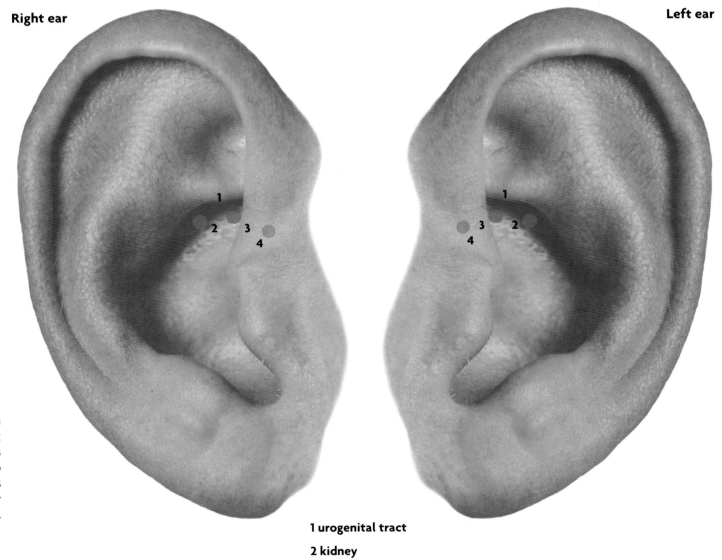

You can massage the reflex zones and points of the ear to alleviate problems in the urinary tract.

1 urogenital tract

2 kidney

3 plexus urogenitalis

4 urethra

Shiatsu

A shiatsu massage of the back with a focus on the sacrum region alleviates the pain that can accompany urinary tract illnesses. The region above the sacrum contains the reflex zones of the bladder and other organs of the lower body. Locate the top hole of the sacrum with both thumbs and place both thumb tips over it. As your partner exhales, apply pressure, adjusting the pressure based on the sensitivity of your partner. As your partner inhales, release the pressure and move your thumbs down toward the feet a little bit. Massage the sacrum point by point in this manner.

Place the heels of your hands on either side of the spine in the sacrum region and apply pressure in synchrony with your partner's breathing. This technique relaxes the area and alleviates pain. Next, interlace your fingers and set the palms of your hands on either side of the spine at the top of the sacrum. As your partner exhales, bring the heels of your hands toward each other, above the sacrum, pushing it "together." Repeat from the top to the bottom of the area. This technique takes weight off the tense sacrum region.

Once you have finished massaging the sacrum, conclude by placing a hot water bottle on the sacrum region. The warmth supports circulation in this area and amplifies the effects of the massage.

Sequence of the Massage

- Apply thumb pressure over the holes of the sacrum.
- Apply pressure with the heels of the hands.
- Move the sacrum "together."

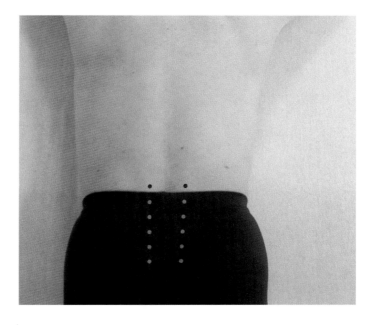

Massage of the sacrum region can relieve urinary tract ailments.

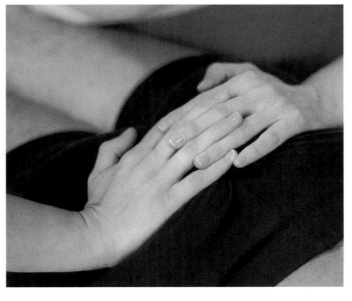

Begin massaging the sacrum using thumb pressure.

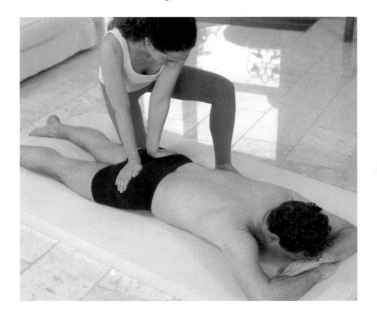

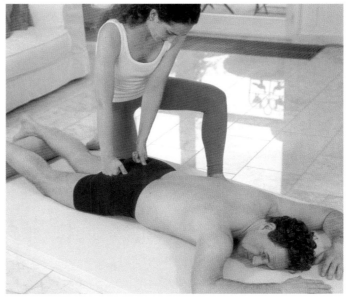

Left: Then switch to applying pressure with the heel of your hand.

Right: Move the sacrum "together" as your partner exhales.

Appendix

Diagrams

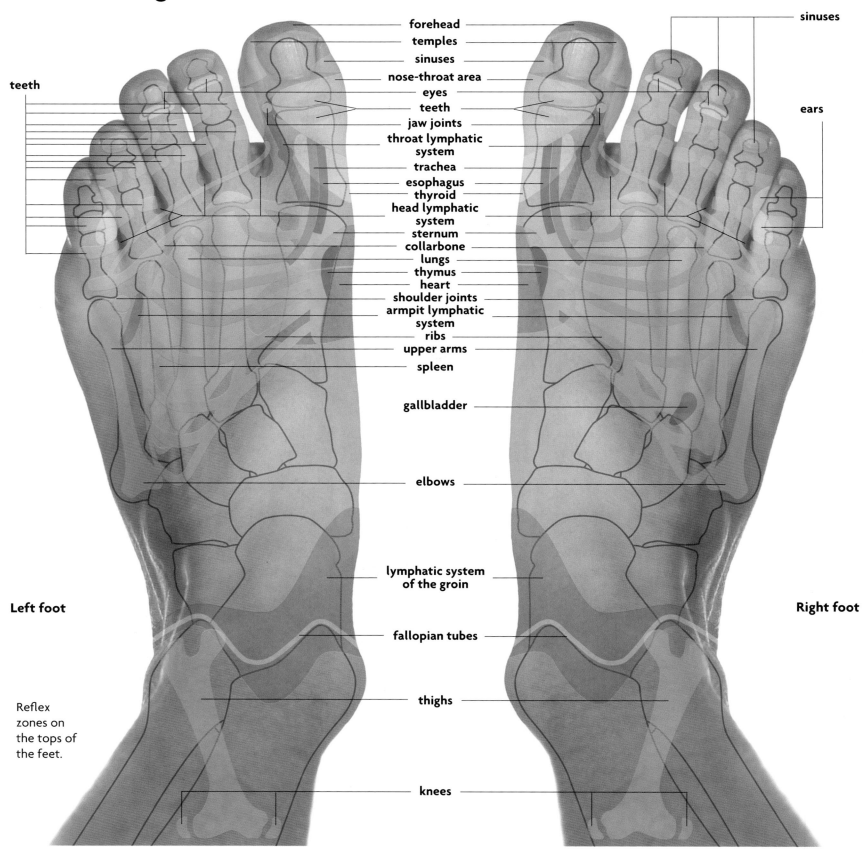

forehead
temples
sinuses
nose-throat area
eyes
teeth
jaw joints
throat lymphatic
system
trachea
esophagus
thyroid
head lymphatic
system
sternum
collarbone
lungs
thymus
heart
shoulder joints
armpit lymphatic
system
ribs
upper arms
spleen

gallbladder

elbows

lymphatic system
of the groin

fallopian tubes

thighs

knees

teeth

sinuses

ears

Left foot

Right foot

Reflex
zones on
the tops of
the feet.

Right foot

Left foot

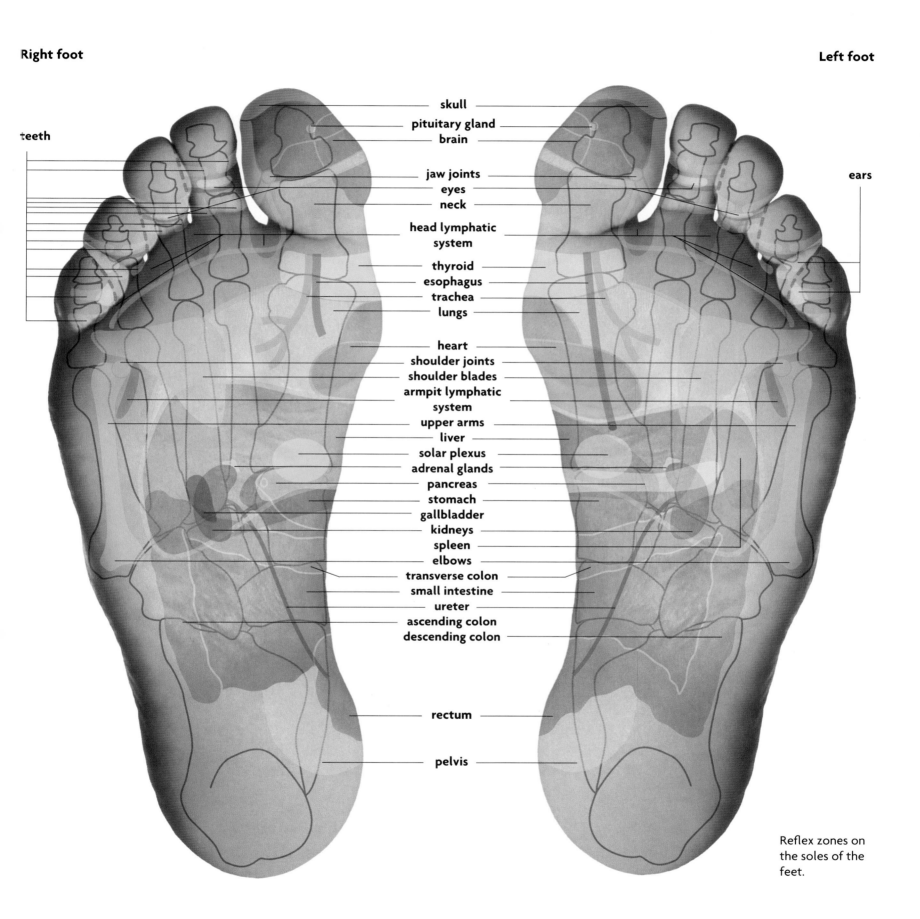

teeth

ears

skull
pituitary gland
brain

jaw joints
eyes
neck
head lymphatic
system
thyroid
esophagus
trachea
lungs

heart
shoulder joints
shoulder blades
armpit lymphatic
system
upper arms
liver
solar plexus
adrenal glands
pancreas
stomach
gallbladder
kidneys
spleen
elbows
transverse colon
small intestine
ureter
ascending colon
descending colon

rectum

pelvis

Reflex zones on
the soles of the
feet.

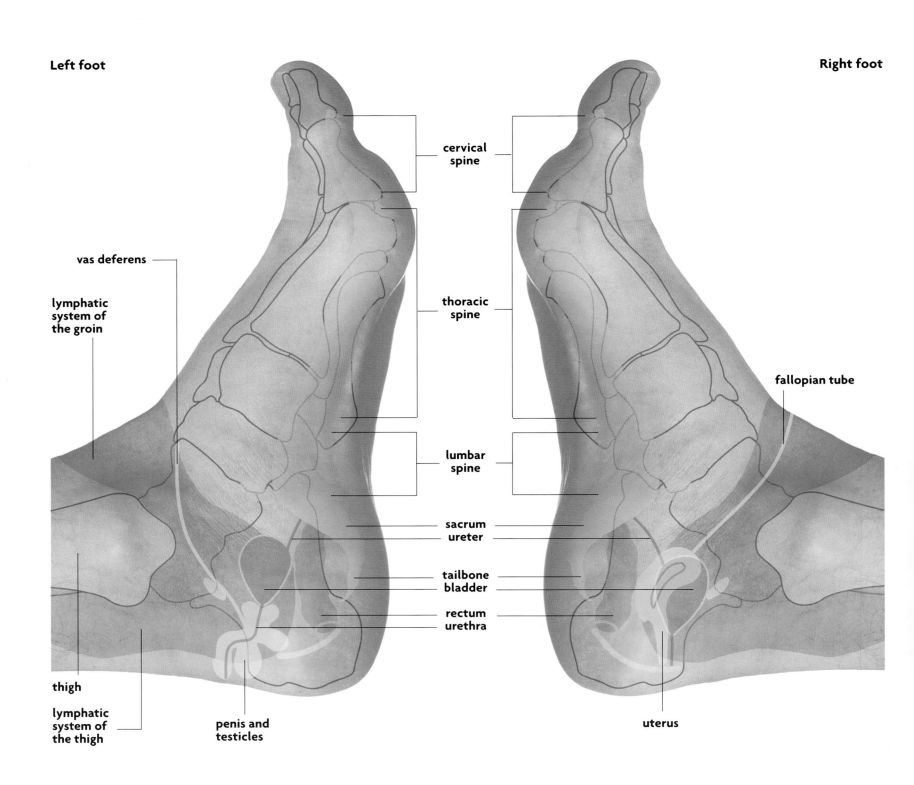

Left foot

Right foot

vas deferens

lymphatic
system of
the groin

cervical
spine

thoracic
spine

fallopian tube

lumbar
spine

sacrum
ureter

tailbone
bladder

rectum
urethra

thigh

lymphatic
system of
the thigh

penis and
testicles

uterus

Reflex zones on
the inner sides
of the feet.

Right foot

Left foot

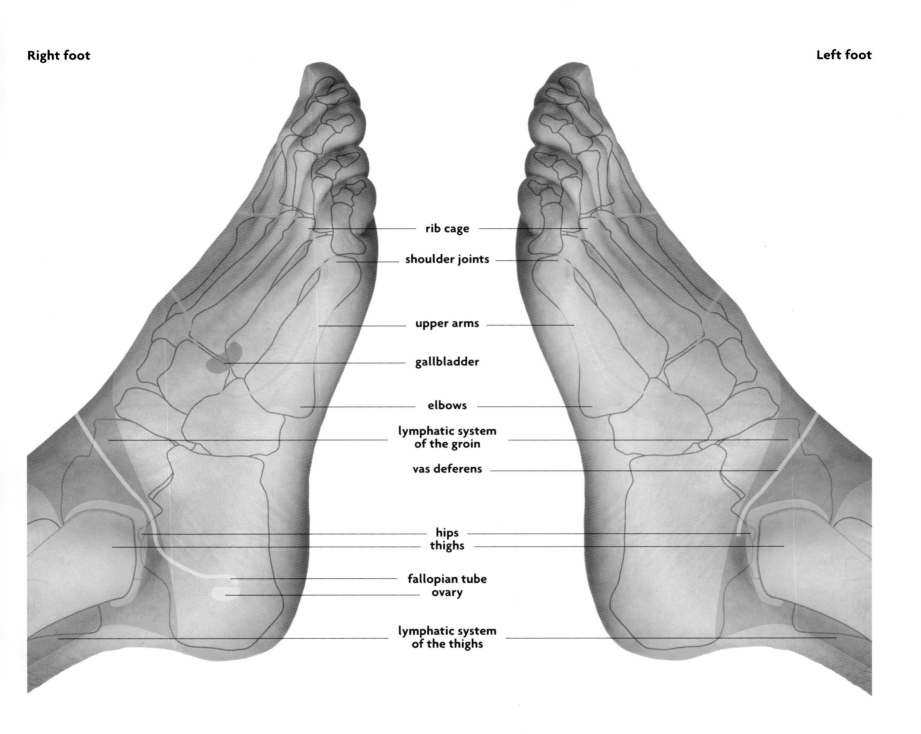

rib cage

shoulder joints

upper arms

gallbladder

elbows

lymphatic system
of the groin

vas deferens

hips
thighs

fallopian tube
ovary

lymphatic system
of the thighs

Reflex zones on
the outer sides
of the feet.

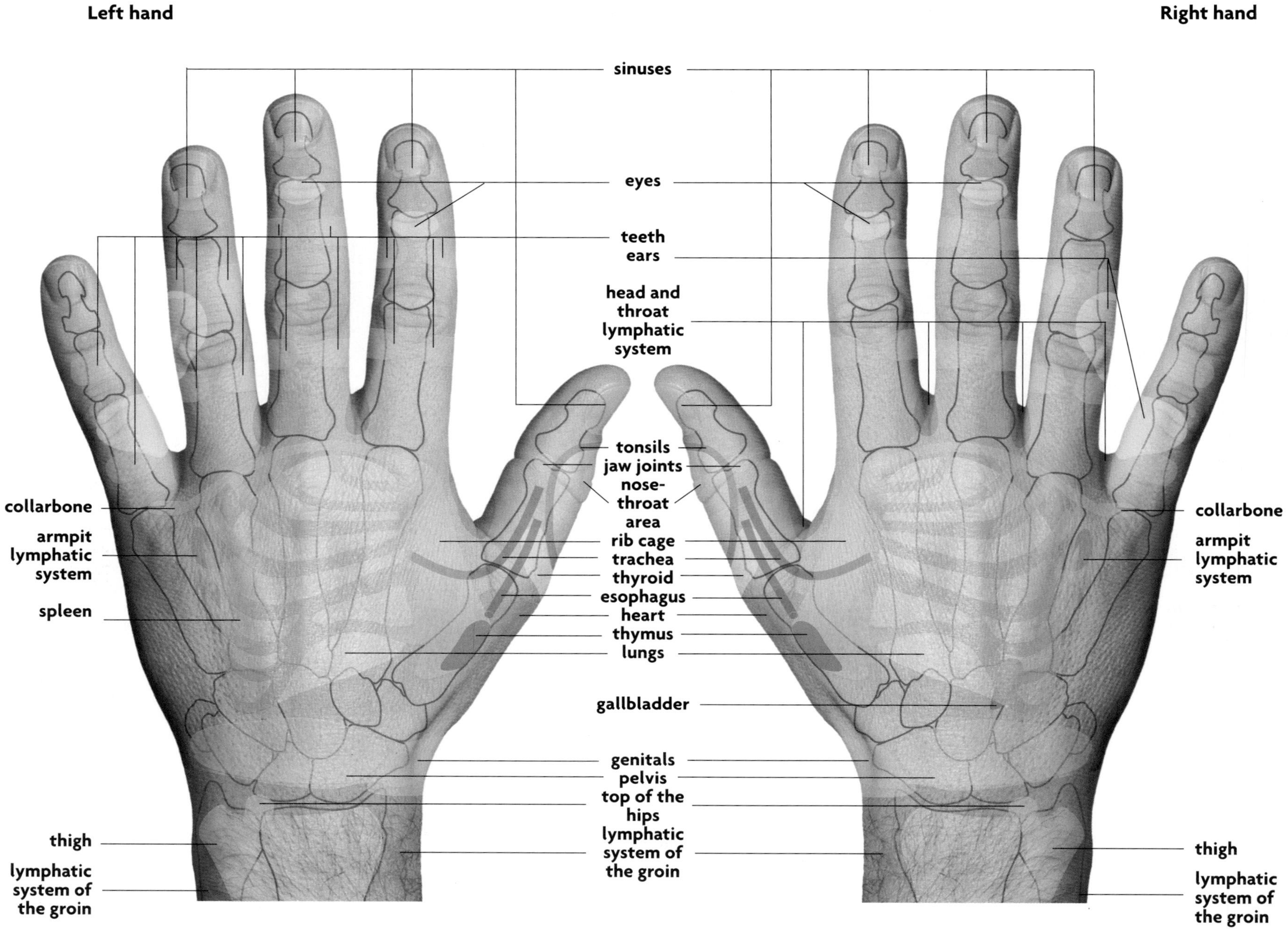

Left hand

Right hand

sinuses

eyes

teeth
ears

head and
throat
lymphatic
system

tonsils
jaw joints
nose-
throat
area
rib cage
trachea
thyroid
esophagus
heart
thymus
lungs

collarbone

armpit
lymphatic
system

spleen

collarbone

armpit
lymphatic
system

gallbladder

genitals
pelvis
top of the
hips
lymphatic
system of
the groin

thigh

lymphatic
system of
the groin

thigh

lymphatic
system of
the groin

Reflex zones
on the backs
of the hands.

Right hand

Left hand

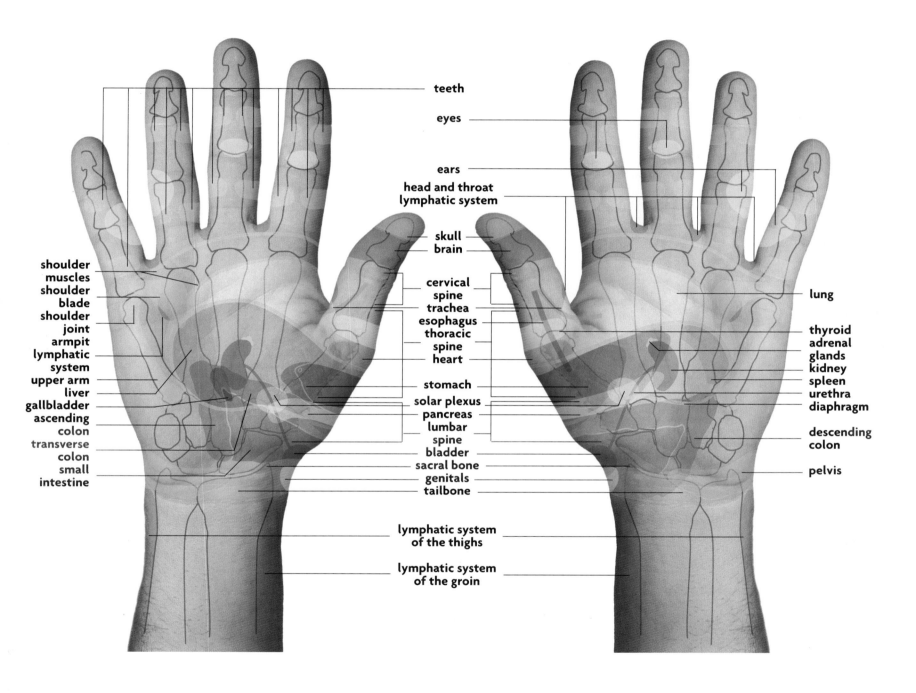

teeth

eyes

ears

head and throat
lymphatic system

skull
brain

cervical
spine
trachea
esophagus
thoracic
spine
heart

stomach
solar plexus
pancreas
lumbar
spine
bladder
sacral bone
genitals
tailbone

lymphatic system
of the thighs

lymphatic system
of the groin

shoulder
muscles
shoulder
blade
shoulder
joint
armpit
lymphatic
system
upper arm
liver
gallbladder
ascending
colon
transverse
colon
small
intestine

lung

thyroid
adrenal
glands
kidney
spleen
urethra
diaphragm

descending
colon

pelvis

Reflex zones
on the palms.

Right ear

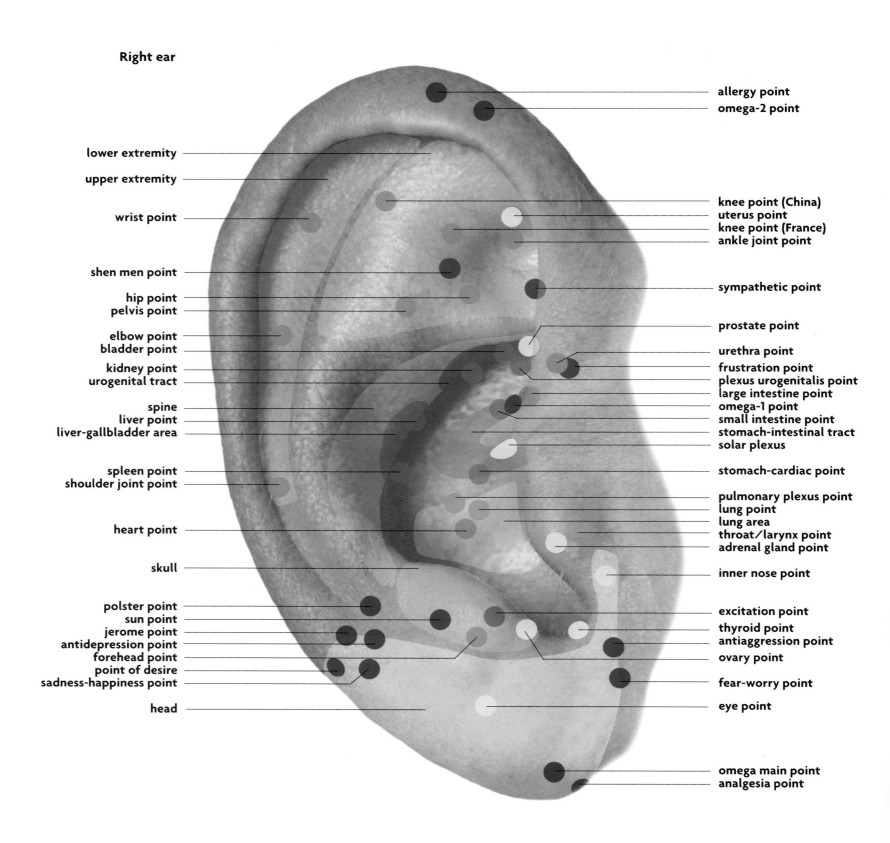

lower extremity

upper extremity

wrist point

shen men point

hip point
pelvis point

elbow point
bladder point

kidney point
urogenital tract

spine
liver point
liver-gallbladder area

spleen point
shoulder joint point

heart point

skull

polster point
sun point
jerome point
antidepression point
forehead point
point of desire
sadness-happiness point

head

allergy point
omega-2 point

knee point (China)
uterus point
knee point (France)
ankle joint point

sympathetic point

prostate point

urethra point
frustration point
plexus urogenitalis point
large intestine point
omega-1 point
small intestine point
stomach-intestinal tract
solar plexus

stomach-cardiac point

pulmonary plexus point
lung point
lung area
throat/larynx point
adrenal gland point

inner nose point

excitation point
thyroid point
antiaggression point
ovary point

fear-worry point

eye point

omega main point
analgesia point

Reflex
zones on
the ear.

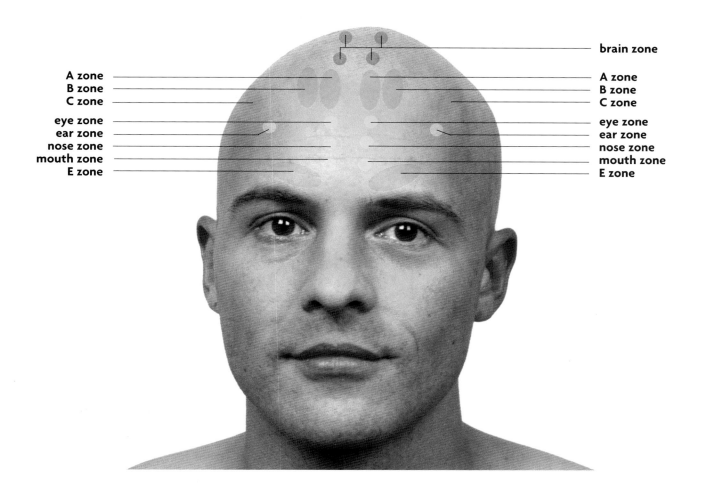

brain zone

A zone — — — — — — — — — — — — — — — — — A zone
B zone — — — — — — — — — — — — — — — — — B zone
C zone — — — — — — — — — — — — — — — — — C zone

eye zone — — — — — — — — — — — — — — — eye zone
ear zone — — — — — — — — — — — — — — — ear zone
nose zone — — — — — — — — — — — — — — — nose zone
mouth zone — — — — — — — — — — — — — — mouth zone
E zone — — — — — — — — — — — — — — — — — E zone

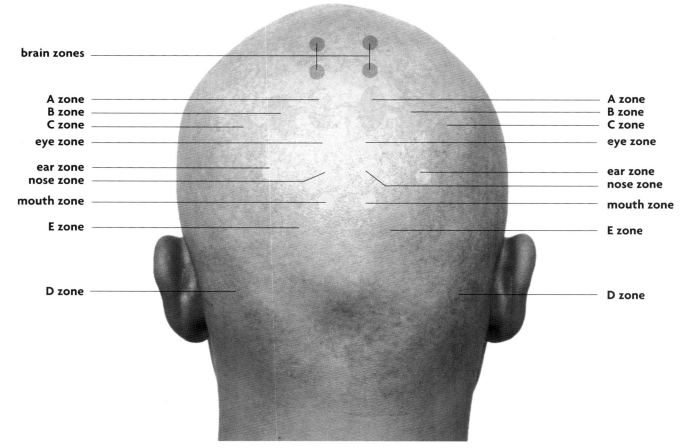

brain zones — — — — — — — — — —

A zone — — — — — — — — — — — — — — — — — A zone
B zone — — — — — — — — — — — — — — — — — B zone
C zone — — — — — — — — — — — — — — — — — C zone
eye zone — — — — — — — — — — — — — — — eye zone

ear zone — — — — — — — — — — — — — — — ear zone
nose zone — — — — — — — — — — — — — — — nose zone

mouth zone — — — — — — — — — — — — — — mouth zone

E zone — — — — — — — — — — — — — — — — — E zone

D zone — — — — — — — — — — — — — — — — — D zone

Reflex
zones of
the head.

Resources

Reflexology

The Reflexology Association of America

Reflexology Association of America
4012 South Rainbow Blvd.
Box K585
Las Vegas, NV 89103-2059
Phone: 978-779-0255
Fax: 978-779-0855
Web site: www.reflexology-usa.org
This national association is a nonprofit organization that promotes the scientific and professional advancement of reflexology. Their Web site offers a state-by-state referral list of reflexology practitioners, a national and international list of reflexology schools, reflexology event listings, and links to other sites related to reflexology.

AboutReflexology.com

This is an informational Web site offering reflexology videos and DVDs; laminated charts for foot, hand, and ear reflexology; a wide selection of reflexology books; a reflexology discussion chat room; a listing of practitioners for the U.S., U.K., Canada, and Australia; and subscription information for *Reflexology World* magazine.

Shiatsu

American Organization for Bodywork Therapies of Asia (AOBTA)

AOBTA National Headquarters
1010 Haddonfield-Berlin Road
Suite 408
Voorhees, NJ 08043-3514
Phone: 856-782-1616
Fax: 856-782-1653
Web site: www.aobta.org
E-mail: office@aobta.org
The American Organization for Bodywork Therapies of Asia is a professional membership organization that promotes Asian bodywork and its practitioners. Their Web site defines several different forms of shiatsu and includes a state-by-state search page for locating certified member practitioners. They also list schools with shiatsu training programs and provide links to other shiatsu-related sites.

Bibliography

Augustin Matthias/Schmiedel, V. *Praxisleitfaden Naturheilkunde.* 2. Aufl. Jungjohann-Verlag. Neckarsulm, 1994.

Beijing College of Traditional Chinese Medicine, Shanghai College of Traditional Chinese Medicine, Nanjing College of Traditional Chinese Medicine, The Acupuncture Institute of the Academy of Traditional Chinese Medicine (Hrsg.). *Essentials of Chinese Acupuncture.* Foreign Languages Press. Beijing, 1980.

Gleditsch, Jochen M. *Reflexzonen und Somatotopien.* 3. Aufl. WBV Biologisch-Medizinische Verlagsges. Schorndorf, 1988.

Ingham, Eunice D. *Geschichten, die die Füße erzählen.* Drei Eichen Verlag. München, 1996.

Kolster, Bernard C./Ebelt-Paprotny, Gisela (Hrsg.). *Leitfaden Physiotherapie.* 2. Aufl. Jungjohann-Verlag. Neckarsulm, 1996.

Kunz, Kevin/Kunz, Barbara. *Durch die Füße heilen.* Ehrenwirth-Verlag. München, 1996.

Marquardt, Hanne. *Reflex Zone Therapy of the Feet.* Healing Arts Press, Rochester, Vt., 1984.

Ogal, Hans P. *Ohrakupunktur I, Grundlagen und praktische Anwendungsgebiete der Ohrakupunktur* (Videocassette). KVM. Marburg, 1996.

Ogal, Hans P. *Ohrakupunktur II, Behandlungskonzepte bei häufigen Erkrankungen des Bewegungsapparates* (Videocassette). KVM. Marburg, 1996.

Ogal, Hans P. *Ohrakupunktur III, Behandlung von funktionellen Erkrankungen* (Videocassette). KVM. Marburg, 1996.

Ogal, Hans P. *Ohrakupunktur IV, Adjuvante Behandlungsmöglichkeiten bei Allergien, bei Sucht und bei psychischen Befindlichkeitstörungen* (Videocassette). KVM. Marburg, 1996.

Ogal, Hans P. *Schädelakupressur,* in: Kolster, Bernard C./Ebelt-Paprotny, Gisela (Hrsg.). *Leitfaden Physiotherapie.* 2. Aufl. Jungjohann. Neckarsulm, 1996.

Ogal, Hans P./Elies, Michael/Herget, Horst F. *Schmerzen des Bewegungsapparates,* in Pothmann Raymund (Hrsg.). *Systematik der Schmerzakupunktur.* Hippokrates-Verlag. Stuttgart, 1996.

Ogal, Hans P./Maric-Oehler, Walburg. *Neue Schädelakupunktur nach Yamamoto (YNSA) II. Behandlung von Erkrankungen des Bewegungsapparates mit den BASIS-Punkten* (Videocassette). KVM. Marburg, 1996.

Ogal, Hans P./Maric-Oehler, Walburg. *Neue Schädelakupunktur nach Yamamoto (YNSA) IV. Behandlung von Erkrankungen des Bewegungsapparates und funktionellen Störungen mit den YPSILON- und BASIS-Punkten* (Videokassette). KVM. Marburg, 1996.

Ogal, Hans P./Kolster, Bernard C. *Kompendium Ohrakupunktur. Der effektive Weg vom Punkt zum Behandlungskonzept.* KVM. Marburg, 1997.

Ogal, Hans P./Kolster, Bernard C. *SEIRIN—Tafel der Neuen Schädelakupunktur nach Yamamoto* (Poster). KVM. Marburg, 1997.

Ogal, Hans P. *Neue Schadelakupunktur nach Yamamoto (YNSA). Einführung in die Halsdiagnostik* (Videocassette). KVM. Marburg, 1999.

Ogal, Hans P./Kolster, Bernard C. *Neue Schädelakupunktur nach Yamamoto (YNSA). Grundlagen, Praxis, Indikationen.* 2. Aufl. KVM. Marburg, 2000.

Pothmann, Raymund (Hrsg.). *Systematik der Schmerzakupunktur.* Hippokrates-Verlag. Stuttgart, 1996.

Rubach, Axel. *Propädeutik der Ohrakupunktur.* Hippokrates-Verlag. Stuttgart, 1995.

Wagner, Franz. *Reflexzonenmassage.* Gräfe und Unzer Verlag GmbH. München, 1999.

Yamamoto, Toshikatsu/Maric-Oehler, Walburg. *Yamamoto Neue Schädelakupunktur.* Chun-Jo-Verlag. Freiburg/Brsg., 1991.

Yamamoto, Toshikatsu. *YNSA—Yamamoto New Scalp Acupuncture.* Springer Japan Publishing Inc., 1997.

Index

Books of Related Interest

The Reflexology Manual
An Easy-to-Use Illustrated Guide to the Healing Zones of the Hands and Feet
by Pauline Wills

Facial Reflexology
A Self-Care Manual
by Marie-France Muller, M.D., N.D., PH.D.

Sexual Reflexology
Activating the Taoist Points of Love
by Mantak Chia and WillIam U. Wei

Trigger Point Therapy for Myofascial Pain
The Practice of Informed Touch
by Donna Finando, L.Ac., L.M.T., and Steven Finando, Ph.D., L.Ac.

Rolfing
Reestablishing the Natural Alignment and Structural Integration
of the Human Body for Vitality and Well-Being
by Ida P. Rolf, Ph.D.

Soft-Tissue Manipulation
A Practitioner's Guide to the Diagnosis and Treatment of
Soft-Tissue Dysfunction and Reflex Activity
by Leon Chaitow, D.O., N.D.

Applied Kinesiology
Muscle Response in Diagnosis, Therapy, and Preventive Medicine
by Tom and Carole Valentine
with Douglas P. Hetrick, D.C.

Body Rolling
An Experiential Approach to Complete Muscle Release
by Yamuna Zake and Stephanie Golden

Inner Traditions • Bear & Company
P.O. Box 388
Rochester, VT 05767
1-800-246-8648
www.InnerTraditions.com

Or contact your local bookseller